T0183023

Water-filtered Infrared A (wIRA) Irradiation

Peter Vaupel

Editor

Water-filtered Infrared A (wIRA) Irradiation

From Research to Clinical Settings

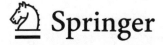

Editor
Peter Vaupel
Department of Radiation Oncology
University Medical Center
University of Freiburg
Freiburg/Breisgau, Germany

This book is an open access publication.

This work was supported by Dr. med. h.c. Erwin Braun Stiftung.

ISBN 978-3-030-92882-7   ISBN 978-3-030-92880-3   (eBook)
https://doi.org/10.1007/978-3-030-92880-3

This Springer imprint is published by the registered company Springer Nature Switzerland AG
The registered company address is: Gewerbestrasse 11, 6330 Cham, Switzerland

"For an understanding of the phenomena the first condition is the introduction of adequate concepts."

Werner Heisenberg
Grifford Lecture, St. Andrew University, 1956/57.

Foreword

Water-filtered infrared A irradiation (wIRA) is a special application of infrared A irradiation. Its preferential induction of thermal, but also nonthermal, effects which have a high tissue penetration and low heat load to the skin surface makes wIRA a promising therapeutic method. Since its introduction in 1989, wIRA has been applied experimentally and clinically to human and animal patients to treat and improve an impressive variety of disease entities.

The editor, Professor Dr. med. Peter Vaupel, an internationally renowned tumor pathophysiologist, has been involved in basic research and preclinical and clinical investigations using wIRA irradiation during the last 30 years.

This book summarizes recent developments by presenting a wide range of up-to-date clinical applications and offers an excellent overview on the topic, which will be of relevance to readers from clinical disciplines and basic researchers alike. The book is organized into two main fields: "Principles" and "Clinical Practice". "Clinical Practice" is the most substantial field being divided into parts on application of wIRA in oncology, psychiatry, neonatology, dermatology, rheumatology, and infectiology. "Principles" summarizes the historic development of wIRA, focusing on the physical basics, body's reaction to hyperthermia, thermography, and thermometry, and recommends clear terminology when applying wIRA.

Part II focuses on the application of wIRA on breast cancer as well as superficial cancers, whole-body application, and combination with gold nanoparticles. In several chapters, the role of wIRA-induced hyperthermia as a radiosensitizer, chemosensitizer, and stimulator of antitumor immune responses as an adjuvant in cancer therapy is described. The role of wIRA in combination with photodynamic therapies (PDT) is also outlined.

Mood enhancement induced by the application of whole-body hyperthermia to treat various diseases led to positive effects being observed following whole-body hyperthermia in depressive patients. Part III elaborates the promising theoretical and practical applications of wIRA in psychiatry.

Hypothermia in neonates born at term or preterm is a serious problem. Part IV presents experimental and clinical evidence describing the advantages of wIRA for delivering direct, remarkable increases in infant-body core temperature, but with lower skin surface warming compared to conventional radiant warmers.

Part V focuses on the effects of wIRA on impaired wound healing, imbalanced fibroblast proliferation, and aberrant scarring and show the potential value of wIRA as an adjuvant therapy. In addition, wIRA has been shown to improve the healing process of acute and chronic wounds and enhance regular wound healing. In principle, wIRA is capable of high tissue penetration accompanied by a low thermal load to the skin surface. In addition, wIRA treatment significantly reduces local pain, wound secretion, inflammation, and infection and, as an example, can significantly accelerate the healing process of second-degree burns.

Part VI describes the results of adding wIRA to the existing multimodal therapy concepts in patients with arthritis and fibromyalgia. In these cases, wIRA again reduces pain by reducing the levels of C-reactive protein (CRP) and of TNF-α and the requirement for analgesics.

Part VII reports the reduction of extra- and intracellular forms of the bacterial genus *Chlamydia*. This is important for treating trachoma, an ocular infection with the species *Chlamydia trachomatis*, which eventually leads to blindness, the treatment of which remains a major challenge using traditional antichlamydial substances. Promising experimental data from the application of wIRA to ocular chlamydial infections of laboratory animals provides good evidence for the efficacy and safety of using wIRA to treat chlamydial infections.

Part VIII focuses on less well-known basic actions of wIRA such as the photobiomodulation, the heat-sensitive transient receptor potential (TRP) ion channels, and its effects on nitric oxide production and infrared (IR) neural stimulation. The intention of the final chapter is to further stimulate the use of wIRA and foster the planning and delivery of additional clinical studies. It should always be kept in mind that wIRA corresponds to the sun's infrared irradiation, completely omitting IR-B, IR-C, and UV spectrum.

In summary, this book provides a unique and excellent overview of the present state-of-the-art use of wIRA and is recommended to readers from medicine, medical physics, physiotherapy, and biology, as well as interested patients.

Andreas Pospischil
University of Zurich,
Institute of Veterinary Pathology,
Zurich, Switzerland

Acknowledgments

As the editor, I feel the strong obligation to express my severe thanks to several enthusiastic supporters and "helping hands" who have enabled the realization of this book project. First of all, I have to thank my wife Lieselotte Vaupel for her tireless efforts and patience during project planning and editing of this book. In addition, thanks go to all authors and co-authors from the Netherlands, Switzerland, Austria, the USA, the UK, South Africa, and Germany for allocating a significant amount of time from their busy schedules to provide their unique and most important contributions.

I am very grateful to Professor Dr. Andreas Pospischil, Zurich (Switzerland), who immediately declared his kind readiness and genuine interest for writing the Foreword as an informative introduction.

Unforgotten should be the initial inspiration and support by Dr. med. h.c. Erwin Braun, Sarnen (Switzerland), relating to the development of water-filtered infrared-A (wIRA) and its medical applications, together with Jerry Rzeznik, Developmental Graduate Engineer, in the 1990s. Both paved the avenue for various applications of wIRA in medicine, as described in this volume.

Furthermore, I must thank Signora Antonella Cerri, Executive Editor Medicine and Life Sciences at Springer Nature, Mr. Vishal Anand (Project Manager) and Ms. Smitha Diveshan, Project Coordinator (Books) for Springer Nature, and the other members of the editorial team whose expertise has been of great help during book production. Many thanks are going to my colleague Professor A. Graham Pockley, PhD (Nottingham, UK). Acting as language editor, he was responsible for "smoothing and styling" the manuscripts. I greatly appreciate the encouragement of Dr. med. h. c. Erwin Braun Foundation, Basel (Switzerland), with its Board of Honorary Trustees (Werner Braun, Jan-Olaf Gebbers, Alexander Gutmans, Mark Hartel, and myself, the Associate Ms. Gabriele Multhoff, and Ms. Sonja Blaser, Administrator of the Foundation). Finally, I am very obliged to Ms. Anna Lisa Braun for her warm welcome in Villa 100, Engelberg (Switzerland), and for generously providing retreats, which have enabled a full and focused revision of all manuscripts in necessarily quiet surroundings.

Peter Vaupel, Mainz, January 2022
Editor

Contents

Part IV Clinical Practice: Neonatology

Part V Clinical Practice: Dermatology

Editor and Contributors

About the Editor

Peter Vaupel studied medicine at the University of Mainz and was awarded the degree of M.D. in 1968 and the degree of Dr. med. in 1969. Thereafter, he underwent training in surgery, internal medicine, obstetrics, and gynecology, and following military service he returned to academic life at the Institute of Physiology, University of Mainz, as a research assistant. His interests turned to the microenvironment of solid tumors. This new area of research proved to be so fascinating and compulsive for Dr. Vaupel that it has kept him occupied for almost 50 years. Initially, Dr. Vaupel carried out theoretical and experimental studies on oxygenation and metabolites in tissue-isolated tumors, for which he was awarded the degree of Dr. med. habil. in 1974. Following promotions to assistant professor (1972) and associate professor (1975), Dr. Vaupel was appointed full professor of physiology in 1977 and became head of the Department of Applied Physiology at the University of Mainz in 1984. In 1987, he left Mainz to take up the newly established Andrew Werk Cook Professorship of Radiation Biology/Physiology at Harvard Medical School. In 1989, Dr. Vaupel assumed the position as professor and chairman of the Department of Pathophysiology at the Institute of Physiology and Pathophysiology at the Johannes Gutenberg-University of Mainz. Since 1998, Professor Vaupel has been a full member of the Academy of Science and Literature at Mainz. Dr. Vaupel has managed to dedicate a great deal of effort to the teaching of physiology, as documented by five standard textbooks of physiology and pathophysiology. He serves in an advisory capacity to many national and international science foundations, is currently a member of several professional societies, serves on the editorial boards of numerous professional journals, and has edited a series of monographs addressing topics in tumor pathophysiology. Over the past 50 years, Dr. Vaupel has published more than 460 well-cited articles and made approximately 560 scientific presentations in which a wide range of therapeutically relevant pathophysiological parameters have been examined. Over the last 40 years, a major focus of Dr. Vaupel's research has been on the effects of hyperthermia, and much of this research has concentrated on the reciprocal influence of microenvironmental parameters and hyperthermia. With these studies, he has made a considerable contribution to our current knowledge of the pathophysiological behavior of solid tumors upon localized heat treatment and the impact of the special tumor pathophysiology on treatment outcome. In cooperation with PD Dr. Debra Kelleher sign for (deceased 17. May 2020), research has been focusing on the development of new treatment modalities such as simultaneously applied combination of localized hyperthermia and photodynamic therapy.

Contributors

N. Auen Department of Psychiatry, Psychotherapy, Psychosomatic and Addiction Medicine, Evangelische Kliniken Essen-Mitte, Essen, Germany

I. Aykara Department of Rheumatology, Clinical Immunology, Osteology and Physical Medicine, Justus-Liebig-University Giessen, Campus Kerckhoff, Bad Nauheim, Germany

A. Bakker Department of Radiation Oncology, Amsterdam University Medical Centers, Cancer Center Amsterdam, University of Amsterdam, Amsterdam, The Netherlands

M. Beck Department of Radiation Oncology, Berlin Institute of Health, Charité-Universitätsmedizin Berlin, Corporate Member of Freie Universität Berlin, Humboldt-Universität zu Berlin, Berlin, Germany

A. S. Bingoel Department of Plastic, Aesthetic, Hand and Reconstructive Surgery, Burn Center, Hannover Medical School, Hannover, Germany

C. Blenn Department of Pathobiology, Vetsuisse-Faculty, Institute of Veterinary Pathology, University of Zurich, Zurich, Switzerland

H. J. G. D. van den Bongard Department of Radiation Oncology, Amsterdam University Medical Centers, Cancer Center Amsterdam, University of Amsterdam, Amsterdam, The Netherlands

N. Borel Department of Pathobiology, Vetsuisse-Faculty, Institute of Veterinary Pathology, University of Zurich, Zurich, Switzerland

C. Borzim Department of Psychiatry and Psychotherapy, Charité Campus Mitte, Charité University Medicine Berlin, Berlin, Germany

J. Crezee Department of Radiation Oncology, Amsterdam University Medical Centers, Cancer Center Amsterdam, University of Amsterdam, Amsterdam, The Netherlands

P. Elsner Department of Dermatology, University Hospital Jena, Jena, Germany

S. Fischer Clinical Psychology and Psychotherapy, Institute of Psychology, University of Zurich, Zurich, Switzerland

A. Frohns Department of Plant Membrane Biophysics, Technical University of Darmstadt, Darmstadt, Germany

F. Frohns Department of Plant Membrane Biophysics, Technical University of Darmstadt, Darmstadt, Germany

J.-O. Gebbers Lucerne, Switzerland

A. L. Grosu Department of Radiation Oncology, University Medical Center, University of Freiburg, Freiburg/Breisgau, Germany

German Cancer Consortium (DKTK) Partner Site Freiburg, German Cancer Research Center (DKFZ), Heidelberg, Germany

J. F. Hainfeld Nanoprobes, Inc, Yaphank, NY, USA

M. R. Hamblin Laser Research Centre, Faculty of Health Science, University of Johannesburg, Doornfontein, South Africa

Radiation Biology Research Center, Iran University of Medical Sciences, Tehran, Iran

K. Hanusch Department of Health Professions, Berne University of Applied Sciences, Berne, Switzerland

S. Heckel-Reusser Heckel Medizintechnik, Esslingen, Germany

A. Heinz Department of Psychiatry and Psychotherapy, Charité Campus Mitte, Charité University Medicine Berlin, Berlin, Germany

U.-C. Hipler Department of Dermatology, University Hospital Jena, Jena, Germany

P. Jauker Department of Dermatology, Medical University of Vienna, Vienna, Austria

S. Kippenberger Department of Dermatology, Venereology and Allergology, University Hospital Frankfurt, Goethe University, Frankfurt/Main, Germany

P. Klemm Department of Rheumatology, Clinical Immunology, Osteology and Physical Medicine, Justus-Liebig-University Giessen, Campus Kerckhoff, Bad Nauheim, Germany

A. Knobel Department of Psychiatry and Psychotherapy, Charité Campus Mitte, Charité University Medicine Berlin, Berlin, Germany

H. P. Kok Department of Radiation Oncology, Amsterdam University Medical Centers, Cancer Center Amsterdam, University of Amsterdam, Amsterdam, The Netherlands

M. W. Kolff Department of Radiation Oncology, Amsterdam University Medical Centers, Cancer Center Amsterdam, University of Amsterdam, Amsterdam, The Netherlands

J. Kuratli Department of Pathobiology, Vetsuisse-Faculty, Institute of Veterinary Pathology, University of Zurich, Zurich, Switzerland

U. Lange Department of Rheumatology, Clinical Immunology, Osteology and Physical Medicine, Justus-Liebig-University Giessen, Campus Kerckhoff, Bad Nauheim, Germany

H. Marti Department of Pathobiology, Vetsuisse-Faculty, Institute of Veterinary Pathology, University of Zurich, Zurich, Switzerland

W. Müller Physical Optics Consultant Office, Wetzlar, Germany

G. Multhoff Project Group Radiation Immuno-Oncology, Central Institute for Translational Cancer Research, Klinikum rechts der Isar, Technical University München, München, Germany

Department of Radiation Oncology, Klinikum rechts der Isar, Technical University München, München, Germany

K. Münch Department of Radiation Oncology, Lindenhofspital, Bern, Switzerland

N. H. Nicolay Department of Radiation Oncology, University Medical Center, University of Freiburg, Freiburg/Breisgau, Germany

German Cancer Consortium (DKTK) Partner Site Freiburg, German Cancer Research Center (DKFZ), Heidelberg, Germany

M. Notter Department of Radiation Oncology, Lindenhofspital, Bern, Switzerland

S. Ohrndorf Department of Rheumatology and Clinical Immunology, Charité-Universitätsmedizin Berlin, Campus Mitte, Humboldt-Universität zu Berlin, Freie Universität Berlin, Berlin, Germany

H. Piazena Department of Anaesthesiology and Intensive Care Medicine, Charité - Universitätsmedizin Berlin, Corporative Member of Freie Universität Berlin and Humboldt Universität zu Berlin, Berlin, Germany

A. Pospischil University of Zurich, Institute of Veterinary Pathology, Zurich, Switzerland

E. A. Repasky Department of Immunology, Roswell Park Comprehensive Cancer Center, Buffalo, NY, USA

F. Rübener Department of Psychiatry, Psychotherapy, Psychosomatic and Addiction Medicine, Evangelische Kliniken Essen-Mitte, Essen, Germany

M. R. Saalmann Department of Radiation Oncology, University Medical Center, University of Freiburg, Freiburg/Breisgau, Germany

M. Schäfer Department of Psychiatry, Psychotherapy, Psychosomatic and Addiction Medicine, Evangelische Kliniken Essen-Mitte, Essen, Germany

G. Schmittat Department of Rheumatology and Clinical Immunology, Charité-Universitätsmedizin Berlin, Campus Mitte, Humboldt-Universität zu Berlin, Freie Universität Berlin, Berlin, Germany

D. Singer Division of Neonatology and Pediatric Critical Care Medicine, University Medical Center Eppendorf, Hamburg, Germany

H. M. Smilowitz University of Connecticut Health Center, Farmington, CT, USA

S. Strauss Department of Plastic, Aesthetic, Hand and Reconstructive Surgery, Burn Center, Hannover Medical School, Hannover, Germany

A. Tanew Department of Dermatology, Medical University of Vienna, Vienna, Austria

A. R. Thomsen Department of Radiation Oncology, University Medical Center, University of Freiburg, Freiburg/Breisgau, Germany

German Cancer Consortium (DKTK) Partner Site Freiburg, German Cancer Research Center (DKFZ), Heidelberg, Germany

G. van Tienhoven Department of Radiation Oncology, Amsterdam University Medical Centers, Cancer Center Amsterdam, University of Amsterdam, Amsterdam, The Netherlands

J. Tittelbach Department of Dermatology, University Hospital Jena, Jena, Germany

P. Vaupel Department of Radiation Oncology, University Medical Center, University of Freiburg, Freiburg/Breisgau, Germany

German Cancer Consortium (DKTK) Partner Site Freiburg, German Cancer Research Center (DKFZ), Heidelberg, Germany

D. Vogler Department of Rheumatology and Clinical Immunology, Charité-Universitätsmedizin Berlin, Campus Mitte, Humboldt-Universität zu Berlin, Freie Universität Berlin, Berlin, Germany

P. M. Vogt Department of Plastic, Aesthetic, Hand and Reconstructive Surgery, Burn Center, Hannover Medical School, Hannover, Germany

C. Wiegand Department of Dermatology, University Hospital Jena, Jena, Germany

P. Wolf Department of Dermatology and Venereology, Medical University of Graz, Graz, Austria

N. Zöller Department of Dermatology, Venereology and Allergology, University Hospital Frankfurt, Goethe University, Frankfurt/Main, Germany

S. Zschaeck Department of Radiation Oncology, Berlin Institute of Health, Charité-Universitätsmedizin Berlin, Corporate Member of Freie Universität Berlin, Humboldt-Universität zu Berlin, Berlin, Germany

Berlin Institute of Health (BIH), Berlin, Germany

R. Zweije Department of Radiation Oncology, Amsterdam University Medical Centers, Cancer Center Amsterdam, University of Amsterdam, Amsterdam, The Netherlands

Part I
Principles

Glossary Used in wIRA-Hyperthermia

1

H. Piazena, W. Müller, and Peter Vaupel

1.1 Introduction

Tissue heating by water-filtered infrared A radiation (wIRA) is based on interactions between radiation and tissues. wIRA-hyperthermia (wIRA-HT) requires an interdisciplinary approach involving photobiological principles and laws, (patho-) physiological tissue responses, and the needs of proper dosimetry. Thus, an exact terminology is crucial to prevent interdisciplinary misunderstanding and to be consistent with the International System of Units (SI). Science-based terms are also the key for traceability and comparability of measured data published by different authors and to prevent misconceptions and confusion of readers/users due to imprecise vocabulary or different denominations of identical parameters. Therefore, a glossary of basic physical terms and of SI-based radiometry units is proposed for consistent use in wIRA-HT. Also provided are terms defined by the European Society of Hyperthermic Oncology (ESHO) which are currently recommended for quality proof of superficial hyperthermia in oncology, and empirical, basic data for wIRA skin exposures in radiation oncology and in physical therapy (Tables 1.1, 1.2, 1.3, 1.4, 1.5, 1.7 and Figs. 1.1, and 1.2).

H. Piazena (✉)
Department of Anaesthesiology and Operative Intensive Care Medicine, Charité - Universitätsmedizin Berlin, Corporative Member of Freie Universität Berlin and Humboldt Universität zu Berlin, Berlin, Germany
e-mail: helmut.piazena@charite.de

W. Müller
Physical Optics Consultant Office, Wetzlar, Germany

P. Vaupel
Department of Radiation Oncology, University Medical Center, University of Freiburg, Freiburg/Breisgau, Germany

German Cancer Consortium (DKTK) Partner Site Freiburg, German Cancer Research Center (DKFZ), Heidelberg, Germany

© The Author(s) 2022
P. Vaupel (ed.), *Water-filtered Infrared A (wIRA) Irradiation*,
https://doi.org/10.1007/978-3-030-92880-3_1

1.2 Recommended Terms

Table 1.1 Terms and tools to characterize the spectrum of infrared radiation [1–3]

Term	Symbol	Spectral range	Note
Electro-magnetic radiation	EMR	10^{-11}–10^8 m	Energy propagating in form of electromagnetic waves
Optical radiation		0.1–1000 μm	Optical radiation is part of EMR responding to the laws of optics regarding refraction, focusing, and reflection. Ranges: Ultraviolet (UV, 0.1–0.4 μm), visible (VIS, i.e., "light," 0.40–0.78 μm), and infrared radiation (IR, 0.78–1000 μm)
Infrared radiation (total)	IR	0.78–1000 μm	IR is a spectral range of optical radiation.
Visible radiation, light	VIS	0.40–0.78 μm	VIS is the visible spectral range of optical radiation. It is usually called "light".
Infrared A radiation	IR-A	0.78–1.40 μm	Sub-range of IR, short-wavelength IR, recommended term for use in medicine
Infrared B radiation	IR-B	1.40–3.00 μm	Sub-range of IR, mid-wavelength IR, recommended term for use in medicine
Infrared C radiation	IR-C	3–1000 μm	Sub-range of IR, long-wavelength IR, recommended term for use in medicine
Water-filtered infrared A radiation[a]	wIRA[a]	0.78–1.40 μm	Short-wavelength IR spectrally filtered by a water layer (= water filter) Recommended term for use in medicine/biomedicine
Near-infrared radiation	NIR	0.78–3.00 μm	Terms are frequently used in physics, geophysics, and astrophysics
Mid-infrared radiation	MIR	3–50 μm	Not recommended for use in medicine due to significant differences in the interaction with biological tissues within the range of IR
Far-infrared radiation	FIR	50–1000 μm	
Optical filter			Object that transmits spectral power selectively or partially
Band-pass filter		$\tau_f \approx 0$	Object that minimizes radiant power outside of a spectral band ($\lambda_{c1} \leq \lambda \leq \lambda_{c2}$), ($\tau_f$ —Transmittance of the filter)
Dichroic filter, Interference filter			Special type of band-pass filter that transmits a defined band of spectral radiant power and reflects the remaining part
Cut-off filter		$\tau_f \approx 0$ for $\lambda \leq \lambda_c$	Object that minimizes transmittance τ_f below a defined "cut-off" wavelength λ_c
Cut-on filter		$\tau_f \approx 0$ for $\lambda \geq \lambda_c$	Object that minimizes transmittance τ_f above a defined "cut-on" wavelength λ_c
Neutral density filter		$\tau_f = f$, ($f < 1$)	Object that reduces spectral radiant power by a factor f (τ_f – Filter transmittance)
Water filter		$\tau_f = \exp(-\mu_{aw} \cdot d_w)$	Object that minimizes spectral power by transmission of a water layer of thickness d_w according to Lambert–Beer's law wherein μ_{aw} defines the absorption coefficient of water, and τ_f the transmittance of the filter
wIRA-radiator (syn.: wIRA-irradiator)			Device to irradiate objects with wIRA. Some types are configured to emit also spectral portions of VIS (syn.: wIRA-irradiator) (i.e., light). This does not enhance their thermal effectiveness.

[a] Note: Effects of wIRA specified in this monograph are based on the use of wIRA-radiators which additionally emit a spectral portion of VIS to enable visual control of the treatment area and visual monitoring of on–off cycles. This does not enhance their thermal effectiveness.

Table 1.2 Terms and parameters to characterize wIRA emitted by a device and incident on the surface of the exposed object [2–7]

Term	Symbol	Unit	Definition and notes	
Emission spectrum			Spectral radiant power or spectral irradiance emitted by the radiation source as a function of the wavelengths	
Exposure			General term to express receiving of radiation by the surface of an object. Do not confuse with → "radiant exposure".	
Exposure time	Δt	[s]	$\Delta t = t_e - t_0$	Duration from the beginning (t_0) to the end (t_e) of exposure
Radiant power[a] Radiant flux[a] Energy flux[a]	Φ, P	[W]	$\Phi = dQ/dt$	Radiant energy emitted, reflected, transmitted, or received per unit of time
Radiant energy[a]	Q	[W s], [J]	$Q = \int_{\Delta t} \Phi \, dt$	Energy of radiation
Radiant exitance[a]	M	[mW cm^{-2}]	$M = d\Phi/dA$	Radiant power emitted per unit area of the source surface. Do not confuse with → "intensity".
Radiant intensity[a]	I	[mW sr^{-1}]	$I = d\Phi/d\Omega$	Radiant power emitted by source surface per unit of solid angle. Do not confuse with → "intensity".
Radiance[a,b]	L	[mW cm^{-2} sr^{-1}]	$L = d\Phi/(d\Omega \, dA)$	Radiant power emitted per unit of solid angle per unit of source area
Irradiance[a,b]	E	[mW cm^{-2}]	$E = d\Phi/dA$	Radiant power received per unit area
Incident irradiance[a,b]	E_s	[mW cm^{-2}]	$E_s = d\Phi_s/dA$	Entering radiant power received per unit area on the surface
Homogeneity criterion of incident irradiance[a,b]	g_2		$g_2 \geq E_{s,min} / E_{s,max}$	Coefficient to evaluate the horizontal distribution of radiant power on the surface of a receiver. For high uniformity of exposure, $g_2 \geq 0.9$ is recommended
Effective size of the irradiated area		[cm^2]	Area on the surface of a receiver where the ratio between minimum and maximum of radiant power exceeds g_2	
Radiant exposure[a,b], Irradiation[a,b] Dose[a,b]	H	[mJ cm^{-2}]	$H = dQ/dA = \int_{\Delta t} E \, dt$	Radiant energy received per unit area. Integral of irradiance over exposure time Δt. Do not confuse with "radiation dose" related to energy of ionizing radiation absorbed per unit of mass.

[a] Note: This quantity depends on the wavelength of radiation and on the spectrum of the irradiation source used.
[b] Note: In case of tilted surfaces, values decrease according to the cosine of angle between the directions of radiation and of the perpendicular on the surface θ, e.g., $E(\theta) = E(\theta = 0) \cdot \cos \theta$ (Lambert's cosine law).

Table 1.3 Terms quantifying interactions of wIRA with tissues [2–7]

(a) *Absorption*				
Term	Symbol	Unit	Definition and notes	
Chromophore			Part of a molecule responsible for absorption of radiation within one or more spectral bands resulting in electronic transition (UV and VIS) or in thermal molecular movements such as vibrations, rotations, and bending (IR). Usually, the absorbing molecule itself is called "chromophore".	
Absorbance[a], Internal absorbance[a]	A		$A = \ln (\Phi_s / \Phi_T)$ $= - \ln \tau$	Logarithmical ratio between the incident radiant power Φ_s and the transmitted radiant power Φ_T. Negative logarithm of ($\rightarrow$) transmittance τ
Absorptance[a]	α		$\alpha = 1 - \tau$	Absorbed part of radiation penetrating the tissue
Absorption[a]			Physical process of radiant energy transfer to tissue	
Absorption coefficient[a]	μ_a	[cm^{-1}]	$\mu_a = A / l$	Absorbance A per path length l
(b) *Transmittance*				
Transmittance[a]	τ		$\tau = \Phi_T / \Phi_s$	Ratio between the transmitted radiant power Φ_T and the incident radiant power Φ_s
Transmission[a]			Physical process of radiant energy transfer passing the tissue	
(c) *Scattering and remittance*				
Scatterers in the tissue			Cells, nuclei, mitochondria, lysosomes, vesicles, striations in collagen fibrils, cross-striations in muscle fibers, macromolecular aggregates, membranes, fluctuations in dielectric constant, density, refractive index	
Scattering[a]			Multiple change of the direction of radiation propagation due to collision with scatterers resulting in prolonging of its retention time in tissue	
Elastic scattering			Scattering without energy loss of the photons	
Inelastic scattering			Scattering with energy loss of the photons	
Rayleigh scattering			Predominately elastic and isotropic scattering of radiation by particles with small or very small diameters as compared to the wavelength	
Mie scattering			Preferred to the forward hemisphere directed and predominately elastic scattering of radiation by particles with diameters similar or larger than the wavelength	
Backscattering			Remission of scattered radiation from the surface of exposed tissue in direction of the backward hemisphere	

Table 1.3 (continued)

Term	Symbol	Unit	Definition and notes	
Scattering coefficient[a]	μ_s	[cm^{-1}]	$\mu_s = N_s \cdot \sigma_s$	Measure of scattering of radiation which depends on volume density N_s and on the scattering cross section σ_s of particles
Reduced scattering coefficient[a]	μ_s'	[cm^{-1}]	$\mu_s' = \mu_s \cdot (1 - g)$	Measure of scattering considering anisotropy (g) of radiation propagation
Attenuation[a]			Decrease of irradiance, radiant fluence rate, and radiance within the tissue due to absorption and scattering of radiation	
Effective attenuation coefficient[a]	μ_{eff}	[cm^{-1}]	$\mu_{eff} = [3\mu_a \cdot (\mu_a + \mu_s')]^{1/2}$	Measure of attenuation of radiation by absorption and scattering
(surface) reflectance[a], Reflectivity[a]	ρ		$\rho = \Phi_{ref} / \Phi_s$	Reflected part Φ_{ref} of incident radiant power Φ_s by reflection at the surface or discontinuity in the tissue
Diffuse reflectance[a], Remittance[a]	R_d		$R_d \approx \exp(-7\mu_a/\mu_{eff})$	Remitted part of incident radiant power by backscattering within the tissue

[a] Note: This quantity depends on the wavelength of radiation and on the spectrum of the radiation source used.

Table 1.4 Terms quantifying propagation of wIRA within tissues [2–7]

Term	Symbol	Unit	Definition and Notes	
Radiant fluence rate[a] Spherical irradiance[a] Scalar irradiance[a]	E_o	[mW m^{-2}]	$E_o = \int_{4\pi sr} L\, d\Omega$	Radiant power received by a target within the tissue from all directions of the surrounding
Radiant fluence[a] Radiant spherical exposure[a]	H_o	[mJ m^{-2}]	$H_o = \int_{\Delta t} E_o\, dt$	Radiant energy received by a target within the tissue from all directions of the surrounding volume during total exposure time
Radiative (effective) penetration depth[a]	δ_p	[cm]	$\delta_p = 1/\mu_{eff}$	Depth of tissue where radiation power or irradiance decreased to 36.77% (= 1/e) of the incident value at the surface

[a] Note: This quantity depends on the wavelength of radiation and on the spectrum of the radiation source used.

Table 1.5 Terms quantifying optical and thermal properties and thermal response of tissues

(a) Optical properties [2–7]				
Term	Symbol	Unit	Definition and notes	
Black body Black body radiation			Idealized non-reflecting body that completely absorbs incident EMR of all wavelengths and emits thermal EMR isotropic and proportional to fourth power of its temperature T according to Stefan–Boltzmann's law	
Emission[a]			Radiation emitted by excited atoms and/or molecules when transitioning into an energetic deeper state	
Emittance[a] Emissivity[a]	$\varepsilon(T)$		$\varepsilon = M(T)/M_{bb}(T)$	Measure to compare thermal radiant exitance from the surface of an object M at temperature T to that of black body M_{bb}
Optical window			Wavelength range where the tissue absorbs optical radiation to a significant lesser extent than at other wavelengths. Based on absorbance of 50%, the optical window ranges at about 600–1300 nm for fair skin and at about 750–1300 nm for black skin.	
Radiant exitance[a]	M	[mW cm^{-2}]	$M = d\Phi/dA$	Radiant power emitted per unit area of tissue surface
Relative refractive index[a]	n		$n = c_1 / c_2 = \sin \theta_1/\theta_2$	Measure of bending of a beam when passing from medium 1 into medium 2 if phase velocities of radiation in both media are different ($c_1 \neq c_2$). θ_1 is the incident angle, and θ_2 is the refracted angle to the normal. The term n is called *absolute refractive index* if the beam transmits from vacuum into a medium.
(b) *Thermal properties and responses* [8–10]				
Temperature	T	[°C]	State variable. Measure of the thermal state of an object	
Temperature difference	ΔT	[K]	$\Delta T = T_1 - T_2$	Measure of the difference between two thermal states
Heating rate[a]	HR	[K min^{-1}]	$HR = \delta T / \delta t$	Increase of tissue temperature after $\delta t = 1$ min of exposure
Heating-up time[a]	Δt_{TSS}	[min]	Exposure time to achieve thermal steady state (TSS)	

Table 1.5 (continued)

Term	Symbol	Unit	Definition and notes	
Specific absorption rate[a]	SAR	$[mW\ g^{-1}]$	$SAR = c_p \cdot HR$	Radiant energy cumulated per unit tissue mass after $\delta t = 1$ min of exposure (under the assumption of negligible heat dissipation due to blood perfusion)
Effective field size	EFS	$[cm^2]$	Size of an area within the tissue at a depth of 1 cm where SAR equals or increases by 50% of its maximum	
Effective penetration depth[a]	EPD	[mm]	Tissue depth at which SAR decreases to 50% of its maximum	
Temperature rise[a]	TR	[K]	Increase of tissue temperature 6 min after start of exposure	
Thermal effective penetration depth[a]	TEPD	[mm]	Tissue depth at which TR decreases to 50% of its maximum	
Thermal effective field size[a]	TEFS	$[cm^2]$	Size of an area within the tissue at a depth of 1 cm where TR equals or increases by 50% of its maximum	
Thermal steady state[a]	TSS	[°C]	Thermal state after achieving balance between heat input and heat loss by dissipation and thermoregulation (i.e., tissue temperature is approx. constant)	
Cumulative thermal equivalent minutes[a]	CEM_{43}	[min]	$CEM_{43} = \int_t R^{(43-T(t))}\ dt$	Thermal dose of treatment performed at temperature T expressed as cumulative equivalent minutes at 43 °C
Cumulative thermal equivalent minutes at T_{90}[a]	$CEM_{43}T_{90}$	[min]	$CEM_{43} = \int_t R^{(43-T90(t))}\ dt$	Cumulative equivalent minutes at 43 °C for the temperature T_{90} during the treatment time
Thermal dose T_x[a]	T_x	[°C]	Thermal dose expressed as tissue temperature exceeded by x% of temperature data measured during the treatment	
Cool-down time	Δt_d	[min]	Time to reach 36.73% (= 1/e) of maximum tissue temperature after finishing wIRA-exposure	

[a] Note: This quantity depends on the wavelength of radiation and on the spectrum of the radiation source used.

1.3 Occasionally Used, Obsolete, and Non-Recommended Terms

Table 1.6 Examples

Non-recommended or obsolete term	Comment	Recommended term
Brightness	Defined to describe physiological perception of visible radiation (light). Not recommended term to characterize radiance of a source emitting ultraviolet or infrared radiation	Radiance
Extinction	Obsolete term	Absorbance
Fluency	Incorrect term to quantify radiant energy received per unit area or by a target within the tissue	Per unit area: radiant exposure, irradiation, dose. By a target: radiant fluence or radiant spherical exposure
Intensity	Term used to describe radiant power, fluence rate, or irradiance. Not recommended for quantitative characterization	Radiant power
Irradiation intensity	Term used in a confuse way to characterize fluence rate or irradiance	Fluence rate or irradiance
Minimal heating dose (MHD)	Not existing as physical parameter due to non-applicability of the *Bunsen–Roscoe* law of reciprocity to tissue heating by infrared radiation or by further (convective or conductive) heat sources	
Near-infrared light, Infrared A light	Wrong and confusing terms	Infrared-A radiation (IR-A)
Radiation strength	Not an official term	Irradiance
VIS/wIRA VIS/wIRA irradiator	Incorrect term for combined use of wIRA and of VIS emitted by a wIRA-irradiator	VIS and wIRA emitted by a wIRA-irradiator (with extended emission spectrum)
VIS/wIRA irradiance	Wrong and confusing term to characterize total irradiance of a wIRA-irradiator	Irradiance (VIS) and irradiance (IR-A) (irradiances of both spectral ranges should be specified separately)
wIRAR	Not an official term	wIRA
wIRA irradiator	Alternative term for specification of a device for irradiation of an object with wIRA	wIRA radiator

Note: A distinction between radiator/radiation and irradiation is proposed according to (1) O.W. Leibiger, I.F. Leibiger, Dictionary for Scientists (1964), Edwards Brothers, Ann Arbor MI, and (2) C. Morris (Ed.) Dictionary of Science and Technology (1992), Academic Press, San Diego, New York. *wIRA radiator*: device emitting water-filtered infrared A; *irradiation*: process by which an object is exposed to radiation.

1.4 Empirical and Basic Data for wIRA Skin Exposures in Radiation Oncology and in Physical Therapy [8, 10–13]

1.4.1 Main Characteristics

Table 1.7 Performance of effective wIRA-hyperthermia (wIRA-HT) in the clinical setting

Parameter	Radiation oncology	Physical therapy	Notes
Incident irradiance (IR-A)	Up to 150 mW cm^{-2}	≤150 mW cm^{-2}	Related to emission within the spectral range of IR-A
Incident irradiance (VIS$_1$)	–	≤50 mW cm^{-2}	Related to emission within the range of 590–780 nm (VIS$_1$)[a]
Incident irradiance (total)	Up to 200 mW cm^{-2}	≤200 mW cm^{-2}	Related to emission within VIS$_1$ and IR-A (590–1400 nm). The use of this quantity is not recommended due to incorrect merging of irradiance of two spectral ranges with different efficacies regarding photochemical and thermal effects.
Diameter of the effective size of the irradiated area	16 cm	16 cm	Using one normally oriented wIRA-irradiator[a] at a distance to skin surface of 33 cm and for required homogeneity of $g_2 ≥ 0.9$
	40 cm	40 cm	For using two parallel and normally oriented irradiators[a] at a distance to skin surface of 33 cm and for required homogeneity of $g_2 ≥ 0.9$. Lateral distance between both irradiators = 23.5 cm
Treatment time	40–60 min	≤60 min	Data presume short preheating times (up to 10–15 min) to reach therapeutically needed tissue temperatures. Times should be adequately prolonged if longer heating-up periods are needed (see Fig. 1.1).
Maximum skin surface temperature	43 °C	≤43 °C	Tissue temperatures ≥43 °C for treatment times >60 min can lead to skin and subcutis toxicity.
Tissue temperature required for effective (adjuvant) HT of superficial cancers	39–43 °C		
Tissue depth with HT ≥ 39 °C in superficial cancers	0–26 mm		HT ≥ 39 °C needed to increase local perfusion, tissue oxygenation, and vascular permeability; stimulation of antitumor immune responses; triggering of abscopal immune responses (see Fig. 1.2)

(continued)

Table 1.7 (continued)

Parameter	Radiation oncology	Physical therapy	Notes
Tissue depth with HT $\geq$ 40 °C in superficial cancers	0–17 mm		HT $\geq$ 40 °C is optimal for thermo-chemotherapy (with little additional increase of sensitization >42 °C).
Tissue depth with HT $\geq$ 41 °C in superficial cancers	0–8 mm		HT $\geq$ 41 °C necessary to inhibit DNA repair (double-strand breaks) (Fig. 1.2)
Tissue depth with HT $\geq$ 43 °C in superficial cancers	Not reached		HT $\geq$ 43 °C can lead to direct cytotoxic effects.

[a]Note: Data related to wIRA-irradiators of type *Hydrosun 750* (Hydrosun Medizintechnik, Müllheim, Germany) equipped with a cut-off filter of type *BTE 595* (BTE Elsoff, Germany).

1.4.2   Heating-up Times Necessary to Reach Thermal Steady-State Temperatures During wIRA-Hyperthermia in Normal Tissues [13]

Fig. 1.1 Mean values and standard deviations of heating-up times necessary to reach steady-state temperatures in the abdominal wall and lumbar region as a function of tissue depth. wIRA skin-exposure using an incident irradiance of 135 mW cm^{-2} (IR-A) [13]

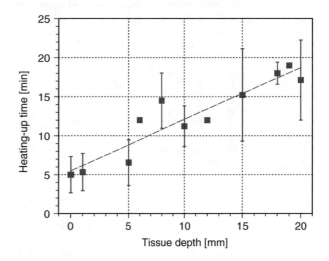

Mean Steady-State Temperatures During wIRA-Hyperthermia in Normal Tissues and Human Cancers [11–13]

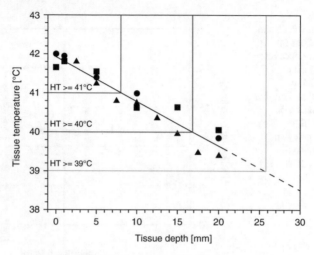

Fig. 1.2 Mean steady-state tissue temperatures during wIRA-HT as a function of tissue depth. Irradiances used for heating of different human tissues: 110–135 mW cm^{-2}. Data assessed in recurrent breast cancer (dots [11]), in various human tumors (triangles [12]), and in abdominal wall and lumbar region (squares [13]). Broken line: extrapolation of the best-fit line (solid). HT levels ≥39 °C: local increase in perfusion, tissue oxygenation, and vascular permeability; stimulation of antitumor immune responses, and fostering of abscopal immune responses (local effects within tissue depths of 0 mm to approx. 26 mm, green border). HT levels ≥40 °C: optimal temperature levels for thermo-chemotherapy with little additional increase of sensitization >42 °C (within tissue depths of 0 mm to about 17 mm, blue border). HT levels ≥41 °C: tissue temperatures necessary to inhibit DNA repair (double-strand breaks, within tissue depths of 0 mm to about 8 mm, red border). Tissue temperatures ≥43 °C for longer treatment times are mandatory for direct cytotoxicity

References

1. Bureau International de Poids and Measures (BIPM). The International system of units (SI). 8th ed. Paris: Organisation Intergouvernementale de la Convention du Métre, BIPM; 2006.
2. Commission International de l'Eclairage (CIE). International lighting vocabulary. Vienna: CIE; 2007.
3. Braslavsky SE. Glossary of terms used in photochemistry. Pure Appl Chem. 2007;79:293–465.
4. Sliney DH. Radiometric quantities and units used in photobiology and photochemistry: recommendations of the commission Internationale de l'Eclairage (international commission on illumination). Photochem Photobiol. 2007;83:425–32.
5. Jacques SL. Brief summary of the major points from a tutorial lecture. Ven: Graduate Summer School; 2003.
6. Piazena H, Kelleher DK. Effects of infrared A irradiation on skin: discrepancies in published data highlight the need for an exact consideration of physical and photobiological laws and appropriate experimental settings. Photochem Photobiol. 2010;86:687–705.
7. Venugupalan V. Tutorial on tissue optics. Optical Society of America BIOMED topical meeting. Beckman laser institute. Irvine: University of California; 2004.
8. Dobsicek Trefna H, Creeze H, Schmidt M, et al. Quality assurance guidelines for superficial hyperthermia clinical trials: I Clinical requirements. Int J Hyperthermia. 2017;33:471–82.
9. Dobsicek Trefna H, Crezee J, Schmidt M, et al. Quality assurance guidelines for superficial hyperthermia clinical trials: II. Technical requirements for heating devices. Strahlenther Onkol. 2017;193:351–66.
10. Vaupel P, Piazena H, Müller W, Notter M. Biophysical and photobiological basics of water-filtered infrared- A hyperthermia of superficial tumors. Int J Hyperthermia. 2019;35(1):26–36.
11. Notter M, Piazena H, Vaupel P. Hypofractionated re-irradiation of large-sized recurrent breast cancer with thermography-controlled, contact-free water-filtered infrared-A hyperthermia: a retrospective study of 73 patients. Int J Hyperthermia. 2016;33:471–82.
12. Seegenschmiedt MH, Klautke G, Walther E, et al. Water-filtered infrared-A-hyperthermia combined with radiotherapy for advanced and recurrent tumours. Strahlenther Onkol. 1996;172:475–84.
13. Thomsen AR, Saalmann MR, Nicolay NH, et al. Temperature profiles and oxygenation status in human skin and subcutis upon thermography-controlled wIRA-hyperthermia. (see Chapter 5, this book).

From Sun to Therapeutic wIRA

W. Müller, H. Piazena, and Peter Vaupel

2.1 Introduction

Everybody realizes intuitively that "sunshine" can be beneficial and invigorating. This also applies to animals and plants. There are first indications that the radiation of the sun was used for therapy and wellness since 1400 B.C. [1]. "Heliotherapy" is one of the oldest treatments humans have intentionally applied for disease prevention and health improvement. The role of the sun for all life on Earth has been recognized at a very early stage. In almost all cultures, people have developed sun cults, which are supposed to be an intuitive appreciation of the importance of the sun. There are profound reasons for this. As part of the solar system, Earth arose after the sun and was always exposed to the solar radiation. As a consequence, whatever happened on Earth took place under the influence of the sun.

Assuming that primeval forms of life arose in water, water was at the same time the element for chemical reactions, and a means of transport for dissolved substances, and environment. Energy available in the radiation of the sun probably acted as a stimulating factor. Fossils in stromatolites of the primeval seas of the archaean verify that cyanobacteria have performed photosynthesis with the aid of

W. Müller (✉)
Physical Optics Consultant Office, Wetzlar, Germany
e-mail: h.-werner.mueller@t-online.de

H. Piazena
Department of Anaesthesiology and Intensive Care Medicine, Charité - Universitätsmedizin Berlin, Corporative Member of Freie Universität Berlin and Humboldt Universität zu Berlin, Berlin, Germany

P. Vaupel
Department of Radiation Oncology, University Medical Center, University of Freiburg, Freiburg/Breisgau, Germany

German Cancer Consortium (DKTK) Partner Site Freiburg, German Cancer Research Center (DKFZ), Heidelberg, Germany

© The Author(s) 2022
P. Vaupel (ed.), *Water-filtered Infrared A (wIRA) Irradiation*,
https://doi.org/10.1007/978-3-030-92880-3_2

the solar radiation billions of years ago [2]. In order to get a better understanding about the nature of this radiation, it is mandatory to have a closer look at how it is produced.

2.2   Generation of the Electromagnetic Radiation in the Sun

The huge amount of energy emitted by the sun is generated by nuclear fusion. The temperature in the core of the sun is about 15×10^6 K, as indicated in Fig. 2.1a. The kinetic energy of atomic particles in this core is correspondingly high. Under these conditions and with the aid of the tunnel effect, by which a particle can pass through a potential energy barrier that is *higher* than its own energy and can overcome mutual repulsions, hydrogen is fused into helium in a multistep process as shown in Fig. 2.1b.

The cycle starts with the collision of two protons to form a deuteron (deuterium nucleus) with the simultaneous creation of a positron and a neutrino. When the positron encounters a free electron, both particles annihilate. Their mass energy is converted into two γ-photons (γ-rays) with high energy, according to Einstein's law:

$$E = \Delta m \cdot c^2 \tag{2.1}$$

where Δm = mass loss in the nuclear fusion, and c = phase velocity of light.

When the deuteron collides with a proton, a helium nucleus is created together with a γ-photon.

The overall equation is as follows:

$$4\,{}^1\mathrm{H} + 2\,e^- \rightarrow {}^4\mathrm{He} + 2\nu + 6\gamma \tag{2.2}$$

and the energy emitted into the space amounts to $\Delta E = 26.2\ MeV$ [4].

2.2.1   The Extra-Terrestrial Solar Spectrum

On its way to the photosphere (see Fig. 2.1a), observable from Earth as the surface of the sun, every γ-photon has its own individual fate. In nearly all cases, it loses energy because of interactions with other atomic particles before it is emitted into the space. Absorptions and re-emissions take place. Photons are also scattered within short distances, and a continuous spectrum of photons, related to their energies, is created. This spectrum of electromagnetic waves can be expressed according to Max Planck's law which connects the energy of a photon with the frequency and the wavelength of an electromagnetic wave, respectively (wave-particle-duality):

$$E = h \cdot \nu = h \cdot \frac{c}{\lambda} \tag{2.3}$$

where E = energy, c = velocity of the light, λ = wavelength, h = Planck's constant, and ν = frequency.

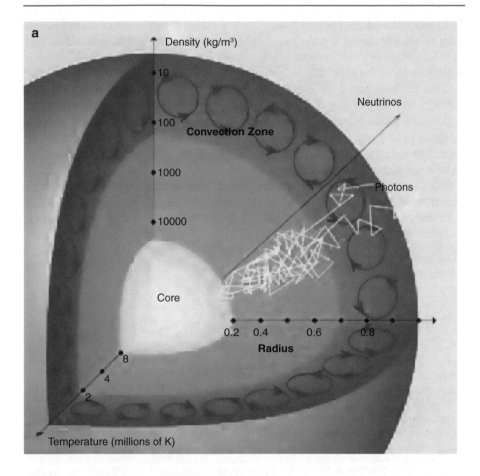

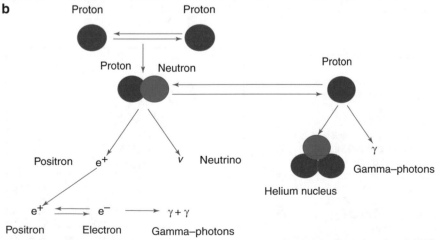

Fig. 2.1 (a) Internal structure of the sun. The radius numbers show the distance from the center related to the total sun radius of about 700,000 km. The way of the γ-photons (γ-rays) from the core to the surface and the decrease of their number is indicated by white zigzag lines (permission granted by Dr. Margarita Metaxa) [3]. (b) Multistep process of the nuclear fusion, in which hydrogen is burned into helium

In this spectrum, the proportion of the γ-photons is small as expected. Photons with less energy cover a wide range, which extends from 10^{-11} m to 10^8 m (see Fig. 2.2). For historical reasons, this spectrum has been arbitrarily subdivided into regions (ranges) based on different wavelengths [5].

This extra-terrestrial solar spectrum has a characteristic shape (see Fig. 2.3, curve 2) and has a maximum at 500 nm (blue-green light). The spectrum is superimposed by emission and absorption lines (Fraunhofer lines) that are mainly caused by gases in the photosphere of the sun at temperatures of about 5800 K. It can be approximated by a black body spectrum at 6000 K and can, therefore, be described mathematically with Planck's radiation law.

Planck's radiation law describes the spectral radiant exitance of electromagnetic radiation emitted by a black body in thermal equilibrium at a given temperature T. In the following form, it mathematically describes the differential spectral radiant exitance of an area A [7]:

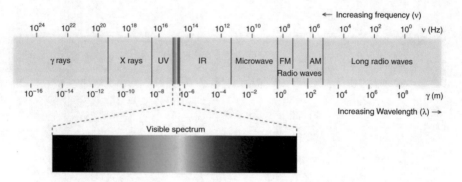

Fig. 2.2 The spectrum of electromagnetic waves emitted from the sun, subdivided into spectral regions. Author: Philip Ronan. Permission granted under the terms of the GNU Free Documentation Licence [5]

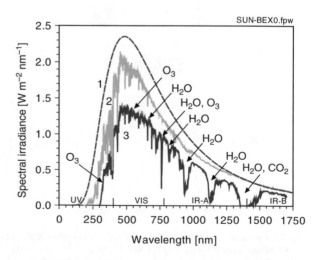

Fig. 2.3 Spectral irradiance as a function of wavelength. Curve 1 (blue): Black body spectral irradiance at 6000 K (data normalized for comparison). Curve 2 (green): Extra-terrestrial solar spectral irradiance [6]. Curve 3 (red): terrestrial solar spectral irradiance measured in Berlin on 2. July 2008 at noontime and clear sky (solar elevation angle = 50°)

$$dM_\lambda = \frac{2\pi hc^2}{\lambda^5} \cdot \frac{1}{e^{\left(\frac{hc}{k\lambda T}\right)} - 1} d\lambda \qquad (2.4)$$

where dM_λ = differential radiant exitance in the wavelength interval $d\lambda$, $c = 2.9979 \cdot 10^8$ ms^{-1} (vacuum velocity of the light), $h = 6.6256 \cdot 10^{-34}$ Ws^2 (Planck constant), and $k = 1.38054 \cdot 10^{-23}$ JK^{-1} (Boltzmann constant).

Other formulas can be derived from this theoretical superstructure. By differentiation, Wien's displacement law is obtained (first described by Wilhelm Wien, independent of Max Planck):

$$\lambda_{max} = \frac{b}{T} \qquad (2.5)$$

where λ_{max}= wavelength of the maximal spectral exitance of a black body, and $b = 2897.8$ µmK (Wien's displacement constant).

Equation (2.5) shows the inverse relationship between the wavelength of the emission maxima and the temperature. At higher temperatures, the maxima are shifted to smaller wavelengths (see Fig. 2.4).

By integration, the Stefan–Boltzmann law can be derived, describing the power radiated from a black body as a function of its temperature (earlier deduced by Josef Stefan and Ludwig Boltzmann):

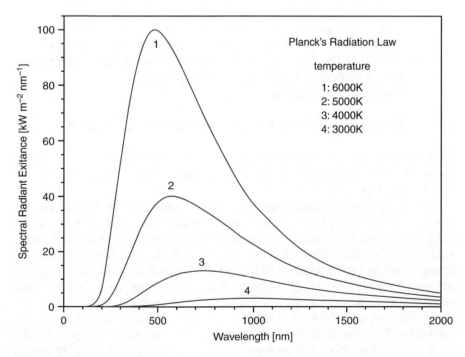

Fig. 2.4 Characteristic radiation curves of a black body at different temperatures covered by Planck's radiation law

$$M = \sigma \cdot T^4 \tag{2.6}$$

where M = radiant exitance, σ = 5.67032·10^{-8} Wm^{-2} K^{-4} (Stefan–Boltzmann constant), and T = absolute temperature [K].

2.2.2   The Terrestrial Solar Spectrum

Before radiation from the sun reaches Earth, it must pass the terrestrial atmosphere.

The solar spectrum on Earth exhibits strong absorption lines and bands indicating interactions of the radiation with gases in the atmosphere (see Fig. 2.3, curve 3).

As soon as water was on Earth, it was also in the atmosphere, mainly as water vapor. The first forms of life in water that were developed during evolution were exposed to solar radiation which was filtered through the water which was contained in the atmosphere and in their environment.

When the first living creatures colonized the land from sea, filtering by their original habitat was lost and they became continuously exposed to the solar radiation which was water-filtered in the atmosphere. Besides atmospheric ozone which absorbs short-wavelength UV radiation, and carbon dioxide which is responsible for thermal buffering in the atmosphere, the water in the atmosphere protects life from overheating by IR-B and IR-C and thereby provides suitable thermal conditions on Earth. Water-filtered IR-A has therefore influenced life during evolution until today.

2.3   The Generation of Absorption Lines and Bands (Water Bands) in the Terrestrial Spectrum, Interaction Between Water Molecules, and Electromagnetic Radiation (Photons)

2.3.1   Structure of the Water Molecule and Hydrogen Bonding

Decisive for the interaction between water molecules and photons is the structure of the water molecule. It consists of two hydrogen molecules and one oxygen molecule forming a triangle (see Fig. 2.5a).

Since the negative electrical charge of an oxygen atom is greater than the positive charge of a hydrogen atom, the electrons of the covalent bonds are drawn to the oxygen molecule. The center of both positive charges is spatially separated from the center of the negative charge, thereby creating a dipole. This dipole can take up energy from an electromagnetic field, and since covalent bonds have a certain amount of elasticity, the energy is converted into kinetic energy, e.g., in the form of *vibrations* along the binding arms and in *rotations* (see below).

Another property of the dipole character allows water molecules to interact with each other. The more positive part (H) approaches the more negative part (O) of a molecule in the neighborhood to create a hydrogen bond [9]. In this way, molecular spatial clusters are formed, and the individual molecules are restricted in their movement (see Fig. 2.5b, c).

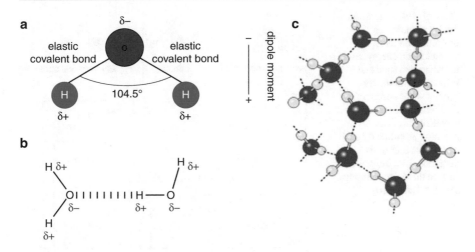

Fig. 2.5 Structure of the water molecule: (**a**) ball and stick model, with the angle between the atoms causing the dipole character of the molecule, (**b**) hydrogen bonds (Author: Benjah-bmm27, public domain [8]), and (**c**) water clusters, discrete hydrogen-bonded assemblies of water molecules. Author: Raimund Apfelbach, public domain [9]

2.3.2   Vibrations of the Water Molecule

2.3.2.1 Fundamental Vibrations

The freely movable water molecule (in water vapor) can vibrate in three basic ways: symmetrical stretching, asymmetrical stretching, and bending (see Fig. 2.6). Transitions from the lowest possible energy state of the molecules to the first excited state in these different vibrational modes are indicated by ν_1, ν_2, and ν_3. Energy required for excitations is supplied - in quanta - by photons, usually expressed in wavelengths [10].

The excited states are characterized by quantum numbers n. $n = 0$ describes the ground state, $n = 1$ the first excited state, etc. (see Fig. 2.6). The wavelengths related to the basic stretch vibrations are in the infrared-B (IR-B) range (1.4–3.0 μm), and the wavelength for bending is in the IR-C range (3–1000 μm). The energy for transitions from the ground state into higher excited states with, for example, two or three times the basic frequency, is taken from photons with smaller wavelengths and can cause absorption lines up into the red region of the visible spectrum (see Fig. 2.7) [10].

According to quantum physics, the higher the step of excitation, the lower the probability that it will occur and the lower the expression of the absorption line. This explains why in the terrestrial solar spectrum the most pronounced absorption bands are in the IR-A range.

2.3.2.2 Combination Vibrations

Vibrations can be composed of basic vibrations like $\nu_1 + \nu_2$ or $\nu_1 + \nu_2 + \nu_3$ or $2\nu_3 + 1\nu_1$. The corresponding energies are added, the absorption lines are shifted to smaller wavelengths. This kind of vibration, called *combination vibration*, provides

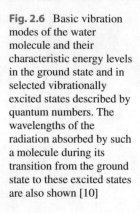
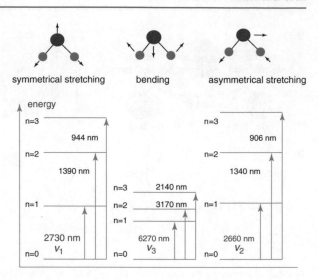

Fig. 2.6 Basic vibration modes of the water molecule and their characteristic energy levels in the ground state and in selected vibrationally excited states described by quantum numbers. The wavelengths of the radiation absorbed by such a molecule during its transition from the ground state to these excited states are also shown [10]

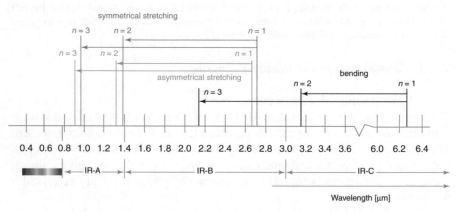

Fig. 2.7 Shift of the basic absorption lines after different steps of excitation

numerous combination possibilities. Combination bands are observed when more than two or more fundamental vibrations are excited simultaneously. Their energies can be close together to form pronounced absorption bands. They are marked by the quantum numbers related to the kinds of vibration $(\nu_1, \nu_2, \nu_3) \rightarrow (2,1,0)$ [11, 12].

2.3.2.3 Rotations

In addition to basic vibrations, rotations can increase the kinetic energy of the water molecule. There are three independent axes of rotation, which all go through the center of gravity close to the oxygen atom (see Fig. 2.8).

The rotation around each of these axes has its own moment of inertia (distribution of the mass related to the axis of rotation). Consequently, the rotational spectrum has no obvious structure. Since the moments of inertia on rotation are very small, the energies required for excitations are correspondingly small and the

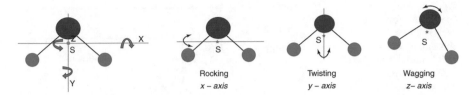

Rocking
x – axis

Twisting
y – axis

Wagging
z– axis

Fig. 2.8 Axes of rotation of the water molecule [13], and the different kinds of rotation related to these axes, with different moments of inertia

absorption lines are in the IR-B and IR-C range, in the microwave range, and in the range of radio waves. In liquid water, the movements of the molecules are considerably restricted by hydrogen bonds. Stretch vibrations require less energy, and rotations are reduced to librations [14, 15], i.e., the molecules no longer rotate, but only oscillate around their axis of rotation: They rotate back and forth. The absorption lines are shifted to longer wavelengths.

Basically, in liquid water each molecule is influenced by its surrounding matrix and creates its own absorption behavior related to the environment in which it is currently located. Summation of all single absorption lines results in a more or less broad absorption band.

The most important conclusions from these processes are as follows: (a) The energy absorbed by water molecules of solar radiation is exclusively converted into kinetic energy that means into heat; since the water content of soft tissues varies between 30–85% [16], *water is the key chromophore/absorber for hyperthermia*; (b) the water content in the tissue allows for detection of locally growing superficial tumors (surrounded by normal tissue) by temperature measurements (e.g., with an IR-camera), because most tumors contain 2–3 times more (interstitial) water than normal tissues [17] and, therefore, can "preferentially" be heated; (c) for thermal therapy (syn. thermotherapy), the water bands are decisive. Before radiation hits the skin, the number of photons within these bands must be reduced. If this would not occur, high irradiation in these bands would preferentially heat up upper tissue layers, which could result in nontolerable heat-induced pain and thereby prevent effective heating of deeper tissue layers. Water-filtered radiation thus reduces the risk of overheating body surfaces and allows for deeper penetration of the rest of the spectrum into the tissue.

In fair skin and underlying tissues, the absorption coefficients of the main chromophores (absorbers) have relative minima in the region between about 600 nm and 1300 nm (visible light and IR-A) (see Fig. 2.9). In this region, called the *optical window*, two effects come together: reduction of the irradiation in the water bands, mainly in the IR-A region and absorption minima of other absorbers. Therefore, the IR-A region is most important for tissue heating.

2.4   Generating Therapeutic wIRA

The generation of therapeutic wIRA requires an electromagnetic spectrum, which aligns with the most important characteristics of the terrestrial solar spectrum:

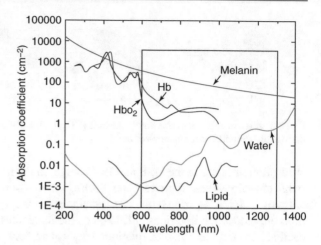

Fig. 2.9 Absorption coefficient spectra of various tissue chromophores ([18] Free PMC article). The spectra within the "optical window" (marked by the rectangle) show relative minima

1. The spectrum should be continuous, similar to the spectrum of a black body.
2. Its maximum should be in the IR-A region.
3. The radiation has to be water-filtered.
4. The radiation power should be higher than that of the sun.

Among all radiation sources, filament lamps best fulfill these criteria, especially halogen lamps. Therefore, in the wIRA-radiator, a 750 W halogen lamp is installed with a correlated color temperature CCT of about 2900 K (see Fig. 2.13a). According to Wien's displacement law, the maximum is at around 1082 nm, approximately in the middle of the IR-A region, as needed (see Fig. 2.10a).

A 7-mm-thick water layer in a hermetically sealed cuvette is used to "water filter" the spectrum. This thickness is an empirical compromise between the need to decrease irradiance within the water absorption bands and achieve the irradiance outside these bands, which is required for therapy.

2.5 Comparison Between Therapeutic wIRA and the Terrestrial Solar Spectrum

There is a great congruence between therapeutic wIRA and the terrestrial solar spectrum (see Fig. 2.11). The small shift of absorption bands to longer wavelengths because of hydrogen bonding is not relevant. The much higher spectral irradiance of wIRA in the IR-A than that of the solar spectrum enables adaptations to specific therapeutic needs as required.

As mentioned above, the water bands are more strongly expressed in the IR-A range due to the higher probability for lower step excitations of the water molecules requiring energy from the IR-A. The absorption lines in the visual part of the spectrum are only slightly pronounced. In principle, they can increase tissue heating, but their contribution, related to those of the bands in the IR-A, is small and can, therefore, be neglected.

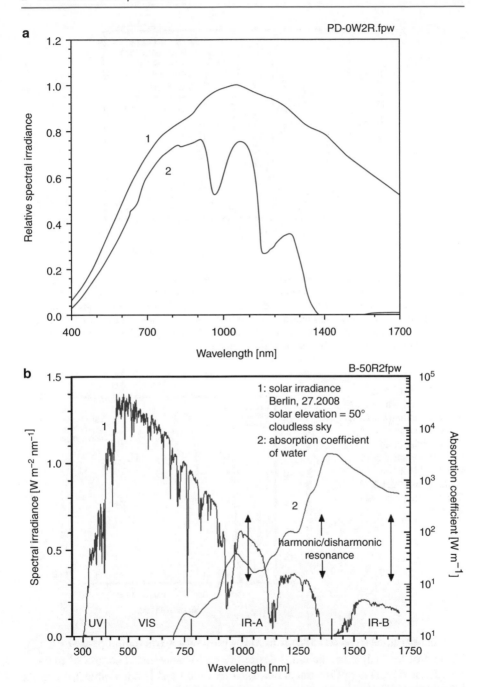

Fig. 2.10 (**a**) Curve 1: spectral irradiance of the 750 W halogen lamp (unfiltered), curve 2: spectral irradiance of the lamp after passing through a 7-mm water filter. (**b**) Comparison of spectra of solar terrestrial irradiance and absorption by water showing that the most significant areas of overlap occur in the region of 800–1300 nm, reducing the irradiance of solar radiation [19]

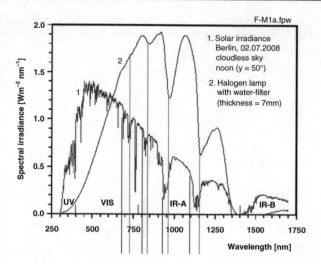

Fig. 2.11 Spectral irradiance of the water-filtered halogen lamp and of the terrestial midday sun in comparison. The shift of the absorption bands to longer wavelengths because of hydrogen bonding is obvious. Vertical red lines indicate the wavelengths of the absorption bands in the solar spectrum, and vertical blue lines indicate those of the halogen radiation filtered by liquid water [11]. It must be considered that additional substances in the atmosphere can influence shape and position of the absorption bands in the terrestrial spectrum

Fig. 2.12 Selection of wIRA spectra with the aid of optical filters. Curve 1: the wIRA spectrum with visible radiation for functional control of the wIRA radiator and marking the target field. Curve 2: the pure wIRA spectrum

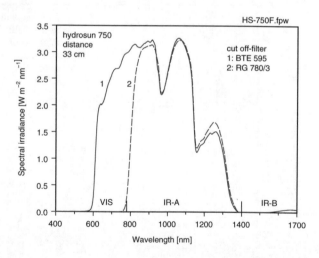

A cut-off filter (type RG 780) is used for pure wIRA irradiation (see Fig. 2.12). If a part of the visible irradiation is desired (e.g., for easy visual control of radiator function and marking of treatment fields. *Note*: Pure IR-A is not visible!), a cut-off filter (type BTE 595) is recommended (see Fig. 2.12).

2.6   The wIRA Radiator

The wIRA radiator (type Hydrosun 750, Hydrosun, Müllheim/Baden, Germany) is schematically shown in Fig. 2.13a. In this wIRA radiator, the halogen lamp is placed in the focal point of a concave mirror collimating most of the radiation. The filter bracket acts as a diaphragm. Because the lamp filament is not a point radiation source and reflection of the concave mirror does not completely create a parallel beam, the main radiation is somewhat divergent (see Fig. 2.13b).

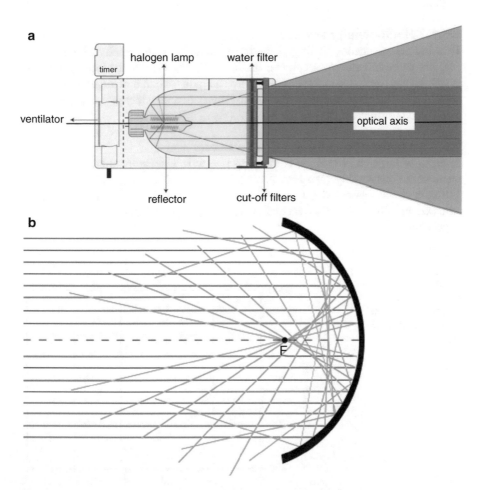

Fig. 2.13 (**a**) Scheme (cross-section) of the Hydrosun wIRA radiator (type *Hydrosun 750,* Hydrosun Medizintechnik, Müllheim/Baden, Germany). Courtesy of Hydrosun Medizintechnik, Müllheim/Baden, Germany), (**b**) collimation of radiation by a concave mirror inside the irradiator. Author: Synkizz. Permission by creative-commons-license 3.0 [20]

2.6.1 Characteristics of Therapeutically Applied wIRA Irradiation

2.6.1.1 Setting the Desired Irradiance

Depending on the therapeutic effect to be achieved, irradiance can be adapted by varying the distance between the wIRA radiator exit and the target area (patient). In this way, the spectrum is not altered. Varying the power supply of the lamp instead would influence the emitted spectrum according to Wien's displacement law (Fig. 2.14).

2.6.1.2 Homogeneity of wIRA

To avoid heterogeneous heating of the target area, the homogeneity of the irradiation has to be monitored. As shown in Fig. 2.15, the size of the homogeneously irradiated area depends on the distance between radiator exit and target. Even in the case of two combined radiators, the homogeneity in a considerably enlarged treatment field is sufficient, despite the overlap (Fig. 2.15b).

2.6.1.3 Combination of Two wIRA Radiators

In cases of large-sized lesions, combining two wIRA radiators enlarges the treatment field considerably (see Fig. 2.15b). The optimal distance between the two radiators can be assessed by real-time thermography. In addition, they can be adjusted in different angles according to individual requirements of the treatment field.

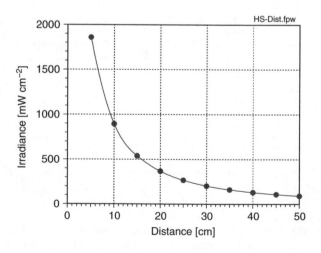

Fig. 2.14 Irradiance of wIRA as a function of the distance between the radiator exit and the target area

Fig. 2.15 Lateral distribution of the irradiance as a function of the distance between the wIRA radiator exit and the target area. (**a**) single radiator [21]. (**b**) Combination of two radiators. The lateral distance of their axes is 23.5 cm, with 33 cm between the radiator exit and the target area [21]

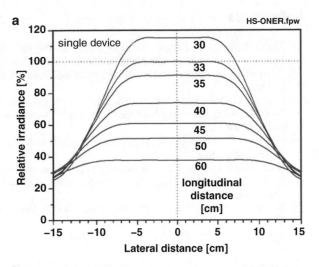

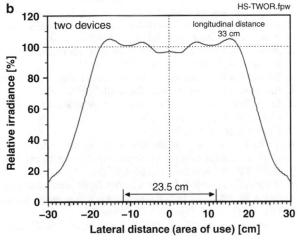

2.7   Conclusions

Compared to other IR radiations used for thermo-therapy such as IR-C radiation, wIRA is approximated (up to a high degree) to the natural IR-A radiation of the sun, filtered by the water vapor in the atmosphere. Humans are adapted to this radiation during evolution. wIRA can be applied contact-free and thus also to ulcerated lesions without any discomfort for patients. Combining wIRA with a part of the visible spectrum clearly indicates the irradiated target field without influencing heating and allows for real-time temperature monitoring in the treatment field; this is unique in the hyperthermia field. The water bands in the spectrum reduce the risk of thermal skin damage yet supply sufficient energy for effective tissue heating (39–43 °C) up to tissue depths of 26 mm [22].

References

1. Krause R, Stange R. (Hrsg): Lichttherapie. Einführung und Geschichte der Lichttherapie. In: Spuren einer Heliotherapie im Altertum. Berlin, Heidelberg: Springer; 2012.
2. Wikipedia. Stromatolite. Text is available under the Creative Commons Attribution-ShareAlike License.
3. Spectr J. The life of stars and their spectra. Under references: The internal structure of the sun (from the book, Astronomy and Space"), in Greek. Permission by Dr. Margarita Metaxa, a co-author of this book.
4. Wikipedia. Proton-Proton-Reaktion. Text is available under the Creative Commons Attribution-ShareAlike License.
5. Wikimedia Commons. File: EM spectrum.svg. This image comes from the English Wikipedia (Original author: Philip Roman. The file is licensed under the Creative Commons Attribution-Share Alike 3.0.
6. Wehrli C. Extraterrestrial solar spectrum. Davos Dorf: Physikalisch-Meteorologisches Observatorium + World Radiation Center; 1985.
7. Magrathea Informatik GmbH. Erstaunliches und Bekanntes beim Planckschen Strahlungsgesetz. Dollinger J. 2014;2:12.
8. Die Chemie-Schule. Wikimedia Commons. Hydrogen bonding of water molecules 2D. Benjah-bmm27. Public domain; 2007.
9. Die Chemie-Schule. Wikimedia Commons. Hydrogen bonds in water. Original author: Raimund Apfelbach. Public domain; 2010.
10. Bogdan W, Jerzy D. Light absorption by water molecules and inorganic substances dissolved in sea water. Cham: Springer; 2007. p. 11–81.
11. Ramasesha K, De Marco L, Mandal A, et al. Water vibrations have strongly mixed intra- and intermolecular character. Nat Chem. 2013;5:935–40.
12. Libre Texts Libraries. Combination vibrations, overtones and fermi resonances. Davis: University of California; 2020.
13. Cruzan J. xactly.com, Water.
14. Verma PK, Kundu A, Puretz MS, et al. The bend+libration combination band is an intrinsic, collective, and strongly solute-dependent reporter on the hydrogen bonding network of liquid water. J Phys Chem B. 2017;122:2587–99.
15. Tong Y, Kampfrath T, Kramer Campen R. Experimentally probing the libration of interfacial water: the rotational potential of water is stiffer at the air/water interface than in bulk liquid. Phys Chem Chem Phys. 2016;18:18424–30.
16. Vaupel P, Schaible HG, Mutschler E. Anatomie, Physiologie, Pathophysiologie des Menschen. In: 7. Auflage. Stuttgart: Wissenschaftliche Verlagsgesellschaft; 2015.
17. Vaupel P. Blood flow, oxygenation, tissue pH distribution and bioenergetic status of tumors. Berlin: Ernst Schering Foundation; 1994.
18. Xia J, Yao J, Wang L. Photoacoustic tomography: principles and advances. NIH Public Access Electromagn Waves. 2014;147:1–22.
19. Tsai S-R, Hamblin MR. Biological effects and medical applications of infrared radiation. J Photochem Photobiol B Biol. 2017;170:197–207.
20. Wikipedia. Datei. Abbildungsfehler am Hohlspiegel (Katakaustik).svg. The file is licensed under the Creative Commons Attribution-Share Alike 3.0 Unported.
21. Vaupel P, Piazena H, Müller W, Notter M. Biophysical and photobiological basics of water-filtered infrared-A hyperthermia of superficial tumors. Int J Hyperthermia. 2018;35:26–36.
22. Piazena H, Müller W, Vaupel P. Glossary used in wIRA-hyperthermia (see Chapter 1, this book).

Physical and Photobiological Basics of wIRA-Hyperthermia

3

H. Piazena, W. Müller, and Peter Vaupel

Abbreviations

ESHO	European Society of Hyperthermic Oncology
HR	Heating rate
SAR	Specific absorption rate
SST	Steady-state (tissue) temperature
TR	Temperature rise
TSS	Thermal steady state
wIRA	Water-filtered infrared A
wIRA-HT	wIRA-hyperthermia

3.1 Introduction

Derived from the primary idea to simulate living tissue heating, as experienced by solar infrared radiation at the surface of our planet, hyperthermia using water-filtered infrared A radiation (wIRA) has been established as a potent method in

H. Piazena (✉)
Department of Anaesthesiology and Operative Intensive Care Medicine, Charité - Universitätsmedizin Berlin, Corporative Member of Freie Universität Berlin and Humboldt Universität zu Berlin, Berlin, Germany
e-mail: helmut.piazena@charite.de

W. Müller
Physical Optics Consultant Office, Wetzlar, Germany

P. Vaupel
Department of Radiation Oncology, University Medical Center, University of Freiburg Freiburg/Breisgau, Germany

German Cancer Consortium (DKTK) Partner Site Freiburg, German Cancer Research Center (DKFZ), Heidelberg, Germany

physical therapy and radiation oncology (see [1–11] and respective chapters in this book). wIRA-hyperthermia (wIRA-HT) is based on tissue heating induced by absorption of water-filtered infrared A radiation by chromophores (mainly water molecules). However, kinetics of heating and resulting heating states depend on several physical and photobiological processes, and on physiological/regulatory responses. These processes interact with each other and should be considered to ensure appropriate hyperthermia levels that are required for special indications.

This article aims to extent and update previous publications on physical and photobiological basics of wIRA-hyperthermia [12, 15] with a special focus on optical interactions of wIRA with tissues, thermal field formation during irradiation within tissues, and the kinetics of temperature decay after completion of wIRA exposure.

The following items will be discussed in more detail: (a) effects of irradiance, exposure time, thermoregulation, and individual responses upon heating, (b) needs for adequate dosage and documentation of wIRA exposures due to the non-applicability of the *Bunsen–Roscoe* law of reciprocity upon tissue heating, (c) evidence of direct conversion of absorbed wIRA irradiation into heat, as assessed by comparison of depth profiles of wIRA penetration and of heating rates, (d) vertical temperature profiles and their dependence on irradiance and individual thermoregulation, and (e) effects of irradiance on tissue heating with respect to the quality assurance criteria of the European Society of Hyperthermic Oncology (ESHO) for adequate heating.

Analyses of the thermal field formation within the tissue have been based on invasive temperature measurements in piglets that had been in vivo irradiated with wIRA using different irradiances [16], supplemented by data derived from analogous measurements in human abdominal wall and breast cancer [17, 18]. Optical interaction data have been derived from measurements on healthy volunteers of different skin color and are discussed using model calculations [19, 20].

3.2   wIRA: Infrared Radiation That Fits into the Optical Window of Tissues

From the optical point of view, human tissues can be considered as turbid media. When optical radiation penetrates the skin, subcutis/fat layer, and muscle, its propagation is characterized by multiple scattering and absorption. Both processes depend on the wavelength. Scatterers with small diameters—as compared to the wavelength—cause *isotropic (Rayleigh) scattering*. Small diameter scatterers include membranes, striations in collagen fibrils and muscle fibers, and macromolecular aggregates with diameters between about 10 nm and 100 nm. However, the greater the diameter of scatterers, the more the scattering passes into forward direction *(Mie scattering)*. Scatterers of the latter type are lysosomes, vesicles, mitochondria, and nuclei having diameters between about 100 nm and 10 μm. Moreover, each interface within the tissue causes scattering if the relative refraction indexes of both media differ. Similarly, fluctuations of the dielectric constant and of density may contribute to scattering. As a consequence, the multiple scattering that appears prolongs the retention time of radiation in the tissue and results mainly in forward propagation of short-wavelength infrared radiation, in deep penetration and transmission, and in backscattering within the tissue and diffuse reflectance (remission) (see Fig. 3.1).

According to the *first law of photobiology* (*Grotthuss–Draper* law), only absorption of radiation (by chromophores) causes photochemical and photophysical effects within tissues. The most important chromophore of human soft tissues is intra- and extracellular water (average water content ≈70–80%). However, as shown in Fig. 3.2, the absorption coefficient of water in the visible spectral range is small. It increases with wavelength up to a factor of about 15 within the range of IR-A, but up to 10^4 for wavelengths above 1400 nm. This causes strong absorption of mid- and long-wavelength infrared radiation (IR-B and IR-C) within the subsurface layer of the skin and defines the long-wavelength edge of the optical window (see Fig. 3.3). The short-wavelength edge of the optical window is mainly defined by absorption of radiation according to the contents of hemoglobin and melanin, and by increasing influence of scattering with decreasing wavelengths (Figs. 3.2 and 3.3).

Presuming values for relative spectral absorbance ≤0.5, the optical window ranges from about 600 nm in fair skin and about 750 in black skin to about 1300 nm. Curve 2 in Fig. 3.3 shows that the spectrum of the wIRA radiator matches

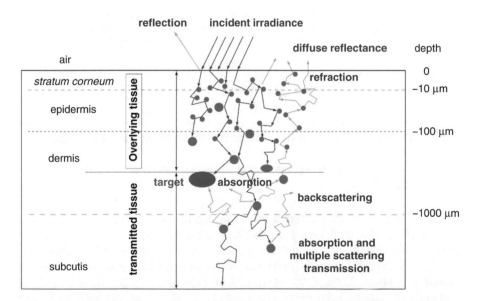

Fig. 3.1 Schematic overview of interactions between optical radiation and skin. Processes of interaction are *reflection* at the surface, *refraction of subsurface irradiance, multiple scattering* and *backscattering*, and *absorption* by chromophores ([14], ©Thieme Gruppe). Layer depths are approximate values for human skin (epidermis and dermis). Individual thicknesses of skin may deviate. Measured values for Caucasians ranged from 0.5 to 2.0 mm with mean values between 0.8 and 1.5 mm [21]. The proportion of the epidermis within the dermis is approx. 4% for Caucasians and up to 8% for Asians [21]. In piglets, thicknesses of skin and fat layer are up to 5 mm each [16]

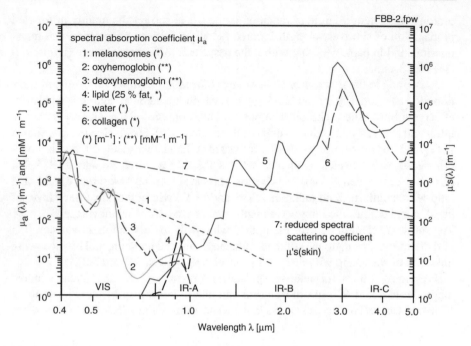

Fig. 3.2 The spectral absorption coefficient (μ_a, left ordinate) of melanosomes, oxyhemoglobin, deoxyhemoglobin, lipids (25% fat), and water, and the reduced spectral scattering coefficient of skin (μ'_s, right ordinate) as a function of wavelength ([14], ©Thieme Gruppe)

the optical window of tissues. It shows minima where spectral absorbance shows maxima, and it is limited to the spectral range inside of the optical window.

3.3 Optical Effects of Interaction Between wIRA and Tissues

3.3.1 Spectral Transmittance and Remittance of wIRA (In vivo Data)

Spectra of transmittance and remittance measured in vivo show characteristic local minima (Fig. 3.4a, b, curves 1a, 1b). These characteristic curves are caused by absorption of radiation within the absorption bands of water (maxima at about 970, 1197, and 1400 nm), of lipids (maxima at about 932 and 1212 nm), of hemoglobin (maxima at about 573 and 758 nm), and of cytochrome-c (maximum at about 840 nm) and can be used for optically based diagnostics. However, since intra- and extracellular water is the main absorbent of infrared radiation in the tissue, the basic concept of wIRA relies on the extracorporeal attenuation of infrared radiation within the spectral absorption bands of water by using a water filter, which minimizes the spectral distribution within these absorption bands and outside of the spectral range of IR-A [13].

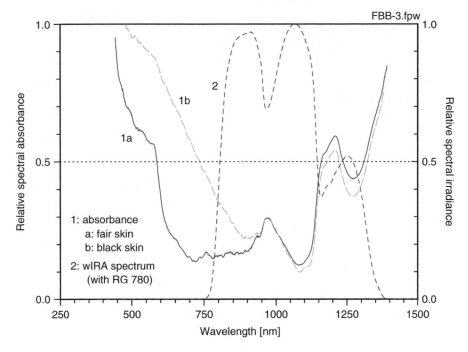

Fig. 3.3 Relative spectral absorbance in fair skin (curve 1a, blue) and in black skin (curve 1b, green) compared to the relative spectral irradiance of a wIRA-radiator (type *Hydrosun 750*, Hydrosun Medizintechnik, Müllheim, Germany, curve 2, red) as a function of wavelength. Relative spectral absorbance data were calculated from in vivo measurements of spectral transmittance at the ear lobes and of spectral remittance at the forearms of volunteers with fair or black skin. Individual thickness of both ear lobes: 2.4 mm [19]. The wIRA-radiator was equipped with a water filter of 7 mm thickness and with a cutoff filter (type: *RG 780/3*, Schott, Mainz, Germany)

Thus, wIRA entering the skin shows a similar spectral distribution as compared to the spectra of transmittance and remittance within the spectral range of IR-A (Fig. 3.4a, b, curves 1a, 1b, and 2). This allows for (a) direct transformation of absorbed energy into heat in deeper tissue layers and (b) reduced heating in the upper tissue layers by absorption of radiation within the absorption bands of water, as compared to unfiltered IR-A (for detailed data, see [19]).

The transmittance of ear lobes (individual thickness: 2.4 mm) is exemplified in Fig. 3.4a: the maximum appears at a wavelength of about 1082 nm with values of 30.0% (fair skin, curve 1a) and approximately 23.4% (black skin, curve 1b), whereas within the total IR-A range, mean values range from 19.4% (fair skin) to 15.3% (black skin).

Weak absorption enabling deeper penetration into the tissue is correlated with a high loss of incident radiation due to backscattering and remission. This results in maximum remittances of 62.4% (fair skin) and 56.5% (black skin) at a wavelength of about 1082 nm and in mean values of 45.4% (fair skin) and 44.0% (black skin) within the total IR-A range (Fig. 3.4b, curves 1a, 1b).

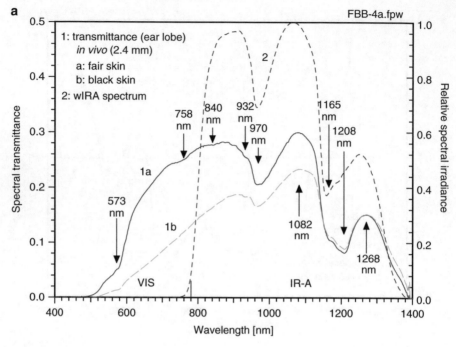

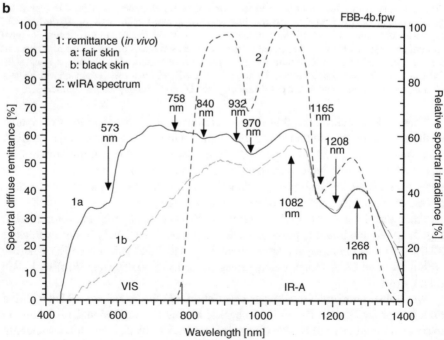

Fig. 3.4 Relative spectral transmittance (**a**) and relative spectral diffuse remittance (**b**) assessed in vivo in fair skin (curve 1a, blue) and in black skin (curve 1b, green) compared to relative spectral irradiance of a wIRA-radiator (type *Hydrosun 750*, Hydrosun Medizintechnik, Müllheim, Germany, curve 2, red) as a function of wavelength. Spectral transmittance data were measured in the ear lobes, and spectral remittance in the forearms of volunteers with fair and black skin. Individual thickness of both ear lobes: 2.4 mm [19]. Arrows show *local minima* due to absorption by hemoglobin (573 nm, 758 nm), cytochrome-c (840 nm), lipids (932 nm, 1212 nm), water (970 nm, 1197 nm, and 1400 nm), and *local maxima* (1082 nm and 1268 nm). The wIRA-radiator was equipped with a water filter of 7 mm thickness and with a cut-off filter (type: *RG 780/3*, Schott, Mainz, Germany)

It is apparent that the effect of absorption by melanin in black skin upon spectral remittance and spectral transmittance within the IR-A range is small. In contrast, mean transmittances (shown in Fig. 3.4a) shift from 13.0% (fair skin) to 5.3% (black skin) and remittances (shown in Fig. 3.4b) from 45.9% (fair skin) to 19.2% (black skin) in the visible range.

3.3.2 Penetration of wIRA into Tissues

Penetration of wIRA into tissues was calculated using a model based on Monte Carlo simulation, which assumes fair, bloodless, plane-parallel oriented skin, and vertical homogeneous distribution of scatterers and chromophores within the tissue [19, 20].

Results depicted in Fig. 3.5 show that incident irradiance (= 100%) decreased to about 53.6% at the immediate subsurface of the skin, indicating a loss of incident irradiance of about 46.4% due to diffuse remission. This calculated value is in very good accordance with the remittance of 45.4% measured in vivo for fair skin using wIRA-exposure (see Fig. 3.4b, curve 1a). Calculated transmittance at a tissue depth of 2.4 mm is about 23.5%, a value that differs from the in vivo measurement (see Fig. 3.4a, curve 1a) by about 20% and is within the ranges of error for the measurement and model calculation.

Considering the 20% margin of error for the model calculation and in vivo conditions, approximated levels of relative irradiances of wIRA in fair skin and underlying tissues (subcutis and muscle) are 36.8% (1/e) at a depth of 2.3 mm, 10% at 5 mm, 1% at 16 mm, and 0.1% at 28.5 mm.

It is noteworthy to mention that the slope of the curve in Fig. 3.5 transitions from a steep to shallow decline with increasing depth at a depth of about 5 mm. This is the result of decomposition of the incident wIRA spectrum with depth due to spectral selective absorption by chromophores (as shown in Fig. 3.2) and in favor of spectral parts where absorption is small.

Fig. 3.5 Relative irradiance of wIRA as a function of tissue depth in fair skin and underlying tissues (subcutis and muscle). Incident irradiance of 100% at skin surface decreased to about 53.6% at the immediate subsurface level due to relative remittance of about 46.4%. Calculated data [20]

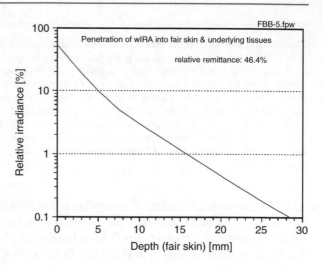

3.4   Thermal Field Formation in Superficial Tissues During wIRA-Hyperthermia

In vivo data reported in this chapter are derived from wIRA-skin exposures of the upper thighs of anesthetized piglets (body weight: 15–20 kg) [16]. To exclude superposing effects of convective or conductive heating upon skin and tissue temperature, wIRA-treatments were performed in a closed room with constant air temperature of 22–24 °C, without airflow, and with humidity monitoring turned on.

3.4.1   Individual Responses to wIRA-Skin Exposures

The thermal state of tissues during wIRA-heating depends not only on spectrum, irradiance, and exposure time, but - according to Pennes' Bioheat equation - also on additional factors such as individual local blood flow, heat conductivity of tissues, and metabolic heat production [20, 22].

This is exemplified in Fig. 3.6 by comparing two identically exposed piglets. Probably due to its higher body core temperature of 39 °C (resulting in decreased vertical temperature gradients in the tissue and in decreased convective heat transport by increased blood flow due to its higher body temperature), piglet p2 was unable to effectively thermoregulate and, thus, showed a continuous increase in temperature during the exposure up to a tissue depth of 10 mm, exceeding 45 °C at a tissue depth of 4 mm after 35 min wIRA-irradiation was consequently stopped. In contrast, piglet p3 initially showed a physiological body core temperature of 37.8 °C. P3 achieved a thermal steady state due to rapidly activated thermoregulation and approximately constant temperatures (up to 43.5 °C) within the upper tissue layers after ≈15 min of wIRA-exposure. Further activation of thermoregulation was started after ≈40 min of exposure to decrease the temperature level.

Fig. 3.6 Temperature at skin surface (1) and at tissue depths of 4 mm (2), 10 mm (3), and 20 mm (4) as a function of treatment time during wIRA-skin exposure of two piglets (p2 and p3) in vivo (a: p3, blue lines, b: p2, red lines). Irradiance used: 126.5 mW cm⁻² (IR-A)

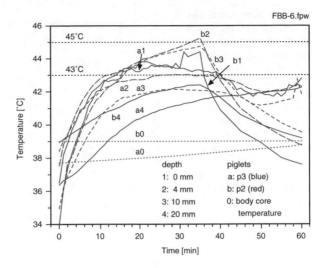

3.4.2   Effects of Irradiance, Exposure Time, and Thermoregulation Upon Heating

During the first 1–2 min of exposure, tissue temperature increases approximately proportionally with exposure time and as a function of irradiance and tissue depth (as shown in Fig.3.6). This is caused by a delayed onset of heat dissipation and thermoregulation and allows for the calculation of heating rates as a crucial measure of heating effectiveness (see Sect. 3.4.3).

Data in Fig. 3.7 A show that after the onset of thermoregulation, i.e., 2–5 min after onset of exposure, irradiance affects the extent of regulatory processes in different ways. Using the smallest irradiance, only moderate regulation is evident resulting in a continuous increase in tissue temperature (curve 3). In contrast, the two higher irradiances caused adequate thermoregulatory responses resulting in a balance between heat input and heat dissipation, i.e., in a thermal steady state (curves 1 and 2).

Note: Limitations in thermoregulation may result in tissue overheating (as discussed above for piglet p2 in Sect. 3.4.1). Therefore, febrile patients and patients with inadequate convective (i.e., blood flow-mediated) heat transfer due to certain peripheral vascular pathologies should be excluded from wIRA-treatment if continuous control/monitoring of skin surface temperatures using thermography is not ensured.

Radiant exposure (dose) H_{wIRA} is calculated according to

$$H_{wIRA} = E_{wIRA} \cdot \Delta t \tag{3.1}$$

where E_{wIRA} denotes the irradiance of wIRA, and Δt denotes the exposure time.

Data in Fig.3.7b show that identical doses result in different levels of tissue hyperthermia. They are inversely related to the exposure time and correlate directly with irradiances. Thus, tissue heating cannot be adequately characterized by specifying the radiant exposure (dose) due to its dependence on the thermal impact

Fig. 3.7 Mean values and standard deviations of skin surface temperatures as a function of exposure time (**a**) and of dose (**b**) calculated according to Eq. (3.1). Skin exposures were performed with wIRA using IR-A irradiances of 126.5 mW cm^{-2} (1, diamonds, four piglets), 103.2 mW cm^{-2} (2, triangles, four piglets), and 85.0 mW cm^{-2} (3, dots, three piglets)

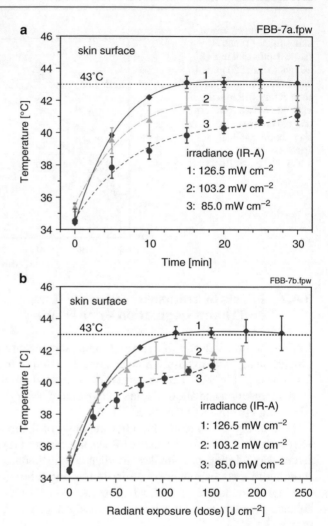

determined by irradiance and exposure time and, additionally, by heat dissipation and metabolic heat production. For this reason, the *Bunsen–Roscoe law of reciprocity* is not applicable in tissue heating and reported data should specify both irradiance and exposure time, instead of the dose only [20].

3.4.3 Effective Tissue Heating by Direct wIRA Absorption and Heat Conduction

To prove effectiveness of wIRA-heating within tissues, vertical profiles of relative heating rates and of relative temperature rises in piglets were compared to the profile of relative wIRA-irradiance (Fig. 3.8a, b).

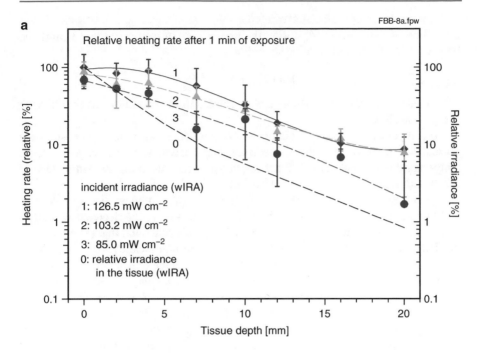

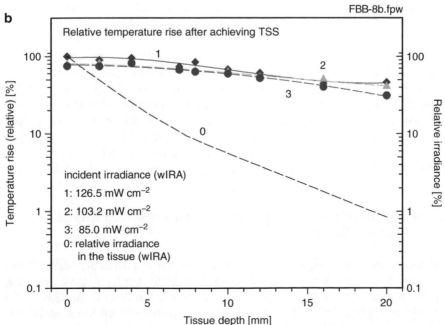

Fig. 3.8 Relative heating rates assessed in piglets after 1 min of wIRA-exposure (**a**), and relative temperature rises during wIRA skin exposure after achieving thermal steady states (**b**) in comparison with relative wIRA-irradiance (0, broken line) and as a function of tissue depth. Piglets were exposed to wIRA-irradiances (IR-A) of 126.5 mW cm^{-2} (1, red diamonds), 103.2 mW cm^{-2} (2, green triangles), and 85.0 mW cm^{-2} (3, blue dots)

Heating rates were calculated using the temperature increase in the tissue (δT) as a function of tissue depth (d) during the first minute of exposure ($\delta t = 1$ min) and before onset of thermoregulation according to:

$$HR(d) = \delta T(d)/\delta t. \tag{3.2}$$

In contrast, temperature rise data were related to the conditions after achieving thermal steady states.

To compare depth profiles, relative wIRA-irradiance data within the tissue were normalized to the value at the skin surface, and relative heating rates and relative temperature rises were related to the respective mean values at the skin surface of piglets exposed to 126.5 mW cm^{-2} (IR-A).

According to Fig. 3.8a, relative heating rates measured at tissue depths of 5–20 mm comparably decrease with depth as compared to the decrease of wIRA-irradiance. This verifies, for the first time by experimental data, that (a) direct conversion of absorbed energy of wIRA into heat occurs significantly in the total depth range observed and (b) absorption of wIRA initially is the only source of heating.

In the skin of piglets (tissue depths of 0–5 mm), the *heating rate* shows a smaller decrease with depth as compared to the decrease in wIRA-irradiance. This is due to a (a) rapid induction of both, conductive (by molecular vibrations) and convective (via blood flowing through U-shaped capillary loops in the papillary and subpapillary layers, thus locally heated by direct radiation absorption), centripetally oriented heat flow, which also contributes to tissue heating in addition to the heating by absorption of radiation and to a (b) heat loss at the skin surface by increased radiant exitance to the environment.

In contrast, after achieving the thermal steady state, relative temperature increments only marginally decreased with depth, as compared to the decrease in relative wIRA-irradiance (Fig. 3.8b). This is caused by the balance between heat input (by wIRA absorption and conductive/convective heat transport from upper to deeper tissue layers) and heat dissipation due to thermoregulatory responses (mainly by an increase in blood flow resulting in convective heating of the body core and by conductive heat transport into deeper tissue layers). Evidence for this interpretation is based on the increased body core temperatures of piglets after skin exposure to wIRA (see [16], Table 3.1).

3.4.4 Vertical Temperature Profiles After Achieving Thermal Steady States

Tissue temperatures in piglets show maxima in the skin at a depth of ≈ 4 mm. These increase skin surface temperatures up to 2 K in individual cases and to about 0.7 K on average, and these ranged from 43.6 °C for 126.5 mW cm^{-2} to 42.6 °C for 85 mW cm^{-2} (Fig. 3.9). Similarly, tissue temperatures assessed in the abdominal wall and the lumbar region of healthy volunteers exceeded skin surface temperatures by about 0.6 K at a depth of 1 mm (see Fig. 3.2 [23]).

In piglets, these maxima result from heat accumulation in the transition region skin/subcutaneous fat layer due to decreased conductive heat transport into deeper

Table 3.1 Mean tissue depth with therapeutically relevant temperature ranges during wIRA-HT after achieving thermal steady states. Means assessed in piglets in vivo exposed to different irradiances and in the abdominal wall of healthy volunteers exposed to wIRA (135 mW cm⁻², IR-A) [16, 23]. Note that skin thickness is different in humans and piglets. Skin thickness is ≈ 5 mm in piglets [16]. In humans, the thickness of the skin (epidermis + dermis) of the abdominal wall and lumbar region ranges from 2 to 2.5 mm [21]

Tissue temperature [°C]	Mean tissue depth with therapeutically efficient HT levels [mm]			
	Piglets exposed to			Humans exposed to
	126.5 mW cm⁻²	103.2 mW cm⁻²	85.0 mW cm⁻²	135 mW cm⁻²
≥39	> 20	>20	>20	≤26
≥40	>20	>20	>20	≤17
≥41	16	16	12	≤8
≥42	11	10	10	≤2
43–44	8	Not reached	Not reached	<1

Fig. 3.9 Mean values and standard deviations of tissue temperatures as a function of tissue depth after achieving a thermal steady state in piglets exposed to wIRA using irradiances of 126.5 mW cm⁻² (1, red diamonds), 103.2 mW cm⁻² (2, green triangles), and 85.0 mW cm⁻² (3, blue dots). Comparison with respective tissue temperatures before heat exposure (0, black squares) [16]

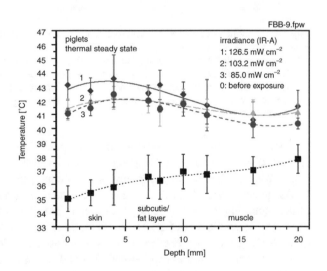

tissue layers when heat passes the fat layer [16], and might, under certain circumstances result in side effects due to overheating of tissues [24].

In both, fat layer and skeletal musculature temperatures continuously decrease with tissue depth. Based on data shown in Fig. 3.9 (and in Fig. 1, presented in Piazena et al. [23]), Table 3.1 provides mean tissue depths with therapeutically relevant temperature levels.

3.4.5 Choice of Irradiance for Adequate wIRA-Hyperthermia in Oncology

Heating rate, as defined in Eq. (3.2), is considered a crucial parameter for characterizing and documenting the performance of heat applicators used in hyperthermia [25].

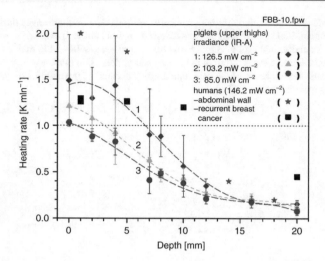

Fig. 3.10 Heating rates assessed in vivo as a function of tissue depth in the upper thigh of piglets exposed to wIRA using IR-A irradiances of 126.5 mW cm^{-2} (curve 1, red diamonds), 103.2 mW cm^{-2} (curve 2, green triangles), and 85.0 mW cm^{-2} (curve 3, blue dots). Data are mean values and standard deviations (curve fits using polynomial regression). Results are compared to published data from preliminary in vivo measurements in human abdominal wall (pink stars, [17]) and in recurrent breast cancer (black squares, [18]) during wIRA skin exposure using 146.2 mW cm^{-2} (IR-A) [26]

For adequate/appropriate performance, the guidelines of the *European Society of Hyperthermic Oncology* (ESHO) require values of HR $\geq$1 K min^{-1} at a tissue depth of 5 mm for applicators used for superficial heating [25].

As shown in Fig. 3.10, heating rates increase with irradiance and decrease with tissue depth. In piglets, the quality criterion of ESHO is not fulfilled at heating rates using wIRA-irradiances of 85.0 mW cm^{-2} and of 103.2 mW cm^{-2}. In contrast, adequate heating rates are reached in piglets exposed to 126.5 mW cm^{-2} and using 146.2 mW cm^{-2} for human abdominal wall and breast cancer [26].

Further data analysis yields an approximately linear increase in mean heating rates with rising irradiances. This results in mean heating rates $\geq$1 K min^{-1} at 5 mm for wIRA-irradiances $\geq$110 mW cm^{-2} (Fig. 3.11).

Figure 3.10 depicts substantial individual variability of HR data, and thus, wIRA-irradiances of 135–150 mW cm^{-2} (IR-A) are currently recommended for wIRA-hyperthermia in the clinical setting to ensure compliance with the quality assurance criteria of ESHO for appropriate heating of patients and to limit the risk of side effects due to overheating. Compliance of wIRA-hyperthermia with temperature rises requested by ESHO for adequate heating has been proven under in vivo conditions after achieving thermal steady state in piglets irradiated with a wIRA-irradiance of 126.5 mW cm^{-2} (IR-A) and in human abdominal wall exposed to 146.2 mW cm^{-2} [26]. Results are provided in Table 3.2, which presents additional data of specific absorption rate (SAR), which is closely related to heating rate by

$$\mathrm{SAR} = c_p \cdot \mathrm{HR}. \tag{3.3}$$

(Data of specific heat capacity: $c_p = 3.662$ Ws g^{-1} K^{-1} for skin, $c_p = 2.387$ Ws g^{-1} K^{-1} for fat, $c_p = 3.639$ Ws g^{-1} K^{-1} for muscle tissue, and $c_p = 3.852$ Ws g^{-1} K^{-1} for tumor tissue [26]). (Eq. 3.3 should be restricted as first estimation of SAR, neglecting the effect of skin blood flow and refers to more accurate models, such as Pennes' Bioheat equation [22].)

Fig. 3.11 Mean heating rates assessed in piglets and in human tissues in vivo at a tissue depth of 5 mm as a function of wIRA-irradiance. Piglets: upper thigh (interpolated data from measurements at a depth of 4 mm and 7 mm, dots). Human tissues: abdominal wall (star) and recurrent breast cancer (square). Linear regression of data

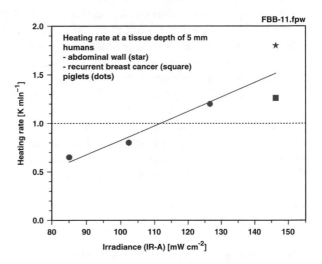

Table 3.2 Summary of in vivo data from superficial tissues of piglets and in humans during wIRA-irradiation with reference to parameters for adequate heating [25]. Tissues investigated: skin/subcutis of the upper thigh (piglets), abdominal wall (humans [17]), and recurrent breast cancers (humans [18])

Quantity	Quality request [1, 18]	Reference depth/exposure time	In vivo data from piglets and humans using wIRA-irradiance (IR-A)		
			Piglets	Humans	
			126.5 mW cm^{-2}	146.2 mW cm^{-2}	
			Upper thigh	Abdominal wall	Recurrent breast cancer
Heating rate [K min^{-1}]	≥ 1[a]	5 mm	1.2 ± 0.5	1.8	1.3
SAR [mW g^{-1}]	≥ 60[a]	5 mm	63 ± 25	110	80
Temperature rise [K]	6[a]	5 mm/ 6 min[a]	5.0 ± 1.0	n.a.	n.a.
		5 mm/ during TSS	8.0 ± 1.3	6.9	n.a.

TSS thermal steady state, *n.a.* not available.
[a] Parameters defined for a muscle tissue equivalent phantom [25].

3.4.6   Post-Heating Temperature Decay Times to Ensure Effective Hyperthermia Levels During Subsequent Radiotherapy

Radiotherapy immediately following hyperthermia (a potent radiosensitizer) must be performed at post-heating temperature levels >39 °C.

Figure 3.12 shows the time periods for post-heating temperature decays to reach effective hyperthermia levels of 39–42 °C. Measurements were performed in anesthetized piglets exposed to an irradiance of 126 mW cm^{-2} (IR-A), i.e., exposed to an irradiance of therapeutic relevance and in accordance with the quality standards of ESHO for appropriate hyperthermia (see Sect. 3.4.5). The shortest times for decays to reach 42 °C were about 1.5 min at the skin surface and approximately 4.5 min at a tissue depth of 8 mm. The longest times for decays to reach 39 °C were about 8 min at the skin surface and 20 min at a tissue depth of 20 mm. The respective mean post-heating decay times for the temperature to reach 40 °C were ≈ 4.5 min and ≈ 11 min. Standard deviations in Fig. 3.12 indicate significant deviations from these mean values in individual cases.

Thus, in radio-oncological (HT-RT) settings, it is strongly recommended/mandatory that, to ensure effective hyperthermia levels (39–42 °C) when following wIRA-HT treatment with radiotherapy (RT), the heated region should be covered with a thermo-isolating blanket between the two treatments (time interval ≤5 min).

3.5   Conclusions

Using irradiances >110 mW cm^{-2} for wIRA-hyperthermia (wIRA-HT) has been proven to comply with the quality standards of ESHO for appropriate tissue heating under in vivo conditions.

Fig. 3.12 Post-heating temperature decay times to reach effective hyperthermia levels of 39 °C (curve 1, red diamonds), 40 °C (curve 2, blue triangles), 41 °C (curve 3, green dots) and 42 °C (curve 4, black squares) as a function of tissue depth. Means and standard deviations were calculated for anesthetized piglets in vivo upon completion of wIRA skin exposure using an irradiance of 126.5 mW cm^{-2} (IR-A)

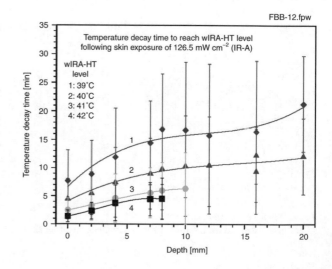

By adjusting the spectrum to the optical window of tissues, wIRA skin exposures allow effective tissue heating (T >39 °C) up to 26 mm in humans (abdominal wall). Direct conversion of absorbed radiation into heat is supplemented by secondarily induced conductive and convective heat transport from upper to deeper tissue layers.

Tissue heating using wIRA should be specified by irradiance and exposure time as wIRA-hyperthermia cannot be sufficiently characterized by the radiant exposure (dose). This is due to heat dissipation by conductive and convective heat transport of individual, different kinetics, and limitations in transport capacity within the tissue. Thus, similar doses result in different heating states if applied irradiances are different, and the *Bunsen–Roscoe* law of reciprocity cannot be applied to describe dosages in schedules of hyperthermia.

The use of hyperthermia in oncology (combined with radiotherapy, chemotherapy, anticancer immunotherapy, or combinations thereof) and in physical therapy should not only consider relevant hyperthermia levels of tissues needed at target depths as shown in Table 3.1 (see also Fig. 3.9 for piglets and Fig. 2 shown for humans by Piazena et al. [23]), but also heating-up times needed to achieve steady state of the target temperature (see Fig. 1, Piazena et al. [23]).

Post-heating temperature decay times (as exemplified for anesthetized piglets in Fig. 3.12) limit eligible intervals between hyperthermia and subsequent radiotherapy to periods ≤5 min to ensure effective hyperthermia levels.

In vivo data from piglets (Fig. 3.9) indicate temperatures within the tissue up to 2 K higher than those measured on the skin surface. This information may be used to protect tissues from overheating and harmful skin effects by controlling skin surface temperature during wIRA-hyperthermia [16]. In humans, comparable temperature increments upon wIRA-exposure have not so far been observed.

References

1. Verein Licht- und Wärmetherapie Abbreviated English Review; 12020. https://www.waerme-therapie.org/infos-und-fachliteratur/wira-therapie/english-abstract.
2. Vaupel P, Kelleher DK, Krüger W.: Wassergefilterte Infrarot-A-Strahlung: Eine neue Technik zur lokalen Hyperthermie oberflächlich liegender Tumoren. In: Wärmetherapie mit wassergefilterter Infrarot-A-Strahlung. Eds.: Vaupel P, Krüger W. Hippokrates, Stuttgart, 1992. p. 57–62.
3. Notter M, Thomsen AR, Nitsche M, et al. Combined wIRA-hyperthermia and hypofractionated re-irradiation in the treatment of locally recurrent breast cancer: evaluation of therapeutic outcome based on a novel size classification. Cancers. 2020;12:606. https://doi.org/10.3390/cancers12030606.
4. Hoffmann G, Hartel M, Mercer JB. Heat for wounds – water-filtered infrared-A (wIRA) for wound healing – a review. Ger Med Sci. 2016;2016:8. https://doi.org/10.3205/000235. eCollection.
5. Künzli BM, Liebl F, Nuhn P, et al. Impact of preoperative local water-filtered infrared-A irradiation on postoperative wound healing: a randomized patient – and observer – blinded controlled clinical trial. Ann Surg. 2013;258:887–94.
6. Rutkowski R, Straburzynska-Lupa A, Korman P, et al. Thermal effectiveness of different IR radiators employed in rheumatoid hand therapy as assessed thermovisual examination. Photochem Photobiol. 2011;87:1442–6.

 7. Lange U, Müller-Ladner U, Dischereit G. Effectiveness of whole-body hyperthermia by mild water-filtered infrared-A radiation in ankylosing spondylitis - a controlled, randomized, prospective study. Akt Rheumatol. 2017;42:122–8.
 8. Klemm P, Eichelmann M, Aykara I, et al. Serial locally applied water-filtered infrared-A radiation in axial spondyloarthritis – a randomized controlled trial. Int J Hyperthermia. 2020;37:965–70.
 9. Xu J, Deng Y, Yu C, et al. Efficacy of wIRA in the treatment of sacroiliitis in male patients with ankylosing spondylitis and its effect on serum VEGF levels. J Orthop Surg Res. 2019;14:313. https://doi.org/10.1186/s13018-019-1322-1327.
10. Borel N, Sauer-Durand AM, Hartel M, et al. wIRA: hyperthermia as a treatment option for intracellular bacteria, with special focus on chlamydiae and mycobacteria. Int J Hyperthermia. 2010;37:373–83.
11. Zöller N, König A, Butting M, et al. Water-filtered near-infrared influences collagen synthesis of keloid-fibroblasts in contrast to normal foreskin fibroblasts. J Photochem Photobiol B. 2016;163:194–202.
12. Cobarg CC, Krüger W, Vaupel P. Physikalische Grundlagen der wassergefilterten Infrarot-A-Strahlung. In: Vaupel P, Krüger W, editors. Wärmetherapie mit wassergefilterter Infraot-A-Strahlung. Stuttgart: Hippokrates; 1992. p. 15–22.
13. Rzeznik J. Eine neue Technik zur loko-regionalen Wärmetherapie mit wassergefilterter Infrarot-A-Strahlung. In: Vaupel P, editor. Wärmetherapie mit wassergefilterter Infrarot-A-Strahlung. Hippokrates, Stuttgart: Krüger W; 1992. p. 23–37.
14. Piazena H, Meffert H, Uebelhack R. Physikalische und photobiologische Grundlagen prophylaktischer und therapeutischer Infrarotanwendungen. Akt Dermatol. 2014;40:335–9.
15. Vaupel P, Piazena H, Müller W, Notter M. Biophysical and photobiological basics of water-filtered infrared-A hyperthermia of superficial tumors. Int J Hyperthermia. 2018;35:26–36.
16. Piazena H, Müller W, Pendl W, et al. Thermal field formation during wIRA-hyperthermia: temperature measurements in skin and subcutis of piglets as a basis for thermotherapy of superficial tumors and local skin infections caused by thermosensitive microbial pathogens. Int J Hyperthermia. 2019;36:938–52. https://doi.org/10.1080/2656736.2019.1655594.
17. Thomsen AR, Saalmann MR, Nicolay NH, et al.: Monitoring of key parameters during thermography-controlled wIRA-hyperthermia in the treatment of superficial tumors. 33rd Annual Meeting, European Society for Hyperthermic Oncology (ESHO), Warshaw; 2019.
18. Notter M, Piazena H, Vaupel P. Hypofractionated re-irradiation of large-sized recurrent breast cancer with thermography-controlled, contact-free water-filtered infrared-A hyperthermia: a retrospective study of 73 patients. Int J Hyperthermia. 2017;33:227–36.
19. Piazena H, Meffert H, Uebelhack R. Spectral remittance and transmittance of visible and infrared-A radiation in human skin – comparison between *in vivo* measurements and model calculations. Photochem Photobiol. 2017;93:1449–61.
20. Piazena H, Kelleher DK. Effects of infrared-A irradiation on skin: discrepancies in published data highlight the need for an exact consideration of physical and photobiological laws and appropriate experimental settings. Photochem Photobiol. 2010;86:687–705.
21. Krackowitzer P, Brenner E. Sonographische Dickenmessungen der Haut (Epidermis & Cutis) an 24 Stellen des menschlichen Körpers. Phlebologie. 2008;37:83–92.
22. Pennes HH. Analysis of tissue and arterial blood temperature in the resting human forearm. J Appl Physiol. 1948;1:93–122.
23. Piazena H, Müller W, Vaupel P. Glossary used in wIRA-hyperthermia. (see Chapter 1, this book).
24. Dobsicek Trefna H, Creeze H, Schmidt M, et al. Quality assurance guidelines for superficial hyperthermia clinical trials: I Clinical requirements. Int J Hyperthermia. 2017;33:471–82.
25. Dobsicek Trefna H, Crezee J, Schmidt M, et al. Quality assurance guidelines for superficial hyperthermia clinical trials: II. Technical requirements for heating devices. Strahlenther Onkol. 2017;193:351–66.
26. Piazena H, Müller W, Vaupel P. wIRA-heating of piglet skin and subcutis *in vivo*: proof of accordance with ESHO criteria for superficial hyperthermia. Int J Hyperthermia. 2020;37:887–96.

Thermography and Thermometry in wIRA-Hyperthermia

4

W. Müller, H. Piazena, A. R. Thomsen, and Peter Vaupel

4.1 Introduction

As the success of locoregional hyperthermia is crucially dependent on the temperature attained in the tissue, e.g., in superficial tumors, reliable temperature measurements are mandatory. The approach for measuring temperature depends on how hyperthermia is performed. In microwave hyperthermia, the skin surface is not directly accessible as a water bolus is used to transfer heat from the microwave applicator to the patient. In this case, thermometry probes are inserted within catheters that are placed in the target region, or a sensor array is pulled through a fixed trajectory during treatment to improve spatial temperature resolution. As recently reported, a 56-sensor thermal monitoring sheet, which is placed on the skin of the patient and provides a spatial temperature resolution of 20 × 25 mm, has been developed [1].

Hyperthermia with water-filtered infrared-A irradiation (wIRA-HT) allows contact-free heating of the tissue and thus also contact-free temperature measurements at the skin surface. This provides the option to use both thermometric and thermographic systems. Although thermometric systems are limited to temperature

W. Müller (✉)
Physical Optics Consultant Office, Wetzlar, Germany
e-mail: h.-werner.mueller@t-online.de

H. Piazena
Department of Anaesthesiology and Operative Intensive Care Medicine, Charité - Universitätsmedizin Berlin, Corporative Member of Freie Universität Berlin and Humboldt Universität zu Berlin, Berlin, Germany

A. R. Thomsen · P. Vaupel
Department of Radiation Oncology, University Medical Center, University of Freiburg, Freiburg/Breisgau, Germany

German Cancer Consortium (DKTK) Partner Site Freiburg, German Cancer Research Center (DKFZ), Heidelberg, Germany

© The Author(s) 2022
P. Vaupel (ed.), *Water-filtered Infrared A (wIRA) Irradiation*,
https://doi.org/10.1007/978-3-030-92880-3_4

measurements within a relatively small measuring spot, the latter have the advantage that thermal variations or heat patterns across a surface can be depicted in a visual image and can be controlled. The spatial temperature resolution is <1 mm. For precise temperature measurements with these systems, some parameters need to be considered. Among these, and probably the most important one, is the *emissivity* of the patient's skin being irradiated. Although IR temperature measurements are basically related to the skin surface of the patient, these data can be used to estimate temperatures in underlying tissue layers and thereby prevent overheating and replace invasive temperature measurements.

4.2 Physical Background of Contact-Free Temperature Measurements

4.2.1 Basic Laws and Parameters

Any material with a temperature above the absolute zero point (0 K, -273.15°C resp.) emits and absorbs electromagnetic radiation, the nature of which strongly depends on its composition and its surface properties, and its description may require complex physical formulae. For simplification, it has proven to be helpful in practice to use an idealized body for which the radiation laws are precisely known and adapt them to those of real bodies [2]. The idealized body is called *black body* or *black body radiator,* which absorbs all incident electromagnetic radiation of all wavelengths and emits it again in a characteristic spectrum, which is only dependent on its temperature, whereas real bodies, called *gray bodies*, emit less radiation than absorbed.

A helpful parameter, which combines the properties of a black body with those of a gray body, is the emissivity, defined as follows:

$$\varepsilon(\lambda,T) = \frac{\text{radiant exitance from a real body at temperature } T}{\text{radiant exitance from a black body at temperature } T} \quad (4.1)$$

Since a black body emits the entire incident radiation again, $\varepsilon(\lambda, T) = 1$, the emissivity of a real body is <1. Further parameters are defined accordingly.

$$\text{Absorption coefficient } \alpha(\lambda,T) = \frac{\text{absorbed radiant power}}{\text{incident irradiant power}} \quad (4.2)$$

$$\text{In the steady state } \varepsilon(\lambda,T) = \alpha(\lambda,T) \text{ applies} \left(\text{Kirchhoff's law} \right) \quad (4.3)$$

$$\text{Reflectance } \rho(\lambda,T) = \frac{\text{reflected radiant power}}{\text{incident radiant power}} \quad (4.4)$$

$$\text{Transmittance } \tau(\lambda,T) = \frac{\text{transmitted radiant power}}{\text{incident radiant power}} \quad (4.5)$$

Because of the conservation of energy

$$\varepsilon(\lambda,T)+\rho(\lambda,T)+\tau(\lambda,T)=1 \qquad (4.6)$$

These are the laws and parameters on which all systems are based and which are used for measuring temperature using infrared radiation, e.g., IR cameras and IR thermometers (pyrometers).

Wien's displacement law can be used to find the optimal range of wavelengths for temperature measurements. Figure 4.1 shows that the wavelengths of the maxima of the curves, indicating maximal spectral radiant exitance, are shifted to smaller wavelengths as temperature increases. This is mathematically expressed by Wien's displacement law:

$$\lambda_{max}=\frac{b}{T}=\frac{2.898\cdot10^{-3}}{T} \qquad (4.7)$$

where $\lambda_{max}=$ maximum wavelength [m], $b=2.898\cdot10^{-3}$ [mK] Wien's displacement constant, and $T=$ absolute temperature [K].

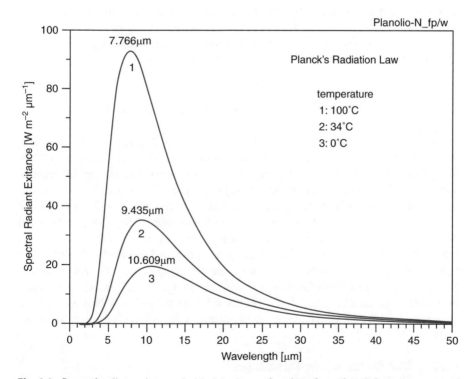

Fig. 4.1 Spectral radiant exitance of a black body as a function of wavelength for temperatures of 100 °C (1), 37 °C (2), and 0 °C (3). According to Wien's displacement law, the maxima of the spectral exitance are at 7.766 μm (100 °C), at 9.435 μm (34 °C), and at 10.609 μm (0 °C). Integration of the spectral data over the wavelengths results in radiant exitance values of ≈316 Wm^{-2} (100 °C), ≈505 Wm^{-2}, and ≈316 Wm^{-2} (0 °C) in accordance with data calculated by using the Stefan–Boltzmann's law (see Eq. 4.8)

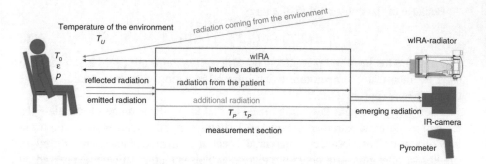

Fig. 4.2 Scheme for measurement of skin surface temperature during wIRA-hyperthermia using an IR camera or a pyrometer. T_0 = temperature of the skin area of the patient that is irradiated, T_P = temperature within the measurement section, T_U = temperature of the environment, ε = emissivity of the patient's skin, ρ = reflectance of human skin, τ_P = transmission of the measurement section

According to this law, the wavelength of electromagnetic radiation emitted by human skin surface with a temperature of 34 °C, at which the maximum of spectral radiant exitance is reached, is at about 9.435 μm (infrared-C range (3–1000 μm)), as shown in Fig. 4.1. The radiant exitance M, emitted from a black body, as a function of its temperature, is described by Stefan–Boltzmann's law:

$$M = \sigma \cdot T^4 \tag{4.8}$$

where σ = 5.67 · 10^{-8} Wm^{-2} ·K^{-4} (Stefan–Boltzmann constant) and T = absolute temperature [K].

Manufacturers of IR systems supply the basic formulae required for measurements with their systems in a general form, as they are interested in applications in many fields [2–4]. Therefore, these formulae need to be adapted to a specific metrological situation. In the following, the arrangement for wIRA-HT in the clinical setting is taken as the basis and the general formulae are adjusted accordingly (Fig. 4.2).

wIRA irradiation (780–1400 nm) is partially absorbed by the patient's skin and partially reflected and remitted into the measurement section, i.e., the space between the patient and the IR system. This directly reflected, and remitted radiation is not perceived by the IR system because its maximal wavelength is at 1.4 μm and the lens of these systems transmits only radiation with wavelengths >7.5 μm. Radiation from objects at room temperature (21 °C), reflected by the patient, is measured, because the wavelength of this radiation is about 10 μm according to Wien's displacement law.

4.2.2 Derivation of the Basic Equation for Temperature Measurement

Assuming human skin would have the properties of a black body, the radiation emitted by the patient could be defined as $\Phi_S(T_0)$. However, as skin is a gray body, it is reduced to $\Phi_\varepsilon = \varepsilon \cdot \Phi_S(T_0)$. Thermal radiation also reaches the patient from the environment and is partially absorbed, contributing to the heating of the patient, and partially reflected. The total radiant power from the environment is assumed to be ΦT_U. A portion of this, $\Phi_\rho = \rho \cdot \Phi(T_U)$, is reflected and enters the measurement section. The total radiant power, $\varepsilon \cdot \Phi(T_0) + \rho \cdot \Phi(T_U)$, entering the measuring section, is attenuated by the transmittance τ_P of the section. It remains

$$\tau_P \left[\varepsilon \cdot \Phi(T_0) + \rho \cdot \Phi(T_U) \right] \tag{4.9}$$

The measurement section with the temperature T_P can also emit radiation $\Phi(T_P)$. As there is no reflection ($\rho = 0$), the additional radiant power is $(1 - \tau_P)\Phi(T_P)$, taking into consideration:

$$\varepsilon + \rho + \tau = 1 \text{ and } \varepsilon = 1 - \tau \tag{4.10}$$

For temperature measurement, the following radiant power is available:

$$\Phi_M = \tau_P \left[\varepsilon \cdot \Phi(T_0) + \rho \cdot \Phi(T_U) \right] + (1 - \tau_P)\Phi(T_P). \tag{4.11}$$

Because of $\varepsilon + \rho = 1$ and $\rho = 1 - \varepsilon$, the formula can be modified to:

$$\Phi_M = \tau_P \left[\varepsilon \cdot \Phi(T_0) + (1 - \varepsilon) \cdot \Phi(T_U) \right] + (1 - \tau_P) \cdot \Phi(T_P) \tag{4.12}$$

This quantity is measured by the IR system, i.e., transferred into an electrical signal. The parameter required is the temperature T_0. Since there is basically no direct measurement of the temperature, the signal needs to be assigned to temperature values in the IR system, taking into consideration that the temperatures in the formulae presented above are absolute temperatures.

Related to (4.12), the following parameters have to be taken into account in order to calculate the patient's skin surface temperature: τ_p, ε, T_U, and T_p.

The transparency of the air in the measurement section, τ_p, depends on the wavelength. Within the region of 8–14 µm, the transparency is constant and high. Since IR measurement systems register wavelengths between 7.5 and 13 µm, one can assume that the radiation from the patient is not influenced by the measurement section.

Because of $\Phi(T_P) = 0$ and $\tau_P = 1$, the formula for $\Phi(T_0)$ is reduced to

$$\Phi(T_0) = \left[\frac{\Phi_M - (1 - \varepsilon) \cdot \Phi(T_U)}{\varepsilon} \right]. \text{ It therefore follows}: T_0 = \Phi^{-1}\left[\frac{\Phi_M - (1 - \varepsilon) \cdot \Phi(T_U)}{\varepsilon} \right] \tag{4.13}$$

where Φ^{-1} is the inverse function of $\Phi(T_0)$.

Emissivity ε of the patient's skin and the temperature of the environment, T_U, are the key parameters. T_U is the mean temperature of the inner surface of the half-sphere around the patient, and it is not the temperature of the ambient air. It is almost impossible to completely eliminate the contribution from the materials/persons surrounding the optical path and the detector. However, due to the relatively high emissivity of the skin, this contribution is low. The emissivity of the patient is the crucial parameter and depends on tissue properties (e.g., normal tissue, tumor tissue) and the skin condition. The emissivity of the skin must be determined and set in the IR system before each measurement (see below).

4.2.3 Determining the Emissivity of Human Skin

4.2.3.1 Reference Temperature

The temperature at a certain point in the target area is measured by a contact thermometer and thereafter at the same place with an IR measurement system. The emission coefficient displayed in the IR measurement system is then adjusted accordingly, until the temperature of the contact thermometer is reached. However, the use of contact thermometers is not practical in cases of ulceration or wet skin surfaces due to the following issues: (a) feedback effect of the contact thermometer on the skin, (b) heat transfer between skin and the contact thermometer, and (c) heat transfer between the contact thermometer and its environment [5].

4.2.3.2 Reference Emissivity

There are materials whose emissivity is known (i.e., lacquer or foil). Such a material must be applied to the skin as a reference area. The emissivity in the IR measurement system is set accordingly. When the reference area has reached the temperature of the skin, the temperature can be measured with the IR measurement system. After that, the temperature is measured at a different spot on the skin and the emissivity in the IR measurement system is adjusted until the same temperature is reached. The displayed emissivity value is the emissivity of the skin.

4.2.3.3 The Use of a Black Body to Measure Skin Temperature

As mentioned above, the emissivity of a black body is 1. The temperature of commercially available black bodies can be reliably set to different temperatures. To calibrate an IR measurement system, the emissivity in the instrument is set to 1 and the system is focused on the reference area of the black body—it should display the same temperature. If not, an internal adjustment of the instruments is necessary. In case of matching, the emissivity in the instrument is set to 0.98, which is generally accepted for healthy skin, and 0.87 for tumor tissue. The general problem is that this could not be the "true" emissivity of the skin.

4.3 The Thermographic Camera (Syn.: Infrared Camera, Thermal Imaging Camera, Thermal Imager)

4.3.1 Basic Mode of Operation

An IR camera is similar to a common digital video camera. Instead of visible radiation (400–700 nm), the thermographic camera creates an image using infrared radiation (1–14 μm). In the medical field, a range between 8 μm and 14 μm is preferred

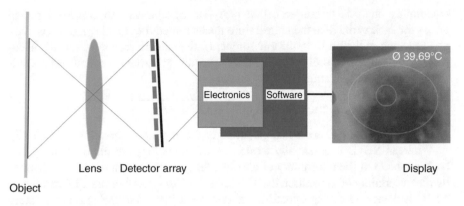

Lens   Detector array   Display

Object

Fig. 4.3   Scheme of a thermographic camera

as explained above. The IR camera consists of a lens that focuses IR onto a focal plane array (FPA) detector, the "heart" of the camera. This detector transforms infrared radiation into an electrical signal and is designed as a chip with microbolometers (resistance thermometers), which are arranged in an array of lines and columns. In this way, the entire thermographic image is subdivided into separated pixels, which allow for access to the respective signals (temperatures). The levels of the measurement signal are assigned to colors for better discrimination of the temperature values (Fig. 4.3).

4.3.2   Performance Criteria

4.3.2.1 The Spectral Region

As mentioned above, the wavelength of radiation from human skin at a temperature of 37 °C, at which maximal irradiation is reached, is at 9.344 µm. To capture all electromagnetic radiation emitted by a patient, the lens of the camera must be transparent for this wavelength, and the whole spectrum that is transmitted should be small to block interfering radiation from the environment.

4.3.2.2 Thermal Resolution, Relative and Absolute Accuracy

Small differences in temperature can be lost due to noise in the detector signal. As a measure of a camera's capacity to differentiate small temperature differences, the noise equivalent temperature difference (NETD) describes the change in temperature, which is equivalent to the effective noise of the system. It can be referred to as the minimal resolvable temperature change. This value only reflects the relative accuracy of the system, not the absolute accuracy. Usually, NETD values are between <30 mK and <40 mK. According to the ESHO Quality Guidelines, the value for IR systems should be <50 mK [6].

The value for absolute accuracy, as specified by the manufacturers, is commonly ±2 K or 2% of the reading. This information is the result of a widely used uncertainty analysis technique called *root sum of squares* and considers partial errors for each variable in the temperature measurement Eq. (4.13) (e.g., emissivity and reflected radiation from the environment), the camera response, and the accuracy of the calibration tool used. The total uncertainty U_T then is calculated according to the error propagation law:

$$\text{Total error} = \sqrt{\Delta T_1^2 + \Delta T_2^2 + \Delta T_3^2 + \ldots}$$

where ΔT_1, ΔT_1, ΔT_1...are the single errors of the parameters mentioned above [7].

Whereas NETD is essentially a question of technology, absolute accuracy is a basic problem of the uncertainty of absolute temperature measurements, enhanced by the uncertainty of the emissivity. This is crucial for hyperthermia applications. If 42 °C is measured during hyperthermia treatment instead of the real temperature $T = 44$ °C, then tissue damage can occur. The only practical way for reliable absolute temperature measurements is for the manufacturer and the operator to calibrate the system as carefully as possible. Uncertainties in the heating concept are to be considered. The ESHO Quality Assurance Guidelines [6] require the precision of the temperature measurement to be 0.1 °C, which can hardly be reached, especially since emissivity is associated with it.

4.3.2.3 Geometric Resolution (Syn.: Optical Resolution, Spatial Resolution)

The geometric resolution indicates the size of the smallest detail (area) on the skin surface, which is visible in the IR image. It can be interpreted as the smallest area on the skin surface related to a single bolometer (pixel) of the camera detector, which can be detected at a set distance, providing temperature data, relevant for the detection of hot spots in, above, and around scars or the separation of two structures close together. This resolution is determined by the number of pixels per area unit on the camera detector and depends on the lens used. Calculation of the resolution is based on the parameter *field of view*, which is the largest area the camera can capture at a set distance and is typically characterized by the vertical and horizontal angle under which the area appears from the camera detector. Since this value is very important, its calculation will be shown using an example.

Camera: optris PI 400 (MTS Messtechnik Schaffhausen, Stein am Rhein, Switzerland), number of pixels on the camera chip: 382 (horizontal) x 288 (vertical), focal length of the lens: 15 mm, horizontal view angle α_h: 38°, and vertical view angle α_v: 29° (data supplied by the camera manufacturer).

The horizontal viewing angle can be expressed as $\alpha_h = 2 \cdot \arctan\left(\dfrac{h}{2 \cdot f}\right)$. According to Fig. 4.4, the following relationships apply:

$$\frac{b}{g} = \tan\frac{\alpha_h}{2} \text{ and } b = g \cdot \tan\frac{\alpha_h}{2} = g \cdot \tan 19° = g \cdot 0.344$$

where g = object distance and b = half the object width.

The width of the area on the skin surface is $2b$, and the distance between the IR camera and the patient is $g = 34$ *cm*. Then, the width of the area on the patient is

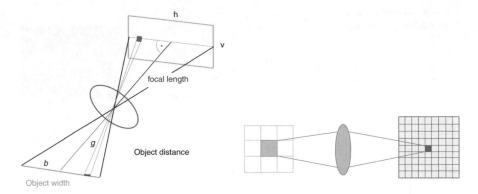

Fig. 4.4 Calculation of the geometric resolution of thermographic cameras [8]

$$2 \cdot 34 \cdot 0,344 \, cm = 23,4 \, cm$$

With 382 horizontal pixels, the smallest width that can be detected is $\dfrac{23.4 \, cm}{382} = 0.6 \, mm$. Since the pixels are squared, the smallest area on the skin surface, which can be captured, thus is 0.6 mm × 0.6 mm.

4.4   Pyrometer (IR Thermometer): Basic Mode of Operation

Compared to IR cameras, IR thermometers are simpler in design, but based on the same physical background, as described above. These thermometers can be characterized as remote thermometers. A lens captures the IR radiation from a measurement spot on the target surface and focuses it onto a detector (see Fig. 4.5). It is important that the emitting area is equal or larger than the measurement spot defined by the system. Different methods are used to mark this spot on the target surface, and these are preferably based on laser technology. For example, a crosshair is projected onto the surface with the size of the measurement spot. As with cameras, the emissivity must be entered [9].

4.5   Special Situations

4.5.1   Curved Surfaces

Two problems arise at curved skin surfaces: (a) wIRA-irradiation—and thus also tissue heating—is reduced by the cosine of the angle between the direction of the radiation and the surface normal, and (b) the area of this less heated surface onto the pixels of the camera is not completely imaged and leads to reduced temperature values (Fig. 4.6).

Fig. 4.5 Scheme of an IR
thermometer (pyrometer)

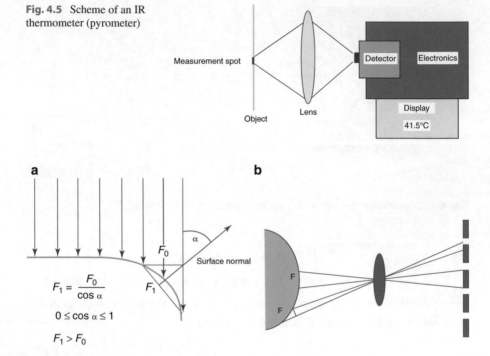

Fig. 4.6 Reduced heating of the tissue at curved skin surfaces (**a**). Incomplete projection of a curved skin area onto the detector array of a thermographic camera (**b**) [8]

4.5.2 Optional Interventions During wIRA-HT

In wIRA-HT, the skin surface remains accessible for interventions. This allows for power deposition modulations by placing shielding sheets on the irradiated area to completely block non-target tissues and for modulations of the temperature measurement procedures. In the cases of ulcerated lesions or wound secretion, heat loss by evaporation can reduce the critical target region below the therapeutically required temperatures. In this case, covering with transparent grease or foils enables more uniform heating (see Fig. 4.7a).

During wIRA-HT in the clinical setting, the highest temperature values (hot spots) within the entire irradiated area are registered automatically and are used for irradiation control to avoid tissue damage. In this case, hot spots outside the target area can be covered with opaque material to eliminate their influence, as shown in Fig. 4.7b.

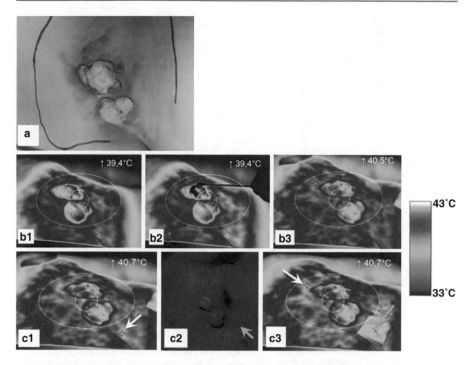

Fig. 4.7 Interventions during wIRA-HT. (**a**) Ulcerated recurrent breast cancer. The nodular tumors are fibrin-coated and permanently produce wound secretion. (**b1**) Due to evaporation, moist surfaces can cool the tissue below the therapeutically relevant temperature level (blue colour). (**b2**) Covering these areas with a thin film of greasy ointment (Bepanthen™) reduces evaporation. (**b3**) A more homogeneous heating is achieved. (**c1**) A hotspot (white arrow) outside the target area may disturb temperature control. (**c2**) The region is covered with opaque material (green arrow). (**c3**) The influence of the hot spot is prevented. Consequently, a hotspot within the target region (white arrow), where it needs to be recorded, is indicated

4.6   Use of Thermographic Cameras for Temperature Measurements on Phantoms

The quality assurance standards of ESHO for water-filtered IR-A hyperthermia require measurements on phantoms [10]. The use of infrared thermography in superficial hyperthermia quality assurance, including measurements on phantoms, has been reported in detail [11]. Currently, there is no recipe for tissue-equivalent phantom materials that adequately consider absorption, scattering, and refraction of IR irradiation in tissues. Even were such a material to be identified, individual patient-related factors influencing heating need to be considered. Thus, the value of phantoms and the significance of measurements made on them must be viewed critically.

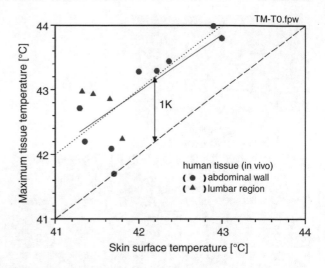

Fig. 4.8 Maximum tissue temperatures in human abdominal wall (dots) and lumbar region (triangles) and corresponding temperatures on the skin surface during wIRA-hyperthermia

4.7 Relationship Between Temperatures Assessed at the Skin Surface and in Deeper Tissue Layers

In hyperthermia, it is crucial to reach the temperatures required to achieve therapeutic effects (39–43 °C). In the clinical setting, this means that (tumor) tissue temperatures at preset depths must reach predefined levels. IR-based temperature measurements can only measure the temperature at the skin surface, and thus, the question arises, whether there are any relationships between the surface temperature and the temperatures in deeper tissue layers. Recent in vivo studies on piglets have shown that maximum tissue temperatures exceeded corresponding temperatures on the skin surface by 1–2 K during wIRA-hyperthermia ([12], Fig. 4.1). Similar relations were found in vivo during wIRA exposure of human abdominal wall and lumbar region (Fig. 4.8). These data can be used for approximate estimations of maximum tissue temperatures if the temperature at the skin surface is monitored during wIRA-hyperthermia.

4.8 Conclusions

In wIRA-HT, contact-free heating enables remote temperature assessments by IR-based devices. The relationship between skin temperatures and temperatures in deeper tissue layers can be used to estimate and control the temperatures in tumors that are needed for therapeutic effects. Since the measurements are contact-free, in the clinical setting physicians can modulate/block heating at locations where it is not needed (e.g., in scar tissues, which tend to become hot spots), with opaque foils. Wet body surfaces can be covered with transparent material to reduce cooling by evaporation. Using software, mean temperature values related to definable areas can be provided and temperature data of individual spots can be displayed. Basically, there is high potential for image analysis to control and interpret the dynamic temperature distribution during heating.

References

1. Bakker A, Zweije R, Kok HP, et al. Clinical feasibility of a high-resolution thermal monitoring sheet for superficial hyperthermia in breast cancer patients. Cancers. 2020;12:3644.
2. Griesinger A. Einführung in die Theorie und Praxis der Infrarot-Thermografie. Dresden: InfraTec GmbH; 2004.
3. Clayton RK. Schulungsunterlagen, Einführung in Theorie und Praxis der Infrarot-Thermografie. 1 Physikalische Grundlagen. Dresden: InfraTec GmbH; 2012.
4. Trankler H-R, Reindl LM. Grundlagen der berührungslosen Temperaturmessung. Berlin: Optris GmbH; 2019.
5. MacRae BA, Annaheim S, Spengler CM, Rossi RM. Skin temperature measurement using contact thermometry: a systematic review of setup variables and their effects on measured values. Front Physiol. 2018;9:20180130. https://doi.org/10.3389/fphys.2018.00029.
6. Trefna HD, Creeze H, Schmidt M, et al. Quality assurance guidelines for superficial hyperthermia clinical trials: I Clinical requirements. Int J Hyperthermia. 2017;33:471–82.
7. Messgenauigkeit und -unsicherheit von Infrarotkameras einfach erklärt, FLIR Nürnberg, Germany; 2016.
8. Schimweg T. Thermographische Temperaturanalyse in Erwärmungsprozessen. Infrared temperature solutions (IST): Fachberichte. Keller HCW; 2017.
9. Infrarot Thermometer Ratgeber. Wie funktioniert ein Infrarot Thermometer (Pyrometer).
10. Trefna HD, Creeze H, Schmidt M, et al. Quality assurance guidelines for superficial hyperthermia clinical trials: II. Technical requirements for heating devices. Strahlenther Onkol. 2017;193:351–66.
11. Müller J. Infrared thermography in superficial hyperthermia quality assurance. Master thesis, Faculty of Physics. Division of Medical Radiation Physics, Department of Radiation Oncology, University Medical Center, Friedrich-Alexander-University Erlangen-Nuremberg; 2015.
12. Piazena H, Müller W, Pendl W, et al. Thermal field formation during wIRA-hyperthermia: temperature measurements in skin and subcutis of piglets as a basis for thermotherapy of superficial tumors and local skin infections caused by thermosensitive microbial pathogens. Int J Hyperthermia 2019;36:938–52.

Temperature Profiles and Oxygenation Status in Human Skin and Subcutis Upon Thermography-Controlled wIRA-Hyperthermia

5

A. R. Thomsen, M. R. Saalmann, N. H. Nicolay, A. L. Grosu, and Peter Vaupel

Abbreviations

HT	Hyperthermia (mild HT, 39–43 °C)
i.v.	Intravenous
pO_2	Oxygen partial pressure, O_2 tension (mmHg)
ROI	Region of interest
RT	Radiotherapy, radiation treatment
stO_2	Oxyhemoglobin (HbO_2) saturation, tissue (%)
T	Temperature (°C)
wIRA	Water-filtered infrared A irradiation

5.1 Introduction

In radiation oncology, localized wIRA-hyperthermia (wIRA-HT) is an effective adjunct for sensitizing superficial tumors to radiation treatment [1]. This sensitization may result from hyperthermia (HT)-induced improvements of tissue oxygenation (i.e., increase in oxygen partial pressure, pO_2, "reversing hypoxia") due to a temporary increase in local blood flow in the temperature range between 39 and 43 °C (exposure

A. R. Thomsen (✉) · M. R. Saalmann · N. H. Nicolay · A. L. Grosu · P. Vaupel
Department of Radiation Oncology, University Medical Center, University of Freiburg, Freiburg/Breisgau, Germany

German Cancer Consortium (DKTK) Partner Site Freiburg, German Cancer Research Center (DKFZ), Heidelberg, Germany
e-mail: andreas.thomsen@uniklinik-freiburg.de

time approx. 1 h). It is noteworthy to mention that in mild hyperthermia, additional mechanisms such as (a) stimulation of anti-tumor immune responses, (b) optimization of chemotherapeutic effects (HT level: 40–43 °C), (c) inhibition of DNA repair (HT level ≥41 °C), and (d) the triggering of liposomal release of drugs (HT level: 41–42 °C; [2]) may also be responsible for improving therapeutic outcomes.

"Probably no area in hyperthermia research is more important than the need to accurately assess the resultant temperature of tumors or normal tissues following heating" [2]. Although skin surface temperatures can adequately be monitored by thermography [3], minimally invasive temperature measurements are required to guarantee effective heating and adequate hyperthermia levels (39–43 °C) in deeper tissue layers [4, 5]. This study thus focuses on assessing temperature distribution in skin and subcutis of healthy volunteers upon localized wIRA treatment. As the tissue oxygen level is a major factor for cellular radiosensitivity [6], HT-induced changes in skin and subcutaneous pO_2 values and oxyhemoglobin (HbO_2) saturations in the microvasculature of the subpapillary tissue and the upper dermis layer are also assessed.

For further orientation, the histomorphology of the human skin and subcutis is schematically shown in Fig. 5.1.

5.2 Materials and Methods

5.2.1 Delivery of wIRA-Hyperthermia

Superficial hyperthermia was applied using the TWH 1500 wIRA-hyperthermia system (Hydrosun®, Müllheim, Germany) with two radiators, controlled independently by two thermographic cameras and safety pyrometers. Radiators were positioned 34 cm between radiator exit and skin surface, resulting in an approximate irradiance of 200 mW/cm².

For the application of hyperthermia, the lower abdominal wall (10 treatment sessions) and the lumbar region (2 treatment sessions) of healthy volunteers (1 female,

Fig. 5.1 Histomorphology of human skin and subcutis (schematic, modified from Beiersdorf-Eucerin). Mean thickness of skin layers according to [7]

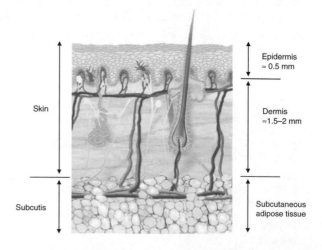

and 2 males, age: 35–49 years) were exposed to wIRA irradiation for approximately 60 min. Participation in this procedure has been found to be ethically sound by the local ethics authority, and volunteers gave their informed consent.

5.2.2 Noninvasive Monitoring of Skin Surface Temperatures (Thermography)

Using this therapeutic approach, maximum skin surface temperature is continuously regulated by a control circuit for each of the two radiators, which is a key element of the TWH 1500 system: When thermography assesses a hot spot and a temperature above a defined maximum (*switch off temperature*: 43 °C), the power supply to the respective radiator is instantly switched off via a relay. As soon as the temperature of the hot spot drops (to *switch on temperature*: 42.5 °C), the radiator is turned back on. In steady-state conditions, between 1 and 4 on–off cycles take place per minute. The resulting peaks in temperature traces are visible in thermography records, but also in superficial skin layers, measured invasively as described below.

A typical example of serially assessed thermographic images during the onset (0–10 min) of wIRA-HT of the skin surface and in situ positioning on the temperature probes is shown in Fig. 5.2. Respective mean region of interest (ROI) temperatures are presented in the upper right corners.

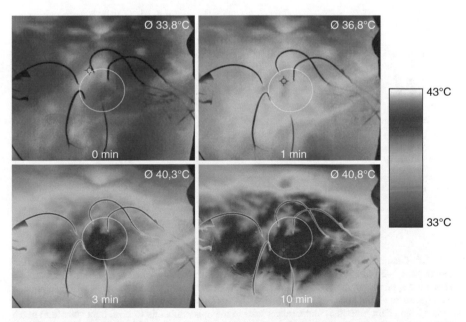

Fig. 5.2 Examples of serially assessed thermography images during the first 10 min of wIRA-HT of the skin surface (abdominal wall). Invasive temperature and pO$_2$ probes are placed in defined tissue depths as shown in Fig. 5.4 Color-coded temperature range: 33–43 °C

5.2.3 Minimally Invasive Measurement of Skin and Subcutis Temperatures (Thermometry)

Tissue temperatures within skin and subcutis of the abdominal wall were measured using fiber-optic sensors (OTG-M600, Opsens, Quebec, Canada). Characteristic and representative traces of skin surface, and intradermal and subcutaneous temperatures before, during, and after wIRA-HT are shown in Fig. 5.3.

5.2.4 Assessment of the Tissue Oxygenation Status

The corresponding tissue oxygen partial pressures (pO_2) were assessed with the Oxylite Pro system (Oxford Optronix, Abington, UK).

Fiber-optic temperature probes (diameter: 0.7 mm) and oxygen sensors (diameter: 0.4 mm) were transepidermally inserted via 1.1 mm i.v. catheters (Vasofix™ Safety, Braun, Melsungen, Germany) down to defined tissue depths (subepidermal ≈0.5 mm, and 1–20 mm within the dermis and subcutis). For positioning of invasive catheters and probes, see Fig. 5.4.

In selected situations, hyperspectral tissue imaging (TIVITA™, Diaspective Vision, Am Salzhaff, Germany) was used to visualize the HbO_2 saturation (stO_2) in the microcirculation of the subpapillary/upper dermis layers [8] of healthy volunteers ($n = 3$) and in superficial chest wall tumors (two patients).

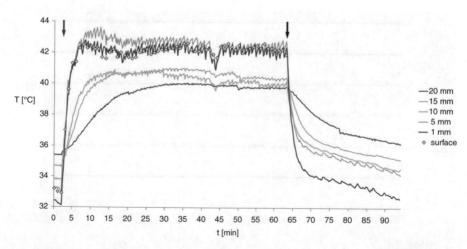

Fig. 5.3 Characteristic traces of subepidermal, intradermal, and subcutaneous temperatures (tissue depths: 1–20 mm; colored lines) and thermographically monitored skin surface temperature (open red symbols) in the region of interest (ROI) of the abdominal wall during wIRA treatment. Start (red arrow) and end (black arrow) of wIRA irradiation are indicated. Subepidermal temperatures (1 mm, dark blue line) and temperatures in the upper subcutis (5 mm, light blue line) reach higher values than the skin surface. On–off cycles due to regulation of the wIRA radiators result in multiple spikes in temperature curves. Spikes are most pronounced in superficial tissue layers, but remain visible down to a tissue depth of 15 mm

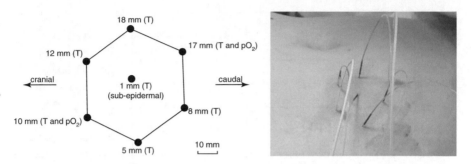

Fig. 5.4 Positioning of invasive catheters and probes in the abdominal wall. Schematic map (left) and actual in situ setup (right) in a representative experiment

Registration of preheating and postheating temperature and oxygen levels completed the data collection upon wIRA exposure.

5.3   Results and Discussion

5.3.1   Temperature Profiles

As shown in Fig. 5.5, upon wIRA irradiation, mean temperature of the skin surface increased from a baseline of 33.4 ± 1.9 °C (mean $\pm$ SD) to 41.7 ± 0.4 °C, with the most superficial invasive probe at 1 mm recording a baseline temperature of 33.1 ± 1.7 °C, increasing to 41.8 ± 0.7 °C (10 experiments). In a tissue depth of 20 ± 1 mm, i.e., in deep subcutis, the mean temperature increased from a baseline of 34.9 ± 1.1 °C to 40.1 ± 0.6 °C (11 experiments). According to these data, wIRA irradiation results in mild hyperthermia with tissue temperatures ≥ 39 °C, extending to tissue depths up to 25 mm, thus confirming earlier, sporadic measurements in superficial cancers [9, 10].

Upon the start of heating, increases in tissue temperatures were steepest close to the body surface, where $T > 40$ °C was achieved within 4 ± 2 min, whereas up to 30 min of wIRA heating were required to reach this temperature at a depth of 20 ± 1 mm. Results in intermediate tissue layers are exemplified in Fig. 5.3.

The highly significant linear correlation between subepidermal and skin surface temperatures for a representative treatment session is shown in Fig. 5.6. There is clear evidence that the maximum tissue (i.e., subepidermal) temperatures can reach 43.5 °C, with the maximum skin surface temperature being 42.5 °C. Considering data collected in all treatment sessions, a reversing of the temperature gradient is observed, as shown in Fig. 5.7. In normothermic conditions and at hyperthermia levels ≤ 42 °C, no substantial gradients between mean subepidermal and skin surface temperature are found (-0.4 to 0 °C, n.s.), which means that both measuring locations yield similar temperatures. With subepidermal temperatures ≥ 42 °C, a temperature gradient is evident, and with subepidermal temperatures ≥ 43 °C, a mean temperature difference of $+0.8$ °C toward skin surface is observed, indicating

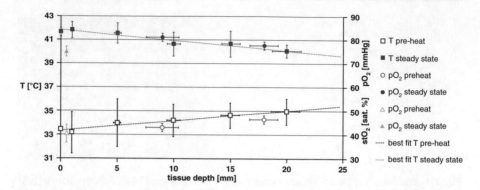

Fig. 5.5 Tissue temperatures T (squares) and pO₂ values (circles) in the skin and subcutis as functions of tissue depth before (lower part) and during steady-state wIRA irradiation (upper part). Baseline and steady-state stO₂ values (triangles) in the upper dermis upon wIRA exposure (values are means ±SD)

Fig. 5.6 Correlation between skin surface temperatures (monitored by thermography) and subepidermal temperatures (measured by invasive probes, thermometry) before, during heating up, and in the steady-state phase of wIRA-hyperthermia. While a fraction of subepidermal values reaches 43.5 °C during HT, all skin surface temperatures stay below 43 °C. Dotted line: best fit

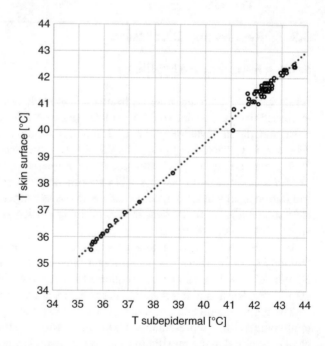

that wIRA-HT yields the highest temperatures in the upper dermis and not at the skin surface (Figs. 5.5 and 5.6). This transepidermal gradient probably relates to increasing heat loss from the skin surface by thermal radiation and convection. Since hemoglobin is a major photochrome for wIRA, HT-induced hyperemia (associated with a higher hemoglobin content) in the subepidermal microvasculature might also contribute to this effect.

When wIRA exposure is terminated, mean temperatures of the uncovered skin surface dropped below 39 °C (i.e., below the lower level of mild HT, obligatory in

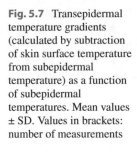

Fig. 5.7 Transepidermal temperature gradients (calculated by subtraction of skin surface temperature from subepidermal temperature) as a function of subepidermal temperatures. Mean values ± SD. Values in brackets: number of measurements

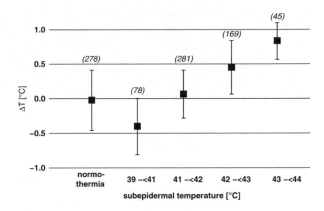

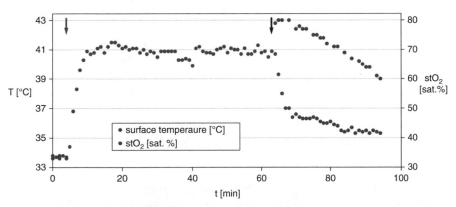

Fig. 5.8 wIRA-hyperthermia causes an increase in the mean subepidermal HbO_2 saturation (stO_2) values starting from a pretreatment level of 33 sat. % up to 80 sat. % at the end of treatment (blue dots), with a steady decline after termination of wIRA exposure. Start (red arrow) and end (black arrow) of wIRA irradiation are indicated. While the surface temperatures (red dots) returned close to baseline within approx. 30 min, stO_2 values remained at significantly elevated levels for more than 40 min. (As wIRA irradiation interferes with hyperspectral imaging, HbO_2 saturations cannot be assessed *during* wIRA exposure)

the oncologic setting) within less than 2 min (Figs. 5.3 and 5.8). In tissue depths of 1–5 mm, mean temperatures dropped to the same extent (see representative examples in Fig. 5.3), whereas at depths of 10 and 20 mm, mean tissue temperature reached 39 °C within 2.5 and 4 min, respectively. These observations demonstrate that effective hyperthermia levels are only maintained for a short period in uncovered skin. This is of relevance for clinical application of superficial HT as a radiosensitizer, for which it is presumed that a simultaneous or quasi-simultaneous application of HT and subsequent radiotherapy provides the most effective synergy [1]. In contrast to the experimental setting applied here, clinical routine aims to maintain tissue temperatures after the wIRA irradiators are switched off. When wIRA-HT is used as a radiosensitizer in the clinical setting, the patient is covered either with a prewarmed dressing gown or with a prewarmed silicone flab when being transferred from the HT unit to the linear accelerator [1]. Therefore, the actual decline in temperature in clinical practice is expected to be significantly slower than observed in the study described herein, where the skin was left uncovered. However, additional investigations are needed to quantify the temperature decline in "heat-insulated" tissues between end of wIRA-HT and subsequent start of RT. In any case, this time interval should be kept very short ($\leq$5 min).

5.3.2 Tissue Oxygenation

5.3.2.1 Oxyhemoglobin Saturations Assessed by Hyperspectral Imaging

Noninvasive monitoring of HbO_2 saturation (stO_2) in the subepidermal microvasculature also confirmed a distinct increase in tissue oxygenation upon wIRA exposure. This effect is visible both in the abdominal wall of healthy volunteers (Fig. 5.9a) and in the skin affected by locally invasive recurrent breast cancer (Fig. 5.9b). The mean HbO_2 saturation (stO_2) in human skin before wIRA exposure was 41%. Upon heating the skin up to 41.7 °C, the saturation almost doubled (Fig. 5.5, green triangles; Fig. 5.10, boxes and whiskers on the left). When wIRA irradiation was terminated, stO_2 values decreased only slightly and thus remained distinctly elevated, even after skin temperatures dropped to baseline, as shown in Figs. 5.8 and 5.10. From these data, it is concluded that improved tissue oxygenation considerably outlasts tissue

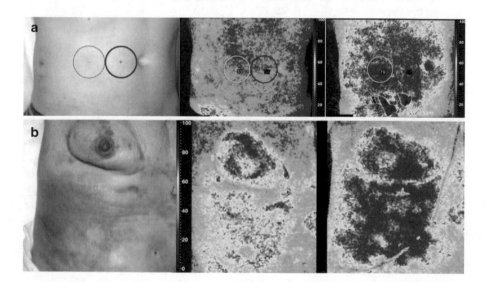

Fig. 5.9 Imaging of HbO_2 saturations in the upper dermis of the abdominal wall of a healthy volunteer (**a**), and in the outer tissue layer ($\approx$1 mm) of a large-size, inflammatory recurrent breast cancer (**b**). Topographic aspect of the treatment area (left panels), stO_2 imaging before (central panels), and at the end of wIRA-hyperthermia (right panels). The malignant inflammatory condition evidently causes higher stO_2 baseline values

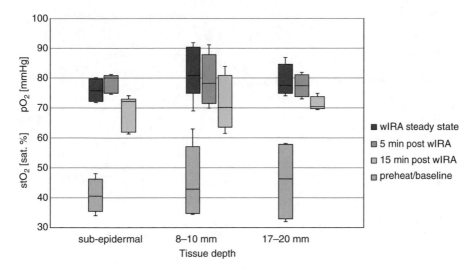

Fig. 5.10 pO_2 and stO_2 values before, during, and following wIRA-hyperthermia. Postheating pO_2 and stO_2 remained at significantly elevated levels within the time frame of subsequent radiotherapy. Subepidermal stO_2 was assessed using hyperspectral skin imaging ($n = 3$), pO_2 in the subcutis with invasive probes ($n = 6$ for 8–10 mm, $n = 4$ for 17–20 mm tissue depths). Boxes show medians with first and third quartiles and whiskers show range

temperature rises upon wIRA-hyperthermia; i.e., oxygenation-dependent radiosensitization is expected to be fully active/maintained during RT in our clinical setting.

Hyperspectral skin imaging was found to be a versatile and noninvasive method to assess HbO_2 saturations in upper skin layers. Since this method only covers the subpapillary microcirculatory vessels in the upper dermis [11], invasive pO_2 measurements are required for oxygenation measurements in the lower dermis down to the subcutis.

5.3.2.2 Assessment of Tissue pO_2 Values

In all tissue depths addressed (subepidermal, 8–10 mm, and 17–20 mm), wIRA-HT caused a marked, highly significant increase in the oxygenation. Mean tissue oxygen tensions in the subcutis rose from 43 to 81 mmHg at tissue depths of 8–10 mm, and from 46 to 77 mmHg at tissue depths of 17–20 mm (Figs. 5.5 and 5.10). Oxygenation reached a maximum within 25–30 min of wIRA-HT and remained at this significantly higher level in the further course of treatment. Upon cessation of wIRA irradiation, oxygenation only slowly decreased and remained at significantly elevated levels within the typical time frame of subsequent radiotherapy protocols (Figs. 5.10 and 5.11).

A similar pattern was observed by Hartel et al. [12] when using wIRA-hyperthermia to improve healing of surgical wounds. These authors have assessed postoperative pO_2 values in a tissue depth of 20 mm. On day 2, the baseline pO_2 before wIRA irradiation was 32 mmHg vs. 42 mmHg after treatment. On day 10, the respective data were 34 mmHg vs. 46 mmHg, both improvements greatly outlasting the actual time of the wIRA exposure.

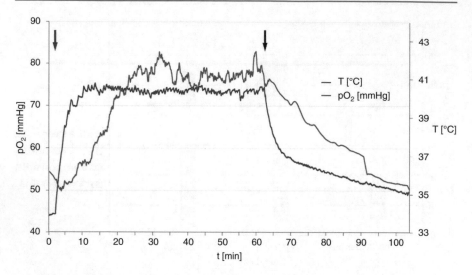

Fig. 5.11 Characteristic tissue temperatures T and pO_2 traces in the subcutis of the abdominal wall during wIRA treatment and post-treatment (tissue depth: 8 mm). Start (red arrow) and end (black arrow) of wIRA irradiation are indicated. Note: tissue pO_2 rises and declines much slower than tissue temperature

As mentioned above, tissue oxygenation status before, during, and after wIRA-hyperthermia was assessed by two different approaches in our experiments:

1. By an indirect, noninvasive approach, using hyperspectral analysis of oxygen saturation (stO_2) of hemoglobin present in subepidermal microvasculatures (Figs. 5.8 and 5.10). Although measurement in deeper tissue layers is technically not possible, this method offers the advantage of noninvasive imaging of larger skin areas (Fig. 5.9).
2. By direct, minimally invasive microsensor measurements of tissue oxygen pressures (pO_2, Figs. 5.10 and 5.11). In principle, this method may be applied at any tissue depth (Fig. 5.4).

Compared to preheating values, wIRA-HT causes a significant improvement of the tissue O_2 status. Both hyperspectral imaging of stO_2 and direct measurement of tissue pO_2 show that this effect outlasts the period needed for subsequent RT (Figs. 5.10 and 5.11).

In Table 5.1, both baseline and steady-state pO_2 values upon superficial wIRA-HT are listed together with known literature data.

5.4   Summary and Outlook

wIRA-HT is a reliable treatment modality for efficiently heating skin and subcutaneous tissue up to a depth of approx. 25 mm. In the set temperature range (mild hyperthermia, 39–43 °C), tissue oxygenation is substantially improved in all tissue

Table 5.1 Mean oxygen partial pressures (pO_2) in different layers of human skin and subcutis under thermoneutral conditions (NT) and steady-state superficial wIRA-hyperthermia (HT). Noteworthy to mention: "Transcutaneous" pO_2 values are assessed from the heated ($\approx$44 °C) skin surface and have been used for monitoring of "arterialized" blood oxygen tensions

Tissue layer	Mean pO_2 (mmHg)	References
Epidermis	8	Wang et al. [13], Carreau et al. [14]
Subepidermal layer	35	Wang et al. [13]
	$\approx$34 (NT @ 33 °C)[a]	This study
	$\approx$50 (HT @ 40 °C)[a]	
Dermis	50 (45–54)[b]	Evans and Naylor [15]
	37 (30–45)[b]	Baumgärtl et al. [16]
	42	Keeley and Mann [17]
Subcutis	56	Keeley and Mann [17]
	50–55	Vaupel et al. [18]
	43 (NT@ 34 °C)[b]	This study
	81 (HT@40.5 °C)	

[a] Estimated from HbO_2 saturation measurements considering the respective shifts of the HbO_2-binding curves at lower or higher temperatures (standard HbO_2 curve refers to 37 °C).
[b] Steady increase with increasing tissue depth.

depths examined ($\approx$0.5–20 mm). Improvement of oxygenation considerably outlasts the wIRA heating period. In the case of superficial tumors reaching into deeper tissue layers, combination of wIRA-HT with microwave HT may broaden the application range [19].

References

1. Notter M, Thomsen AR, Nitsche M, et al. Combined wIRA-hyperthermia and hypofractionated re-irradiation in the treatment of locally recurrent breast cancer: evaluation of therapeutic outcome based on a novel size classification. Cancers (Basel). 2020;12:3. https://doi.org/10.3390/cancers12030606.
2. Hall EJ, Giaccia AJ. Radiobiology for the radiologist. 8th ed. Philadelphia, Baltimore, New York, London, Buenos Aires: Wolters Kluwer; 2019.
3. Vaupel P, Piazena H, Müller W, et al. Biophysical and photobiological basics of water-filtered infrared-a hyperthermia of superficial tumors. Int J Hyperthermia. 2018;35:26–36. https://doi.org/10.1080/02656736.2018.1469169.
4. Dobšíček Trefná H, Crezee J, Schmidt M, et al. Quality assurance guidelines for superficial hyperthermia clinical trials : II. Technical requirements for heating devices. Strahlenther Onkol. 2017;193:351–66. https://doi.org/10.1007/s00066-017-1106-0.
5. Trefná HD, Crezee H, Schmidt M, et al. Quality assurance guidelines for superficial hyperthermia clinical trials: I Clinical requirements. Int J Hyperthermia. 2017;33:471–82. https://doi.org/10.1080/02656736.2016.1277791.
6. Vaupel P. Tumor microenvironmental physiology and its implications for radiation oncology. Semin Radiat Oncol. 2004;14:198–206. https://doi.org/10.1016/j.semradonc.2004.04.008.
7. Krackowizer P, Brenner E. Dicke der Epidermis und Dermis. Phlebologie. 2008;37:83–92. https://doi.org/10.1055/s-0037-1622218.
8. Wild T, Becker M, Winter J, et al. Hyperspectral imaging of tissue perfusion and oxygenation in wounds: assessing the impact of a micro capillary dressing. J Wound Care. 2018;27:38–51. https://doi.org/10.12968/jowc.2018.27.1.38.
9. Notter M, Piazena H, Vaupel P. Hypofractionated re-irradiation of large-sized recurrent breast cancer with thermography-controlled, contact-free water-filtered infra-red-A hyperthermia: a

retrospective study of 73 patients. Int J Hyperthermia. 2017;33:227–36. https://doi.org/10.108 0/02656736.2016.1235731.

10. Seegenschmiedt MH, Klautke G, Walther E, et al. Water-filtered infrared-A-hyperthermia combined with radiotherapy in advanced and recurrent tumors. Initial results of a multicenter phase I-II study. Strahlenther Onkol. 1996;172:475–84.

11. Lu G, Fei B. Medical hyperspectral imaging: a review. J Biomed Opt. 2014;19:10901. https://doi.org/10.1117/1.JBO.19.1.010901.

12. Hartel M, Hoffmann G, Wente MN, et al. Randomized clinical trial of the influence of local water-filtered infrared A irradiation on wound healing after abdominal surgery. Br J Surg. 2006;93:952–60. https://doi.org/10.1002/bjs.5429.

13. Wang W, Winlove CP, Michel CC. Oxygen partial pressure in outer layers of skin of human finger nail folds. J Physiol. 2003;549:855–63. https://doi.org/10.1113/jphysiol.2002.037994.

14. Carreau A, El Hafny-Rahbi B, Matejuk A, et al. Why is the partial oxygen pressure of human tissues a crucial parameter? Small molecules and hypoxia. J Cell Mol Med. 2011;15:1239–53. https://doi.org/10.1111/j.1582-4934.2011.01258.x.

15. Evans N, Naylor P. Steady states of oxygen tension in human dermis. Respir Physiol. 1966;2:46–60. https://doi.org/10.1016/0034-5687(66)90037-5.

16. Baumgärtl H, Ehrly AM, Saeger-Lorenz K, et al. Initial results of intracutaneous measurements of pO_2 profiles. In: Ehrly AM, Hauss J, Huch R, editors. Clinical oxygen pressure measurement: Tissue oxygen pressure and transcutaneous oxygen pressure. Berlin Heidelberg: Springer; 1987. p. 121–8.

17. Keeley TP, Mann GE. Defining physiological normoxia for improved translation of cell physiology to animal models and humans. Physiol Rev. 2019;99:161–234. https://doi.org/10.1152/physrev.00041.2017.

18. Vaupel P, Mayer A, Höckel M. Impact of hemoglobin levels on tumor oxygenation: the higher, the better? Strahlenther Onkol. 2006;182:63–71. https://doi.org/10.1007/s00066-006-1543-7.

19. Crezee J, Zweije R, Bakker A et al. Combining 70MHz and 434MHz or wIRA hyperthermia applicators for optimal coverage of demi-deep tumour sites. In: 2019 49th European Microwave Conference: 1–3 October 2019, Paris, France. IEEE, Piscataway, pp. 164–167; 2019.

Part II

Clinical Practice: Oncology

Thermography-Controlled, Contact-Free wIRA-Hyperthermia Combined with Hypofractionated Radiotherapy for Large-Sized Lesions of Unresectable, Locally Recurrent Breast Cancer

6

M. Notter, A. R. Thomsen, A. L. Grosu, K. Münch, and Peter Vaupel

6.1 Introduction

In 75% of all cases of primary breast cancer, tumor tissue is removed by breast-conserving surgery (BCS) to avoid mastectomy. In standard procedure, BCS is followed by adjuvant radiotherapy (RT) using a total dose of 50–60 Gy in order to eradicate remaining cancer cells and decrease the risk of locoregional recurrence. Improved approaches for the early detection of breast cancer and surgical techniques and RT protocols have decreased the median incidence rate of locoregional recurrence in high-income countries to 0.6% per year. However, the increasing number of longtime breast cancer survivors increases the number of patients at risk of developing a local recurrence later, thereby leading to a median cumulative local recurrence rate of 6.2% [1]. In subgroups of patients, such as triple-negative breast cancer in premenopausal patients, cancer recurrence occurs considerably more often and after a shorter time interval. The first manifestation of locally recurrent breast cancer (LRBC) after BCS is generally treated by mastectomy, in some cases even by a second BCS. The option of a second adjuvant radiotherapy of 50–60 Gy must be weighed against the risk of severe side effects due to cumulative radiotoxicity.

M. Notter (✉) · K. Münch
Department of Radiation Oncology, Lindenhofspital, Bern, Switzerland
e-mail: markus.notter@lindenhofgruppe.ch

A. R. Thomsen · A. L. Grosu · P. Vaupel
Department of Radiation Oncology, University Medical Center, University of Freiburg, Freiburg/Breisgau, Germany

German Cancer Consortium (DKTK), Partner Site Freiburg and German Cancer Research Center (DKFZ), Heidelberg, Germany

© The Author(s) 2022
P. Vaupel (ed.), *Water-filtered Infrared A (wIRA) Irradiation*,
https://doi.org/10.1007/978-3-030-92880-3_6

If the recurrent tumor cannot completely be removed by mastectomy with an adequate safety margin or if the pathologist finds cancer cells in the margin of the removed tissue, then the so-called "microscopic disease" carries a high risk of macroscopic recurrence. Furthermore, locoregional recurrences at the chest wall in the pre-irradiated area are often irresectable and/or resection would require complicated surgical procedures that would be associated with major mutilations. Another RT at a standard dosage, which is required for effective tumor control, must be denied due to expected unacceptable toxicity for heart, lung, and rib bones. An inflammatory subgroup of locoregional recurrences, lymphangiosis carcinomatosa, even tends to recur repeatedly after short time gaps. In these final stages of unresectable locally recurrent disease in pre-irradiated sites, the ambition for tumor control is often abandoned, and patients suffer from a tremendous loss of quality of life caused by uncontrolled local tumor growth with symptoms such as pain, constriction, bleeding, ulceration, and infection. These symptoms also often lead to social isolation.

Mild hyperthermia (HT) as a potent radiosensitizer (Thomsen et al., Chap. 5, this book) enables a reduced RT dose and toxicity. In combined HT/RT schedules, good tumor control can be achieved using total re-irradiation doses of 20–39 Gy with very different fractionation schedules. A systematic review and meta-analysis have demonstrated the efficacy of combined HT/RT in the treatment of LRBC, with an especially high benefit for pre-irradiated patients [2]. In most of the published studies, HT was applied by microwave (MW) devices consisting of a microwave antenna and a water bolus, which is directly applied to the target region. Superficial HT using MW can achieve effective hyperthermia temperatures >39 °C up to a depth of approx. 30–40 mm. However, the MW technique has considerable limitations as the treatment of large-sized diffuse tumor spread cannot be covered by one applicator, especially in the case of heterogeneous body contours. With ulcerating lesions, the applicator contact may be uncomfortable and painful. In addition, the incidence of thermal skin damage is high [3].

6.2 Patients and Treatments

So far, tumor response and local control have been documented in 280 patients presenting with LRBC in pre-irradiated sites and treated with thermography-controlled, superficial wIRA-HT. In 2020, an intermediate analysis of the outcome data of 201 patients was published [4]. Since tumor size has been described as being the most significant prognostic factor [5], the evaluation has been stratified into 4 size classes of macroscopic disease, ranging from tumors <10 cm (rClass I), up to carcinoma en cuirasse with extensions to the back (rClass IV, as shown in Fig. 6.1). In addition, the microscopic disease is classified as rClass 0.

6.2.1 Basic Characteristics of the Patients

In the intermediate analysis, 170 patients presented with macroscopic disease and 31 patients with microscopic disease. Most patients were heavily pretreated and

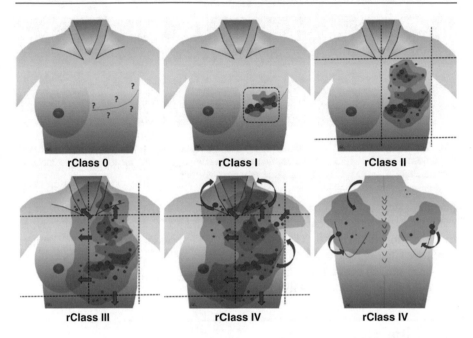

Fig. 6.1 Size classification for locally recurrent breast cancer, as suggested by Notter et al. (modified from [4])

sent to thermography-controlled wIRA-hyperthermia since no other therapeutic option remained. All patients had previously received radiotherapy, with 116 patients having received more than 2 systemic chemotherapies. Of the patients with macroscopic disease, 141 (83%) had large-sized tumors (rClass II–IV), 49 of whom had 2 or more regions to be treated. Poor prognostic factors were prominent in these patients: 50 patients (25%) presented with triple-negative breast cancer, 115 patients (57%) presented with inflammatory LRBC (lymphangiosis carcinomatosa), and 70 patients (35%) with ulcerating lesions. More than half of the patients with macroscopic disease presented with additional distant metastasis, which is the decisive factor for limited life expectancy. However, effective control of local tumor growth is crucial, even for patients with a life expectancy of just a few months, in order to achieve a satisfying palliative effect, and to improve the quality of life during the remaining lifetime.

6.2.2   Treatment Schedule

The basic treatment protocol was thermography-controlled, superficial wIRA-hyperthermia directly followed by hypofractionated re-irradiation of 5×4 Gy, once a week, as introduced by Notter et al. [6]. The total re-irradiation dose of 20 Gy is the lowest RT dose ever applied in a protocol aiming for effective tumor control. Since wIRA-HT works with a contact-free energy input, the treatment allows the

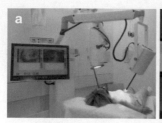
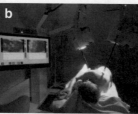
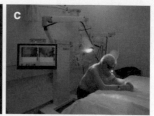

Fig. 6.2 (**a–c**) Treatment of patients using the Hydrosun®-TWH1500 hyperthermia device (Hydrosun Medizintechnik, Müllheim, Germany): various positions are supported to meet the requirements of extended lesions, e.g., carcinoma en cuirasse

patient to stay in a comfortable position (see Fig. 6.2a–c). Automatic control of the maximum surface temperature between 42 °C and 43 °C achieves effective hyperthermic temperatures >39 °C up to a depth of approximately 25 mm (Thomsen et al.; see Chap. 5) and overheating leading to thermal skin damage can be avoided. The time interval between HT and RT is <5 min for the transport of the patient from HT to the RT room and RT delivery.

6.3 Results

6.3.1 Tumor Response and Toxicity

The assessment of a new treatment method is based on the ratio of efficacy and toxicity. High toxicity is especially unacceptable in a therapy with palliative intent. Tumor response rates are shown in Table 6.1. As expected, rates of complete response (CR) decrease with increasing tumor size. Correspondingly, rates of partial response (PR) develop in opposite directions. In patients with large-sized LRBC and distant metastasis, the purely palliative treatment was often deliberately confined to regions where the tumor caused debilitating symptoms. With an overall clinical response (CR + PR) of 95% only very few patients experienced no benefit from the treatment.

As shown in Table 6.2, toxicity is extremely low. All grade I acute side effects did not require any medical intervention and had almost no impact on quality of life. Radiation dermatitis grade II and scurfs only occurred in 14 patients. Thermal skin damage (a rather common side effect in microwave hyperthermia [3]) occurred in only 1 patient. Hyperpigmentation had only a cosmetic impact and was not relevant for these patients.

Figure 6.3 (a–d) show an example of a patient with CR (rClass 2), and Figs. 6.4 and 6.5 (a, b) demonstrate patients with PR (rClasses III and IV)

6.3.2 Local Control and Re-Recurrence

In the majority of patients, the local tumor remained controlled during lifetime. Some patients with a formerly fatal prognosis of local tumor growth, but without

Table 6.1 Tumor response rates (modified from [4])

| | rClass 0 | Macroscopic All | Macroscopic Size | | | | Macroscopic Other Factors | |
			rClass I	rClass II	rClass III	rClass IV	Lymphangiosis	Ulceration
Patients	31 (100%)	170 (100%)	29 (100%)	56 (100%)	44 (100%)	41 (100%)	115 (100%)	70 (100%)
CR		73 (43%)	22 (76%)	34 (61%)	16 (36%)	1 (2%)	41 (36%)	12 (17%)
PR		88 (52%)	7 (24%)	20 (36%)	27 (61%)	34 (83%)	68 (59%)	52 (74%)
NC		6 (4%)		2 (3%)		4 (10%)	4 (3%)	4 (6%)
PD		3 (2%)			1 (2%)	2 (5%)	2 (2%)	2 (3%)

Table 6.2 Toxicity of water-filtered infrared A hyperthermia (wIRA-HT) and re-irradiation (re-RT) (modified from [4])

No. of patients	201 (100%)
No acute side effects	114 (57%)
Acute side effects	87 (43%)
− Radiodermatitis grade I	65
− Radiodermatitis grade II	4
− Scurfs	10
− Hyperpigmentation	64
− Burn with blistering	1
No chronic side effects	145 (72%)
Chronic side effects	56 (28%)
− Grade I: Hyperpigmentation	53
− Grade II: New telangiectasia	7

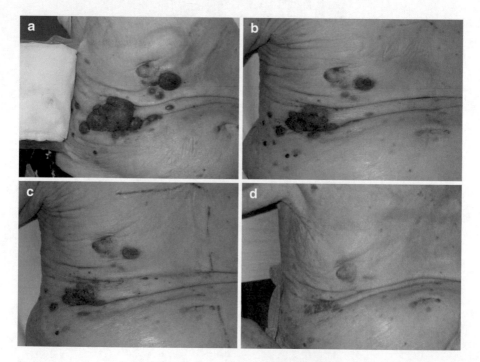

Fig. 6.3 Treatment response of a patient with extended triple-negative LRBC, rClass II, treated with combined wIRA-HT and re-RT: (**a**) before treatment, (**b**) after 2 × 4 Gy, (**c**) after 4 × 4 Gy, and (**d**) CR 2 months after 5 × 4 Gy

metastasis could even be cured. However, the progressed stage of disease and especially the characteristics of inflammatory lymphangiosis carcinomatosa are associated with a high risk of repeat recurrences and new local progression, respectively, distant metastasis. Local control rates after CR and locally progression-free rates after PR are shown in Tables 6.3 and 6.4.

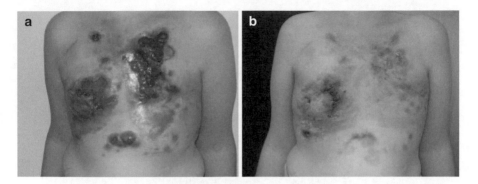

Fig. 6.4 Treatment response of a patient with LRBC, rClass III, treated with combined wIRA-HT and re-RT: (**a**) before treatment and (**b**) PR 9 weeks after 5 × 4 Gy

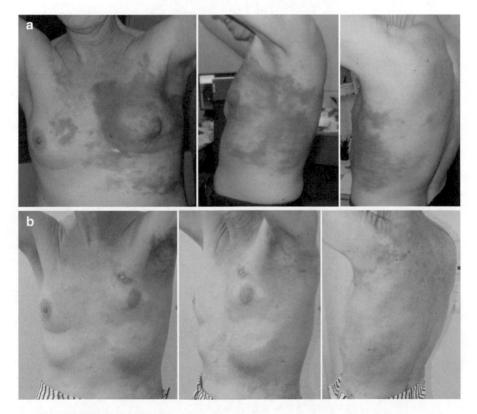

Fig. 6.5 Treatment response of a patient with LBRC, rClass IV, treated with combined wIRA-HT ad re-RT: (**a**) before treatment, (**b**) after treatment of anterior left chest wall, infraaxillary region, and infrascapular region and left supraclavicular region; each volume received 5 × 4 Gy

Table 6.3 Local control during lifetime and infield/border recurrences after complete response (CR). LFU = lost to follow-up (modified from [4])

	rClass 0	Macroscopic all	Macroscopic size				Macroscopic other factors	
			rClass I	rClass II	rClass III	rClass IV	Lymphangiosis	Ulceration
Patients	31 (100%)	73 (100%)	22 (100%)	34 (100%)	16 (100%)	1 (100%)	41 (100%)	12 (100%)
LC	21 (68%)	49 (67%)	17 (77%)	21 (61%)	11 (69%)		24 (59%)	7 (58%)
Local re-rec	2 (6%)	21 (29%)	2 (9%)	12 (36%)	5 (31%)	1 (100%)	17 (41%)	5 (42%)
LFU	8 (26%)	3 (4%)	3 (14%)	1 (3%)				

Table 6.4 Progression-free rate during lifetime and new infield/border progression after partial response (PR) (modified from [4])

| | Macroscopic all | Macroscopic size | | | | Macroscopic other factors | |
		rClass I	rClass II	rClass III	rClass IV	Lymphangiosis	Ulceration
Patients	88 (100%)	7 (100%)	20 (100%)	27 (100%)	34 (100%)	68 (100%)	52 (100%)
Locally progression-free	48 (55%)	3 (43%)	8 (40%)	14 (52%)	23 (71%)	37 (56%)	27 (54%)
New local progression	40 (45%)	4 (57%)	12 (60%)	13 (48%)	11 (29%)	31 (44%)	25 (46%)

The extremely low toxicity of combined thermography-controlled wIRA-HT and re-RT with a total dose of 20 Gy allows for repeat re-irradiation(s) in case of repeat recurrence(s). Of the 21 patients presenting with re-recurrences after CR, 19 were treated with the same schedule again. Among these 19 patients, 13 achieved another CR, and 6 patients had a PR. Repeat re-irradiation was also applied in 24 of 40 patients presenting with new local progression after PR. Two patients achieved a CR, and 16 patients achieved a PR. In some patients, a formerly desperate situation could be turned into a sustainable management of tumor control throughout several subsequent re-recurrences with good quality of life for several years. An example of this scenario is shown in Fig. 6.6.

The Kaplan–Meier estimates are commonly used for comparing a new therapeutic method with an existing standard therapy in comparative clinical trials. Unfortunately, the characteristics of unresectable, large-sized LRBC in pre-irradiated regions do not allow for the design of comparative studies since there is no standard therapy available. Therefore, the comparison of a promising therapeutic intervention with a non-treatment-responsive best supportive care strategy cannot be justified ethically [7, 8]. Nevertheless, the Kaplan–Meier estimates can be used to compare overall survival with respect to tumor size and to the presence of metastasis (Fig. 6.7). As expected, overall survival progressively reduces with increasing tumor size (Fig. 6.7a). The high mortality in the first 18 months is primarily caused by death due to metastatic disease. In our analysis, the presence of metastasis has the most significant impact on overall survival. The upper curve in Fig. 6.7b (including all patients) and in Fig. 6.7c (including patients with macroscopic disease) shows a relevant proportion of long-term survivors. By using combined HT/re-RT in the treatment of inoperable LRBC in pre-irradiated areas, a curative intent should not be excluded. Figure 6.7d shows survival of patients with initially microscopic disease, only very few of whom had distant metastasis.

6.4 Conclusion and Outlook

Combining HT and re-RT at considerably reduced RT doses has shown an excellent efficacy/toxicity ratio in the treatment of unresectable LRBC in pre-irradiated sites and offers a new option for patients in formerly desperate situations of uncontrollable tumor growth. Thermography-controlled superficial wIRA-HT is mainly indicated in the treatment of large-sized lesions, lymphangiosis carcinomatosa, and ulcerated lesions up to a tissue depth of approximately 2.5 cm (Thomsen et al., Chap. 5 in this book). Clinical experiences have shown a comparable efficacy in the treatment of other superficial tumors (e.g., malignant melanoma, skin carcinomas, radiation-induced angiosarcoma, and Merkel cell carcinoma).

In addition to the described combination with radiotherapy, combined treatment schedules including chemotherapy and immunotherapy should be considered in the future.

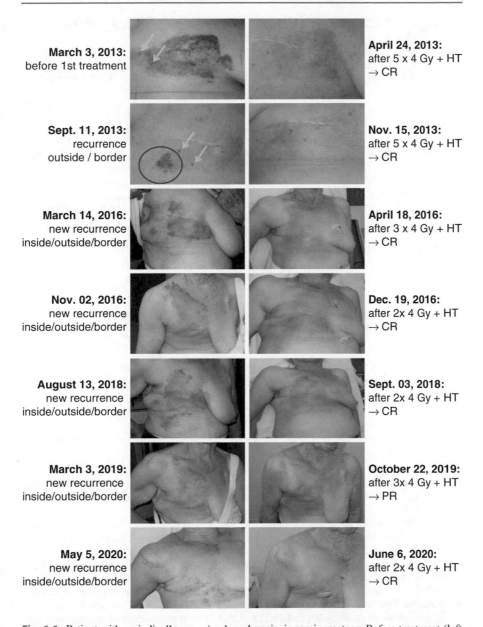

Fig. 6.6 Patient with periodically recurring lymphangiosis carcinomatosa. Before treatment (left column) and after treatment (right column). Schedule of some treatments was interrupted after 2 or 3 therapeutic sessions due to an independently occurring urinary bladder infection and unavailability of the patient

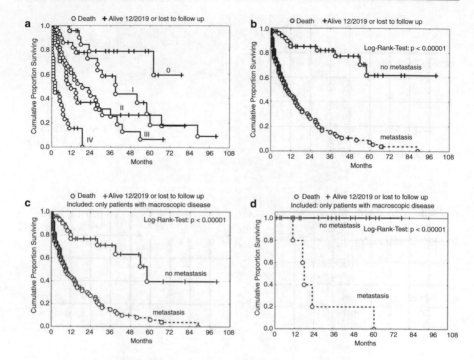

Fig. 6.7 Kaplan–Meier estimates of overall survival stratified into size classes (**a**), in patients with and without metastasis including all patients (**b**), including only macroscopic disease (**c**), and including only microscopic disease (**d**)

References

1. Spronk I, Schellevis FG, Burgers JS, de Bock GH, Korevaar JC. Incidence of isolated local breast cancer recurrence and contralateral breast cancer: a systematic review. Breast. 2018;39:P70–9.
2. Datta NR, Puric E, Klingbiel D, Gomez S, Bodis S. Hyperthermia and radiation therapy in locoregional recurrent breast cancers: a systematic review and meta-analysis. Int J Radiat Oncol Biol Phys. 2016;94:1073–87.
3. Bakker A, van der Zee J, van Tienhoven G, Kok HP, Rasch CRN, Crezee H. Temperature and thermal dose during radiotherapy and hyperthermia for recurrent breast cancer are related to clinical outcome and thermal toxicity: a systematic review. Int J Hyperth. 2019;36(1):1024–39.
4. Notter M, Thomsen AR, Nitsche M, Hermann RM, Wolff H, Habl G, Münch K, Grosu AL, Vaupel P. Combined wIRA-hyperthermia and hypofractionated re-irradiation in the treatment of locally recurrent breast cancer: evaluation of therapeutic outcome based on a novel size classification. Cancers. 2020;12, 606. https://doi.org/10.3390/cancers12030606.
5. Oldenborg S, Griesdoorn V, Os RV, Kusumanto YH, Oei BS, Venselaar JL, Paul J, Vörding ZVS, Heymans MW, Kolff MW. Reirradiation and hyperthermia for irresectable locoregional recurrent breast cancer in previously irradiated area: size matters. Radiother Oncol. 2015;117:223–8.

6. Notter M, Piazena H, Vaupel P. Hypofractionated re-irradiation of large-sized recurrent breast cancer with thermography-controlled, contact-free water-filtered infra-red-A hyperthermia: a retrospective study of 73 patients. Int J Hyperth. 2017;33:227–36.
7. Thomsen AR, Vaupel P, Grosu AL, Notter M. Hyperthermia plus re-irradiation in the management of unresectable locoregional recurrence of breast cancer in previously irradiated sites. J Clin Oncol Sep. 2020;8:JCO2001857. https://doi.org/10.1200/JCO.20.01857.
8. Buchholz TA, Ali S, Hunt KK. Reply to Thomsen A (2020). J Clin Oncol. 2020;8:JCO2002247. https://doi.org/10.1200/JCO.20.02247.

Combined Use of wIRA and Microwave or Radiofrequency Hyperthermia

7

J. Crezee, A. Bakker, R. Zweije, M. W. Kolff,
H. J. G. D. van den Bongard, G. van Tienhoven, and H. P. Kok

7.1 Introduction

Clinical results of hyperthermia treatment at 40–43 °C for 1 h applied in combination with chemotherapy and/or radiotherapy are excellent. The reported increase in tumor response for various tumor sites is in the order of 15–20%, without significant increase in radiotherapy or chemotherapy-related side effects [1–3]. An important application is superficial hyperthermia, as part of the treatment of recurrent breast cancer, chest wall recurrences, or melanoma. Clinical outcome is strongly correlated with the achieved tumor temperatures [4]. Achieving sufficiently high and uniform tumor temperatures of approximately 41–43 °C is therefore important, but at the same time excessive normal tissue temperatures exceeding approximately 43 °C must be avoided to reduce the risk of toxicity [5]. Treatment guidelines for superficial hyperthermia recommend achieving a median tumor temperature exceeding 41 °C and achieving temperatures exceeding 40 °C in 90% of the tumor volume [6].

Dedicated heating devices are available for specific tumor sites, e.g., deep-seated versus superficial tumor locations [7]. Tumor sites located close to the skin surface can be heated adequately with infrared (up to 1.5 cm depth) or microwave radiation (up to 4 cm depth) [8]. However, a different approach is required when the tumor size and shape are such that the entire target region cannot be covered adequately using a single technique. This issue occurs for instance for tumors with large surface areas with partially superficial and partially more deep-seated tumor and semi-deep-seated tumors, which start at the skin and extend deep, beyond 4 cm of depth. This chapter describes the approach used at Amsterdam UMC of treating the complete

J. Crezee (✉) · A. Bakker · R. Zweije · M. W. Kolff · H. J. G. D. van den Bongard ·
G. van Tienhoven · H. P. Kok
Department of Radiation Oncology, Amsterdam University Medical Centers, Cancer Center
Amsterdam, University of Amsterdam, Amsterdam, The Netherlands
e-mail: h.crezee@amsterdamumc.nl

P. Vaupel (ed.), *Water-filtered Infrared A (wIRA) Irradiation*,
https://doi.org/10.1007/978-3-030-92880-3_7

target region for challenging tumor geometries by sequential or simultaneous application of different hyperthermia devices, each covering another part of the target volume. Our clinical protocols and system combinations are presented, followed by two examples of clinical application of infrared combined with microwave or radio-frequency hyperthermia, including tumor temperatures measured at various depths to monitor and guide treatment quality.

7.2   Available Equipment for Different Tumor Depths

Superficial chest wall recurrences of breast cancer or melanoma generally extend a few cm down from the skin surface [6] and are treated with different suitable commercially available devices, including water-filtered Infrared-A (wIRA) applicators [9], 915 MHz antennas [10], and 434 MHz microstrip and lucite cone applicators [11]. When treating chest wall recurrences, the skin is always part of the target region, and thus, normal tissue and tumor tissue are heated to similar temperatures. Temperatures beyond 40 °C are required to ensure treatment quality [6], but at the same time temperatures should not exceed 43 °C to avoid thermal toxicity [5]. Therefore, the temperatures in the target volume are limited to a narrow 40–43 °C therapeutic temperature range.

Advantages of using infrared heating include the lack of need for a water bolus between applicator and skin, the ability to heat large and irregularly shaped body surfaces, and high-resolution skin surface temperature monitoring by using infrared cameras. This means that a comparatively fast workflow can be realized, combined with optional surface temperature control. Limitation is that therapeutic heating cannot be guaranteed beyond ≈1.5 cm depth.

More deep-seated lesions up to ca 2–3 or 4 cm depth are generally heated using 915 MHz or 434 MHz antennas, respectively. A water bolus containing temperature-controlled circulating deionized water (typically in the 40–43 °C range) is placed between the antenna and the skin to couple the energy into the skin. A slightly lower water temperature is chosen when a relatively large penetration depth is required. A lower, but still therapeutic, skin temperature permits increasing the amount of applied power to achieve deeper heat penetration up to ≈4 cm [12].

Even more deep-seated tumors, i.e., starting at the skin surface and extending more than 4 cm at depth, require antennas operating at 70–150 MHz to achieve sufficient penetration depth. Dedicated systems have been developed and applied for this category, consisting of either a single or two 70 MHz applicators [13, 14]. A challenge for semi-deep-seated tumors is the need to heat both the surface and at depth, which can create conflicting optimal system settings for each goal. Heating at depth requires the use of more aggressive surface cooling with temperatures below 40 °C to maximize penetration depth [12], thus potentially underdosing the skin surface.

Our department uses three different devices for recurrent breast cancer and melanoma, each representing device categories suitable for one of the aforementioned different tumor depths:

1. The water-filtered infrared-A (wIRA) Hydrosun® 1500 system (Hydrosun Medizintechnik, Müllheim/Baden, Germany) combines a high color temperature halogen lamp (type HPL, Ushio, Tokyo, Japan) with water filtering, resulting in emission of IR-A radiation (wavelength 0.6–1.4 μm). This heating device has the advantage of being contact-free and suitable for more irregularly shaped and very large skin surfaces.
2. Microstrip applicators operating at 434 MHz are available in 5 different sizes with largest aperture size of 20 × 30 cm (Medlogix, Rome, Italy; and Istok, Fryazino, Russia). A rubber water bolus integrated with the applicator is placed between applicator and patient skin to ensure that the emitted electromagnetic energy is coupled effectively into the patient. This water bolus is a plastic bag containing circulating distilled water to provide warming of the skin surface to the therapeutic range. Power is generated by the ALBA 4000 Double-ON system (Medlogix, Rome, Italy), which supports optional simultaneous use of two applicators to cover larger tumor surfaces.
3. An in-house developed water-filled 70 MHz double waveguide system for semi-deep-seated breast tumors. Depending on the target size and location, waveguides with aperture sizes of 34 × 21 cm, 34 x 15 cm, or 34 x 8.5 cm can be selected [14]. A water bolus placed between waveguide and patient skin ensures that the emitted electromagnetic energy is coupled effectively into the patient. This water bolus contains circulating distilled water to provide either warming or cooling of the skin, depending on whether the skin is part of the tumor target or not. The generator system is an 8-channel DDS-based phase and amplitude-controlled RF generator system (SSB Electronic, Iserlohn, Germany) combined with 500 W solid-state 70 MHz amplifiers (Restek, Rome, Italy).

Single applicators or combinations of these three systems are deployed, depending on tumor size and depth. We use wIRA for different subgroups of patients: the first is patients with very widespread cancer en cuirasse type of disease, often spreading to both the ventral and dorsal sides of the patient. Consequently, patients are sometimes heated in seated position with wIRA-radiators on either side of the body to achieve simultaneous heating of the entire target region. A second application of wIRA is for patients with silicone breast prosthesis with tumor recurrence in the narrow strip of skin tissue overlaying the prosthesis. In both aforementioned applications, wIRA may be combined with the other two methods if some tumor sections are too deep-seated to be covered by wIRA. A third application of wIRA involves patients with semi-deep-seated tumors, for instance when an intact breast is the target region, including the skin surface and extending more than 4 cm deep into the breast. In that case, wIRA heating is applied for the skin, and a MW or RF antenna is used for the more deep-seated parts of the tumor. In case of combined use of devices, we select either simultaneous use during a single hyperthermia session, or separate hyperthermia sessions per device/region.

7.3   Temperature Control and Thermometry

Thermal monitoring during hyperthermia treatments is essential to ensure treatment quality. Amsterdam UMC uses extensive thermometry during hyperthermia treatment of recurrent breast cancer, which includes both noninvasive measurements on the skin surface and invasive intra-tumoral measurements. During RF or MW heating, skin temperatures are monitored using a number of 6–15 thermocouple probes, distributed evenly over the skin surface. Typically, an additional 1–3 probes are placed invasively (if possible) and 2–6 probes on scar tissue. The invasive thermometry catheters are in principle left in situ for the 3- to 4-week duration of the treatment series, unless contraindicated or at signs of inflammation. The Amsterdam UMC uses 7-sensor and 14-sensor copper constantan thermocouple probes (Volenec RD Inc., Hradec Králové, Czech Republic) with an outer diameter of 0.5 mm or 0.9 mm, respectively, and either 5 or 10 mm spacing between consecutive temperature sensors. An in-house developed 196-channel thermometry system is used to measure every 30 sec undisturbed temperatures during a short power-off interval of the RF or MW antenna [15]. During hyperthermia treatments with the wIRA system, skin temperature measurements are performed using an IR camera. The control program provides real-time temperature control by switching off and on the wIRA radiation to maintain the maximum skin temperature in a predefined range of 42–43 °C. When sections of the tumor extend beyond 1 cm depth, catheters are inserted for additional invasive thermometry, prior to the first hyperthermia session. If wIRA is used in conjunction with 434 MHz microstrip applicators, then the thermocouple probes are preferably placed in the direction perpendicular to the dominant field direction of the 434 MHz applicator to minimize the risk of picking up MW energy.

In more simple cases, implantation of thermometry catheters is performed by the staff at the Radiation Oncology Department. Implantation at more challenging locations, e.g., close to blood vessels, is performed under ultrasound guidance by an interventional radiologist. After implantation, the catheter position and insertion depth are determined using a CT scan. Information on the probe positions is important to assist the staff in interpreting temperature data during the hyperthermia sessions and perform adjustments in system settings when needed. A number of relevant thermal dose parameters are derived from the temperature data in accordance with QA guidelines [6]. Target temperatures during treatment are reported as T10, T50, and T90, i.e., the temperature at least achieved in 10%, 50%, and 90% of the target representative measurements during the steady-state period. The thermal dose parameters CEM43 T90 and CEM43 T50 can be derived, which represent the thermal dose given in equivalent number of minutes at 43 °C. This allows inter-comparison of treatment data.

7.4   Treatment Schedules

Patients with superficial chest wall recurrences of breast cancer are treated with radiotherapy and hyperthermia at Amsterdam UMC. The hyperthermia target volume follows the re-irradiation target volume, and this also applies in case of elective re-irradiation after local tumor resection. Different fractionation schedules are used. The standard schedule consists of 23 daily fractions of 2 Gy for radiotherapy, with hyperthermia given once a week, for 5 weeks, within one hour after radiotherapy that day. The latter is based on preclinical and clinical data, demonstrating better treatment outcome for shorter time intervals between radiotherapy and hyperthermia [16–18]. Two hyperthermia sessions are given each week in case parts of the target zone need to be heated in separate sessions, one session using wIRA for the most superficial part and one session using RF/MW antenna(s) for remaining deeper-seated parts of the tumor. Time between those two hyperthermia sessions is at least 48 h to prevent the occurrence of thermotolerance [19].

For frail and very elderly patients an alternative, hypofractionated 8 x 4 Gy schedule is used with radiotherapy twice a week and hyperthermia once a week, again within one hour after radiotherapy. For cancer en cuirasse patients, a hypofractionated 5 x 4 Gy schedule is used, with once a week radiotherapy and once a week hyperthermia. In this case, hyperthermia is given first, followed by radiotherapy aiming at an ultrashort time interval shorter than 5 min [9].

7.5 Clinical Application of wIRA Combined with Other Hyperthermia Devices

This section covers two clinical applications where wIRA is combined with RF or MW hyperthermia for tumor sections, which are too deep-seated to be covered by wIRA alone. The first case is a patient with a semi-deep breast tumor in an intact breast, and the second case is a patient with silicone breast prosthesis and a laterally extending semi-deep tumor lesion. Selection of RF versus MW depends on the heating depth required.

Case 1 Semi-deep-seated tumor in an intact breast. A typical case for an intact breast is the target region as schematically illustrated in Fig. 7.1. Here, the target region starts at the skin surface and extends more than 4 cm deep into the breast, which requires the use of our 70 MHz system to reach the entire tumor. To heat the skin surface, we used the wIRA system (Fig. 7.1b), and to heat the deeper-seated part of the tumor, we used 70 MHz applicators with water bolus temperatures set to low temperatures (20–30 °C) to provide skin cooling (Fig. 7.1c). The wIRA and RF hyperthermia are applied in separate sessions.

In a patient case described in [20] and illustrated in Fig. 7.1, hyperthermia treatment of a semi-deep-seated breast tumor extending 6 cm below the skin was performed using wIRA combined with a single 20x34 cm 70 MHz waveguide in five weekly sessions. The patient received 23 daily radiotherapy fractions of 2 Gy, with two weekly hyperthermia fractions, one for the superficial part and one for the deeper part of the tumor. Invasive thermometry was performed using a catheter placed at maximum tumor depth. Surface thermometry during wIRA sessions was performed using the IR camera. We achieved median tumor temperatures T50

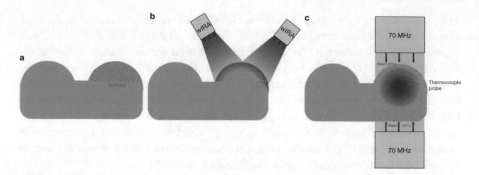

Fig. 7.1 (**a**) patient with a semi-deep-seated tumor in an intact breast. (**b**) the breast surface is treated with two wIRA applicators. (**c**) the more deep-seated tumor section is heated with one ventral (not shown) or a ventral and a dorsal 70 MHz applicator with bags with circulating cool water between antenna and skin. The blue dotted line indicates invasive thermometry present to guide the treatment

between 40.8 °C and 42.2 °C measured at depth during the 70 MHz sessions and skin temperatures between 42 °C and 43 °C during the wIRA sessions [20]. Thus, therapeutic temperatures were achieved in the entire treatment volume by applying two different hyperthermia devices in two separate sessions, and the treatment was successful and resulted in complete tumor control.

Case 2 Tumor lesion near silicone implant. A 58-year-old patient with a retro-pectoral silicone breast prosthesis directly under the skin had a tumor lesion in the skin, which was extending laterally. The tumor depth was about 1 cm in the skin overlying the prosthesis and up to 4 cm in the lateral section. The patient was treated with 23×2 Gy plus hyperthermia. Simultaneous application of combined wIRA and microwave hyperthermia was applied. We heated the skin over the breast with the wIRA system and the lateral section of the tumor with a 434 MHz applicator, as shown in Fig. 7.2.

Prior to treatment, an interventional radiologist placed three catheters for invasive thermometry close to the prosthesis edge at medial, cranial, and caudal locations with respect to the prosthesis, a fourth catheter was placed lateral to the prosthesis for measurement underneath the 434 MHz applicator as illustrated in Fig. 7.3. In addition, multiple thermocouple probes were placed on the skin just prior to each treatment session.

The catheters are left in situ for the duration of the treatment series, usually 3–5 weeks. After a treatment session, each catheter is covered with patches for hygiene as shown in Fig. 7.4.

The patient received four hyperthermia sessions of one hour each with simultaneous use of the wIRA system and a 434 MHz applicator. The part of the 434 MHz applicator that was in the field of view of the wIRA system was covered with a white towel to prevent IR temperature measurement artifacts: See Figs. 7.5 and 7.3.

Treatment was well-tolerated and recorded temperatures were in the therapeutic range. Median surface and invasive temperatures T50 for the area treated with the

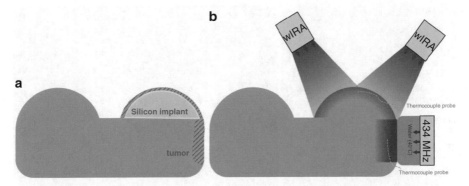

Fig. 7.2 (**a**) A patient with tumor lesions in the skin overlying a silicone breast prosthesis and extending laterally. (**b**) Schematic setup for simultaneous wIRA heating for the breast, combined with a 434 MHz applicator for the more deep-seated lesions. Blue dotted line indicates invasive thermometry present to guide the treatment

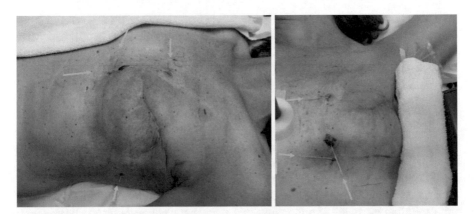

Fig. 7.3 Location of catheters for invasive thermometry at medial, lateral, cranial, and caudal locations with respect to the prosthesis. Green arrows indicate the entry points of the catheters. Right-hand panel shows the 434 MHz applicator covered with a white towel positioned lateral to the breast

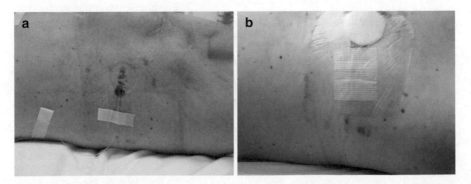

Fig. 7.4 (**a**) A ca 3-cm section of the thermometry catheter extends outside the skin. (**b**) External sections of catheters are covered with patches between consecutive hyperthermia sessions

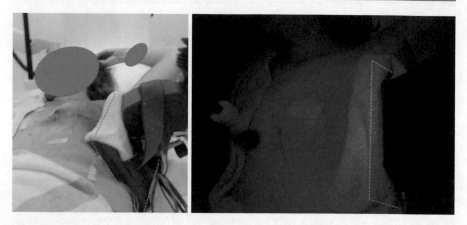

Fig. 7.5 Simultaneous use of the wIRA system and a 434 MHz applicator (indicated by green dotted outline) for tumor heating

wIRA system ranged between 42.5 °C and 43 °C, and between 38.0 °C and 39.9 °C, respectively. Median surface and invasive temperatures T50 under the 434 MHz applicator ranged between 40.4 °C and 41.4 °C, and between 39.9 °C and 40.9 °C, respectively. The treatment was successful and resulted in complete tumor control.

7.6 Conclusions

Our results demonstrate that a good heating quality can be achieved for heating superficial versus deep subsections of a tumor, when using treatment protocols, which combine the use of wIRA, MW, and RF systems. These combination protocols were successfully applied for different challenging clinical cases, and they permit extending the range of tumor sites and sizes that can be adequately heated with existing hyperthermia devices.

References

1. Cihoric N, Tsikkinis A, van Rhoon G, Crezee H, Aebersold DM, Bodis S, et al. Hyperthermia-related clinical trials on cancer treatment within the ClinicalTrials.gov registry. Int J Hyperthermia. 2015;31(6):609–14.
2. Datta NR, Gomez Ordonez S, Gaipl US, Paulides MM, Crezee H, Gellermann J, et al. Local hyperthermia combined with radiotherapy and−/ or chemotherapy: recent advances and promises for the future. Cancer Treat Rev. 2015;41(9):742–53.
3. Peeken JC, Vaupel P, Combs SE. Integrating hyperthermia into modern radiation oncology: what evidence is necessary? Front Oncol. 2017;7:132.
4. Bakker A, van der Zee J, van Tienhoven G, Kok HP, Rasch CRN, Crezee H. Temperature and thermal dose during radiotherapy and hyperthermia for recurrent breast cancer are related to clinical outcome and thermal toxicity: a systematic review. Int J Hyperthermia. 2019;36(1):1024–39.

5. Bakker A, Kolff MW, Holman R, van Leeuwen CM, Korshuize-van Straten L, R. Oldenhof-de kroon et al., "Thermal skin damage during reirradiation and hyperthermia is time temperature dependent". Int J Radiat Oncol Biol Phys. 2017;98(2):392–9.
6. Trefná HD, Crezee H, Schmidt M, Marder D, Lamprecht U, Ehmann M, et al. Quality assurance guidelines for superficial hyperthermia clinical trials: I. Clinical requirements. Int J Hyperthermia. 2017;33(4):471–82.
7. Kok HP, Cressman ENK, Ceelen W, Brace CL, Ivkov R, Grüll H, et al. Heating technology for malignant tumors: a review. Int J Hyperthermia. 2020;37(1):711–41.
8. Dobšíček Trefná H, Crezee J, Schmidt M, Marder D, Lamprecht U, Ehmann M, et al. Atzelsberg research group quality assurance guidelines for the application of superficial hyperthermia clinical trials: II. Technical requirements for heating devices. Strahlenther Onkol. 2017;193(5):351–66.
9. Notter M, Piazena H, Vaupel P. Hypofractionated re-irradiation of large-sized recurrent breast cancer with thermography-controlled, contact-free water-filtered infra-red-A hyperthermia: a retrospective study of 73 patients. Int J Hyperthermia. 2017;33(2):227–36.
10. Johnson JE, Neuman DG, Maccarini PF, Juang T, Stauffer PR, Turner P. Evaluation of a dual-arm Archimedean spiral array for microwave hyperthermia. Int J Hyperthermia. 2004;22(6):475–90.
11. Lamaitre G, van Dijk JD, Gelvich EA, Wiersma J, Schneider CJ. SAR characteristics of three types of contact flexible microstrip applicators for superficial hyperthermia. Int J Hyperthermia. 1996;12(2):255–69.
12. Van der Gaag ML, de Bruijne M, Samaras T, van der Zee J, van Rhoon GC. Development of a guideline for the water bolus temperature in superficial hyperthermia. Int J Hyperthermia. 2006;22(8):637–56.
13. Crezee J, Zweije R, Sijbrands J, Kok HP. Dedicated 70 MHz RF systems for hyperthermia of challenging tumour locations. Int J Microw Wirel Technol. 2020;12:839–47.
14. van Stam G, Kok HP, Hulshof MC, Kolff MW, van Tienhoven G, Sijbrands J, et al. A flexible 70MHz phase-controlled double waveguide system for hyperthermia treatment of superficial tumours with deep infiltration. Int J Hyperthermia. 2017;33(7):796–809.
15. De Leeuw AA, Crezee J, Lagendijk JJ. Temperature and SAR measurements in deep-body hyperthermia with thermocouple thermometry. Int J Hyperthermia. 1993;9(5):685–97.
16. Van Leeuwen CM, Oei AL, Chin KW, Crezee J, Bel A, Franken NA, et al. A short time interval between radiotherapy and hyperthermia reduces in-field recurrence and mortality in women with advanced cervical cancer. Radiat Oncol. 2017;12:75.
17. Overgaard J. Simultaneous and sequential hyperthermia and radiation treatment of an experimental tumor and its surrounding normal tissue in vivo. Int J Radiat Oncol Biol Phys. 1980;6(11):1507–17.
18. Crezee J, Oei AL, Franken NAP, Stalpers LJA, Kok HP. Response to: the impact of the time interval between radiation and hyperthermia on clinical outcome in patients with locally advanced cervical cancer. Front Oncol. 2020;10:528.
19. Overgaard J, Nielsen OS. The importance of thermotolerance for the clinical treatment with hyperthermia. Radiother Oncol. 1983;1(2):167–78.
20. Crezee J, Zweije R, Bakker A, van Tienhoven G, Kok HP. Combining 70MHz and 434MHz or wIRA hyperthermia applicators for optimal coverage of semi-deep tumour sites. In: 49th European Microwave Conference (EuMC). Paris: IEEE; 2019. p. 164–7.

Whole-Body Hyperthermia in Oncology: Renaissance in the Immunotherapy Era?

8

S. Zschaeck and M. Beck

Abbreviations

CT	Computed tomography
FRWBH	Fever-range whole-body hyperthermia
HNSCC	Head and neck squamous cell carcinomas
HPV	Human papillomavirus
HT	Hyperthermia
MRI	Magnetic resonance imaging
PET	Positron emission tomography
TER	Thermal enhancement ratio
WBH	Whole-body hyperthermia

8.1 Introduction

A key property of malignant tissue is its potential to metastasize. The major obstacle to obtain long-term curation in cancer entities with the highest incidence of metastasis such as breast, prostate, colorectal, and lung is distant metastases. Approximately

S. Zschaeck (✉)
Department of Radiation Oncology, Berlin Institute of Health, Charité-Universitätsmedizin Berlin, Corporate Member of Freie Universität Berlin, Humboldt-Universität zu Berlin, Berlin, Germany

Berlin Institute of Health (BIH), Berlin, Germany
e-mail: Sebastian.zschaeck@charite.de

M. Beck
Department of Radiation Oncology, Berlin Institute of Health, Charité-Universitätsmedizin Berlin, Corporate Member of Freie Universität Berlin, Humboldt-Universität zu Berlin, Berlin, Germany

© The Author(s) 2022
P. Vaupel (ed.), *Water-filtered Infrared A (wIRA) Irradiation*,
https://doi.org/10.1007/978-3-030-92880-3_8

90% of cancer-related deaths are due to metastatic disease. Metastases can occur synchronously at the time of tumor diagnosis or metachronously, i.e., during follow-up after initial treatment with curative intent. Hyperthermia (HT) is well known to enhance the therapeutic ratio of radiotherapy and chemotherapy. The term "hyper-thermia" is often not clearly defined. The most frequently applied *capacitive* or *radiative hyperthermia* devices aim for a local or locoregional improvement of tumor control and potentially also a moderate decrease of metachronous distant metastases by stopping the formation of metastases at its source. In contrast, whole-body hyperthermia (WBH) aims to increase the temperature within the whole organism. Consequently, this mode of action could improve locoregional and also systemic therapies. Three levels of WBH can be distinguished, depending on the targeted body core temperature: mild WBH temperatures below 38.5 °C, moderate WBH temperatures between 38.5 and 40.5 °C, which is also denoted as fever-range WBH (FRWBH), and extreme WBH temperatures above 40.5 °C.

Out of the plethora of investigated agents, platin derivates, especially cisplatin, are the most comprehensively studied chemotherapeutic agents regarding thermo-enhancement. Urano et al. were able to show that thermal enhancement can already be observed with slight temperature increases up to 39 °C, but that a much stronger ther-mal enhancement ratio (TER) was observed with temperatures above 41 °C [1]. This was the rationale to implement WBH into early clinical trials in which an enhanced cytotoxic effect against distant metastases was envisaged. Since most trials focused on TER, the aim was to achieve body core temperatures as high as clinically achievable. Therefore, most clinical trials on WBH investigated extreme WBH, i.e., with targeted body core temperatures of 41–41.5 °C. However, extreme WBH is difficult to apply, bears important risks, and is quite expensive. Patients need to be sedated and often even ventilated. Close, invasive cardiovascular monitoring and narcosis must be per-formed by experienced anesthesiologists. At the same time, patients with cancer often present with poor general health and relevant cardiovascular comorbidities. Extreme WBH has therefore only been investigated in non-randomized phase I or phase II clinical trials and does not appear to deliver practice-changing results. Lassche et al. summarized the available evidence for this kind of treatment in a recent review and concluded that "...as modern oncology offers many less invasive treatments options, it is unlikely WBH will ever find its way in routine clinical care" [2].

Given these data, extreme WBH currently does not seem to have a major role in oncology. However, FRWBH might be an attractive adjunct to modern oncological treatment strategies as this kind of treatment is usually well tolerated. In the follow-ing, we will therefore mainly focus on FRWBH, since preclinical studies and early clinical trials in oncology and in non-oncological diseases showed promising results for this approach.

8.2   Techniques for Whole-Body Hyperthermia (WBH)

Various methods can be used to induce WBH in patients. Some authors argue that fever induction by mistletoe can also be regarded as a method to induce fever-like temperatures. However, an important difference between inducing WBH by technical devices and mistletoe is that the latter induces endogenous fever, whereas externally induced WBH induces the body to activate a plethora of processes to maintain homeostasis. These two approaches should therefore have distinctly different effects on organ-specific perfusion rates.

There are three frequently applied methods to induce WBH by medical devices, the most common of which being used currently is water-filtered Infrared-A irradiation (wIRA) (see Chap. 11, this book).

8.3   Effects of Fever-Range WBH

FRWBH has highly pleiotropic effects, many aspects of which, especially those relating to the tumor microenvironment (TME) and the immune system, are tightly interwoven. This might also be the case for its psychological effects and the influence of these on immune function. Nonetheless, for didactical reasons, we propose the following subdivision for the FRWBH effects.

8.3.1   Effects on the Tumor Microenvironment (TME)

FRWBH has been studied in various preclinical models. The laboratories of Elizabeth Repasky and Sharon Evans in Buffalo, NY (USA), have provided substantial data on the mechanisms of FRWBH in preclinical oncology models. They showed that FRWBH reduced the interstitial fluid pressure within an established head and neck squamous cell carcinoma (HNSCC) and in a patient-derived xenograft model. The reduced interstitial fluid pressure is followed by an increased tumor perfusion and thus oxygen supply, and consecutively reduced tumor hypoxia. Since tumor hypoxia is a well-known negative prognostic factor in oncology, especially given its ability to confer resistance to radiotherapy, FRWBH increased the efficacy of radiotherapy in vivo [3]. The same effect could be demonstrated in vivo using murine models of colon cancer and melanoma. The decreases in interstitial fluid pressure and tumor hypoxia were relatively long-lasting and were still apparent 24 hours after the application of FRWBH [4]. Another group was able to show that local heating with mild temperatures decreases tumor hypoxia in a murine breast cancer model, as measured by dedicated small animal positron emission tomography (PET) scans [5]. However, it is difficult to draw a conclusion for the impact of FRWBH from this study since the influence on perfusion is probably very different for local or whole-body heating. Nonetheless, the effect of FRWBH on tumor perfusion has been shown in a case report of a patient with a huge (14 cm) head and neck squamous cell carcinoma lymph node metastasis of an unknown primary. The patient was treated within a prospective pilot trial of FRWBH (Clinicaltrials.gov ID: NCT0189677) and received curatively intended definitive chemoradiation. Additional computed tomography (CT) scans to assess tumor perfusion were performed and showed a pronounced increase in tumor perfusion immediately after FRWBH which remained on a higher level for 5 days following FRWBH treatment [6]. The patient showed rapid tumor shrinkage and remained locoregionally controlled at the last follow-up visit 2 years after the end of treatment. One limitation of this case, besides being only one case, is that tissue immunohistochemistry (IHC) revealed cells with positive p16 staining. p16 is a surrogate for human papillomavirus (HPV)-induced HNSCC. These tumors present relatively favorable outcome, even in locally advanced stages, especially due to their high sensitivity to radiation. Therefore, it cannot be ruled out that the observed effect is, at least partly, tumor-specific and not related to FRWBH.

Although HPV-associated HNSCCs have relatively good prognosis even in locally advanced stages, the opposite holds true for HPV-negative HNSCC that recur after initial radiotherapy/chemoradiation. In this setting, re-irradiation is a frequently chosen approach, but is usually only able to achieve short-term palliation since the re-irradiation dose is limited due to prior dose exposure of surrounding at-risk organs and due to the usually high radioresistance of recurrent tumors. This was the rationale to initiate a prospective trial on re-irradiation of locally recurrent HNSCC in combination with FRWBH (Clinicaltrials.gov ID: NCT03547388). The trial included sophisticated hypoxia-PET examinations and perfusion imaging by magnetic resonance imaging (MRI). The intention was to repeat hypoxia-PET-MRI during treatment to provide clinical data on the anti-hypoxia effect of FRWBH. The trial recruited all 10 planned patients, eight of which had additional PET and seven additional MRI imaging. Surprisingly, baseline examinations revealed an absence of PET-detectable hypoxia and very heterogeneous blood flow behavior in recurrent tumors [7]. Figure 8.1 shows representative patient examples. Therefore, no conclusions on the effect of FRWBH on tumor hypoxia and perfusion could be drawn in this cohort. Nonetheless, in an exploratory analysis, patients who received at least three FRWBH treatments concomitant with re-irradiation showed a potential improvement of locoregional tumor control [8].

8.3.2 Effects on the Immune System

Temperature is a key element for the immune system of vertebrates, and a large amount of preclinical data have shown the importance of HT and FRBWH on anti-tumor immunology. HT enhances both cellular and humoral immune responses by several mechanisms. It increases natural killer (NK) cell function, the trafficking of cytotoxic T cells to tumors, the functional activity of macrophages and dendritic cells (DCs), and the production of pro-inflammatory cytokines. The data are comprehensively summarized in two review articles [9, 10]. Various groups have been able to demonstrate that FRWBH positively influences immune responsiveness, especially in cancer. Preclinical in vivo studies by the group of Joan Bull in Houston, TX (USA), were able to show that fever-range hyperthermia has the potential to foster anti-tumor immune responses without increasing normal tissue toxicity— short-term extreme WBH caused severe damage to normal tissue [11]. This led to a first clinical trial to investigate the efficacy of combining cytostatic agents plus interferon-alpha with FRWBH in patients with different metastatic diseases [12]. This trial was performed in the pre-immune checkpoint era, and this approach was

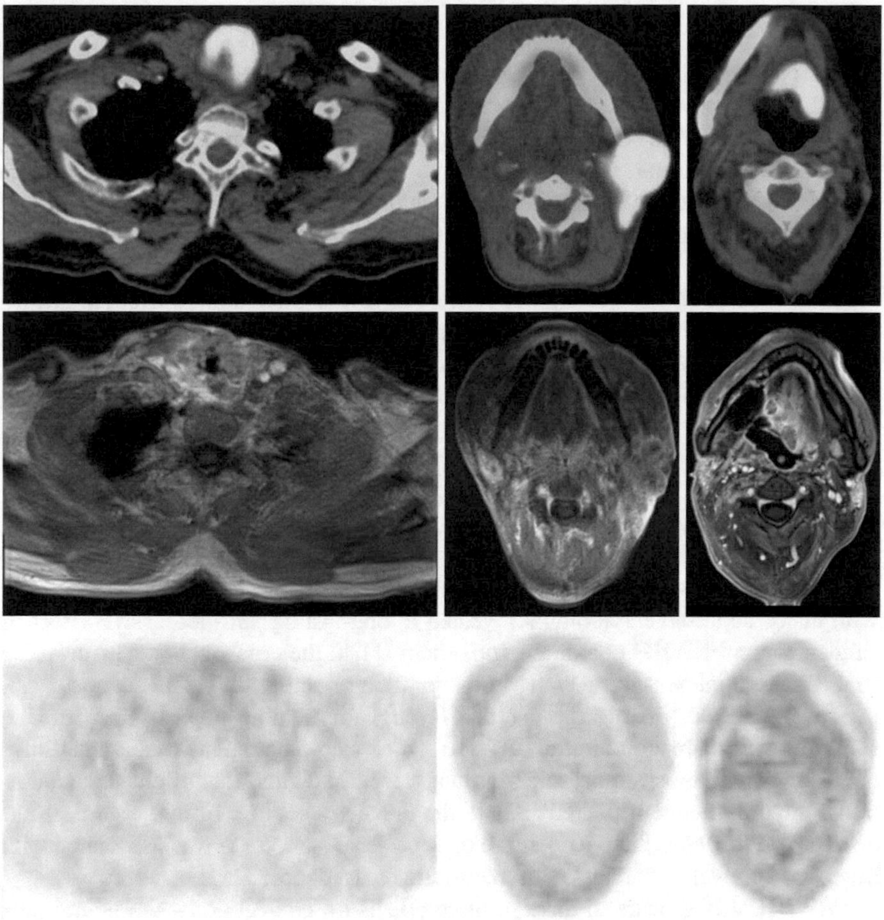

Fig. 8.1 Example of three patients treated with FRWBH plus re-irradiation for recurrent head and neck squamous cell carcinomas. FDG-PET CT (upper row) shows high glucose uptake of all tumors, while MRI (middle row) and hypoxia-related PET (lower row) do not show relevant tumor hypoxia or perfusion restriction. Image taken from [7]

unfortunately not pursued despite promising results regarding response rate and patient-reported quality of life. A recent retrospective analysis of 131 patients with stage IV solid cancers that had failed to respond to all conventional therapies and were treated with checkpoint inhibition and FRWBH has shown that the treatment was well tolerated, and response and progression-free survival rates were very promising, especially considering the unfavorable prognosis of the patient cohorts. However, one important limitation is the magnitude of interventions within these patients: Patients did not receive standard doses of checkpoint inhibition, only low-dose ipilimumab (CTLA-4, 0.3 mg/kg instead of 1.0 mg/kg). In addition, several other co-interventions were performed: additional locoregional HT and also inter-leukin 2 administration [13]. Although this hampers any conclusions on the potential use of each single intervention, it does highlight the potential to improve current immunotherapeutic approaches.

Prospective trials that combine immunotherapy with HT are therefore warranted. With respect to combining immunotherapy and HT, currently three studies have investigated this combination. Two studies are non-randomized trials undertaken in China that have used the Thermotron RF-8EX capacitive hyperthermia device. Both studies combine checkpoint inhibition, cellular immunotherapy, and HT in either mesothelioma or various abdominal/pelvic malignancies (Clinicaltrials.gov ID: NCT03757858 and NCT03393858). Another non-randomized phase-Ib/II clinical study in France has investigated intraperitoneal checkpoint inhibition in combination with hyperthermic intraperitoneal chemotherapy in patients with advanced ovarian carcinoma (Clinicaltrials.gov ID: NCT03959761). So far, no clinical trial on combining checkpoint inhibition and FRWBH has been started.

8.3.3 Psychoneurological Effects

In the non-oncology setting, a small, randomized, double-blind study in patients with major depressive symptoms revealed a long-lasting anti-depressive effect of single-session FRWBH compared with sham HT in the control [14]. This positive trial increased interest in FRWBH in the psychiatry community, and several ongoing trials are investigating the use of FRWBH for treating depressive disorders, some of which are combining FRWBH with pharmacological treatment. Since depressive symptoms are prevalent among cancer patients, this might be an additional important benefit of FRWBH in the oncology setting. In this regard, it has been shown that an effective decrease of depressive symptoms was associated with improved survival in patients with metastatic breast cancer [15].

FRWBH also appears to have positive effects on nociception—the neural processes of encoding and processing noxious stimuli. A small randomized clinical trial has shown FRWBH to significantly alleviate nonspecific lumbar back pain in patients receiving multimodal pain therapy [16]. Two other studies, one of them randomized, have also shown the potential of FRWBH to improve symptoms of fibromyalgia [17, 18]. Since pain is a frequent symptom of advanced-stage cancer, this might be another desirable effect of FRWBH in the oncology setting (see Chap. 11, this book).

8.3.4 Other Effects Possibly Relevant in Oncology

An interesting preclinical study in mice revealed the potential of FRWBH to *ameliorate severe neutropenia* and induce a more rapid recovery from neutropenia after total body irradiation compared to control mice [19]. This is a very encouraging finding given that neutropenia is one of the most frequently observed severe side effects of chemotherapy and chemoradiation which is potentially life-threatening

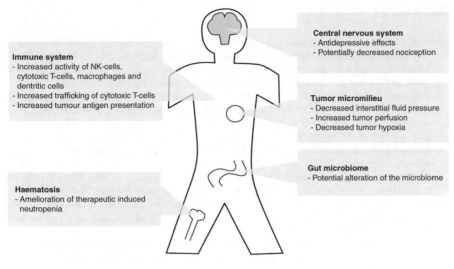

Immune system
- Increased activity of NK-cells, cytotoxic T-cells, macrophages and dentritic cells
- Increased trafficking of cytotoxic T-cells
- Increased tumour antigen presentation

Central nervous system
- Antidepressive effects
- Potentially decreased nociception

Tumor micromilieu
- Decreased interstitial fluid pressure
- Increased tumor perfusion
- Decreased tumor hypoxia

Gut microbiome
- Potential alteration of the microbiome

Haematosis
- Amelioration of therapeutic induced neutropenia

Fig. 8.2 Overview of pleiotropic FRWBH effects in oncology

and hampers the administration of additional cycles of chemotherapy. However, this finding has not yet been corroborated in clinical trials.

Although FRWBH is also very likely to have a strong impact on the composition of the *gut microbiome* [20] which is known to influence therapeutic response to conventional cancer therapy and immunotherapy, preclinical and clinical data in this area are currently lacking. Figure 8.2 summarizes the pleiotropic effects of FRWBH in the oncology setting.

8.4   Conclusions

We are currently witnessing dramatic changes in the paradigms for the treatment of cancer. Although radiotherapy has always been regarded as a local treatment that aims to kill all viable tumor cells within the irradiated target volume, the advent of novel immunotherapies has somewhat shifted this paradigm. Abscopal radiation responses, i.e., responses outside the irradiated field, and radiation-induced boosting of immunotherapy by generating neoantigens are gaining interest and have led to several ongoing clinical trials that pursue this unconventional radiotherapy approach. The same might be the case with (whole-body) hyperthermia. In 1987, van der Zee summarized the knowledge of that time as follows: "*In view of the fact that immunological factors in tumor therapy do not play a significant role..., it is likely that the elevated temperatures have been instrumental*" [21]. This reflects the strong impact of hyperthermia on classical TER of cytostatic drugs and radiotherapy in the past. Nowadays, we know that immunological factors play a pivotal role in oncology and it is noteworthy to mention that the pioneers of preclinical FRWBH were immunologists or oncologists having a strong focus on tumor immunology.

References

1. Urano M, Kahn J, Kenton LA. The effect of cis-diamminedichloroplatinum(II) treatment at elevated temperatures on murine fibrosarcoma, FSa-II. Int J Hyperthermia. 1990;6:563–70.
2. Lassche G, Crezee J, van Herpen CML. Whole-body hyperthermia in combination with systemic therapy in advanced solid malignancies. Crit Rev Oncol Hematol. 2019;139:67–74.
3. Winslow TB, Eranki A, Ullas S, et al. A pilot study of the effects of mild systemic heating on human head and neck tumour xenografts: analysis of tumour perfusion, interstitial fluid pressure, hypoxia and efficacy of radiation therapy. Int J Hyperthermia. 2015;31:693–701.
4. Sen A, Capitano ML, Spernyak JA, et al. Mild elevation of body temperature reduces tumor interstitial fluid pressure and hypoxia and enhances efficacy of radiotherapy in murine tumor models. Cancer Res. 2011;71:3872–80.
5. Myerson RJ, Singh AK, Bigott HM, et al. Monitoring the effect of mild hyperthermia on tumour hypoxia by Cu-ATSM PET scanning. Int J Hyperthermia. 2006;22:93–115.
6. Rich LJ, Winslow TB, Alberico RA, et al. Enhanced tumour perfusion following treatment with water-filtered IR-A radiation to the thorax in a patient with head and neck cancer. Int J Hyperthermia. 2016;32:539–42.
7. Rogasch J, Beck M, Stromberger C, et al. PET measured hypoxia and MRI parameters in re-irradiated head and neck squamous cell carcinomas: findings of a prospective pilot study. F1000Res. 2021;9:1350.
8. Zschaeck S, Weingärtner J, Ghadjar P, et al. Fever range whole body hyperthermia for re-irradiation of head and neck squamous cell carcinomas: final results of a prospective study. Oral Oncol. 2021 May;116:105240. https://doi.org/10.1016/j.oraloncology.2021.105240.
9. Repasky EA, Evans SS, Dewhirst MW. Temperature matters! And why it should matter to tumor immunologists. Cancer Immunol Res. 2013;1:210–6.
10. Evans SS, Repasky EA, Fisher DT. Fever and the thermal regulation of immunity: the immune system feels the heat. Nat Rev Immunol. 2015;15:335–49.
11. Sakaguchi Y, Makino M, Kaneko T, et al. Therapeutic efficacy of long duration-low temperature whole body hyperthermia when combined with tumor necrosis factor and carboplatin in rats. Cancer Res. 1994;54:2223–7.
12. Bull JMC, Scott GL, Strebel FR, et al. Fever-range whole-body thermal therapy combined with cisplatin, gemcitabine, and daily interferon-alpha: a description of a phase I-II protocol. Int J Hyperthermia. 2008;24:649–62.
13. Kleef R, Nagy R, Baierl A, et al. Low-dose ipilimumab plus nivolumab combined with IL-2 and hyperthermia in cancer patients with advanced disease: exploratory findings of a case series of 131 stage IV cancers - a retrospective study of a single institution. Cancer Immunol Immunother. 2020;70(5):1393–403.
14. Janssen CW, Lowry CA, Mehl MR, et al. Whole-body hyperthermia for the treatment of major depressive disorder: a randomized clinical trial. JAMA Psychiatry. 2016;73:789–95.
15. Giese-Davis J, Collie K, Rancourt KMS, et al. Decrease in depression symptoms is associated with longer survival in patients with metastatic breast cancer: a secondary analysis. J Clin Oncol. 2011;29:413–20.
16. Ettrich U, Konrad B, Prate K, et al. Mild whole body hyperthermia in combination with inpatient multimodal oriented pain therapy: evaluation in patients with chronic unspecific lumbar back pain. Orthopade. 2014;43:165–74.
17. Romeyke T, Scheuer HC, Stummer H. Fibromyalgia with severe forms of progression in a multidisciplinary therapy setting with emphasis on hyperthermia therapy-a prospective controlled study. Clin Interv Aging. 2015;10:69–79.
18. Brockow T, Wagner A, Franke A, et al. A randomized controlled trial on the effectiveness of mild water-filtered near infrared whole-body hyperthermia as an adjunct to a standard multimodal rehabilitation in the treatment of fibromyalgia. Clin J Pain. 2007;23:67–75.

19. Capitano ML, Nemeth MJ, Mace TA, et al. Elevating body temperature enhances hemato-poiesis and neutrophil recovery after total body irradiation in an IL-1-, IL-17-, and G-CSF-dependent manner. Blood. 2012;120:2600–9.
20. Hylander BL, Repasky EA. Temperature as a modulator of the gut microbiome: what are the implications and opportunities for thermal medicine? Int J Hyperthermia. 2019;36:83–9.
21. Field SB, Franconi C, editors. Physics and technology of hyperthermia. Amsterdam: Springer; 1987.

Gold Nanoparticles and Infrared Heating: Use of wIRA Irradiation

9

J. F. Hainfeld and H. M. Smilowitz

9.1   Introduction

There is intense interest in using hyperthermia (HT) as a therapeutic strategy to directly treat tumors by extreme heating (>43 °C for expanded heating times) or, preferentially, using mild hyperthermia (39–43 °C) to sensitize tumors to other therapies such as X-irradiation and/or chemotherapy. Despite considerable effort in this area, the promise of using hyperthermia to treat human tumors has not yet been fully realized. The holy grail would be an injectable that can access metastatic tumors with a high degree of specificity allowing sufficient heating of the tumor to cause necrosis or sensitization to other therapies while sparing normal tissues. To our knowledge, such an injectable is not yet widely available—despite major efforts to develop such reagents—particularly those efforts using iron nanoparticles and electromagnetic heating. The prospect of using nanoparticles to heat superficial and/or localized tumors in humans seems closer at hand.

This review focuses on the preclinical use of gold nanoparticles and water-filtered infrared A (wIRA) heating using a special wIRA radiator (Model 09.06.00, Hydrosun, Müllheim, Germany). This is discussed in the context of other nanogold constructs (e.g., nanoshells, nanorods, and nanotubes) that have been used for the heating of superficial and/or localized tumors and, with fiber-optic light guides, deeper tumors.

Near-infrared irradiation (NIR and wIRA) has photons of longer wavelength and less energy enabling the irradiation to penetrate deeper into living tissue. Gold nanostructures provide a mechanism for photothermal effect mechanisms whereby wIRA irradiation is converted into heat. A number of investigators have tried to take

J. F. Hainfeld
Nanoprobes, Inc, Yaphank, NY, USA

H. M. Smilowitz (✉)
University of Connecticut Health Center, Farmington, CT, USA
e-mail: smilowitz@uchc.edu

© The Author(s) 2022
P. Vaupel (ed.), *Water-filtered Infrared A (wIRA) Irradiation*,
https://doi.org/10.1007/978-3-030-92880-3_9

advantage of the known collective plasmon modes of metal nanoparticles in which the optical properties of gold molecules shift when gold molecules are brought into close apposition to one another [1, 2]. For example, Souza et al. [3] cleverly used phage display methodology to generate networks of gold-filamentous fd (also known as f1 or M13) phage constructs that targeted cells and also functioned as signal reporters for fluorescence, dark-field, and near-infrared (NIR) surface-enhanced Raman scattering (SERS) spectroscopy, since they formed tangled clusters that brought gold molecules close together. Nam et al. [4] designed "smart" 10 nm gold nanoparticles that were designed to clump together under mild acidic intracellular space where electrostatic interactions between nanoparticles form aggregates inside acidic cell organelles, such as lysosomes; once becoming trapped due to their large size, the aggregates of gold nanoparticles exhibited an absorption shift to far-red and near-infrared that could be exploited for therapy since these wavelengths have maximal tissue penetration properties.

Nanoprobes, Inc., and collaborators developed tumor-cell receptor-targeted spherical gold nanoparticles with net negative charge designed to enter cells by receptor-mediated endocytosis and then aggregate in the acidic and proteolytic environment of the lysosome [5, 6]. Once aggregated by adjusting the pH to 5 in the presence of proteases, they undergo the aforementioned spectral shift, illustrated in Fig. 9.1, in which absorption in the 800 nm range is greatly increased. The extinction amplification factor (extinction after aggregation divided by extinction before aggregation) was $\approx$20 at 800 nm. This resulted in increased heating. Three different gold nanoparticle constructs were synthesized (Fig. 9.2).

9.1.1 Construct I

AuNPs had antibodies to epidermal growth factor receptor (EGFR) adsorbed to them; adsorption of antibodies to the AuNPs was via electrostatic interactions. Many tumors overexpress EGFR. After binding to EGFR, the antibody-coated AuNPs were endocytosed. Endocytic vesicles then fused with lysosomes where the proteolytic enzymes of the lysosome degraded the adsorbed antibodies; the low pH of the lysosome resulted in AuNP aggregation. In cell studies, AuNPs were found to accumulate in punctate spots that were distributed in cytoplasmic structures largely around the cell nucleus that likely represented endocytic vesicular structures (endosomes) and lysosomes.

9.1.2 Construct II

AuNPs were coated with lipoic acid which provided a free carboxyl group and dithio(succinimidyl propionate) (DSP) used to covalently couple anti-EGFR antibodies. Again, after binding to EGFR receptors, endosomal internalization resulted in lysosomal antibody degradation and AuNP aggregation; protonation removed negative charges that kept AuNPs apart. Degradation of antibodies removed steric hindrance to van der Waals-mediated aggregation.

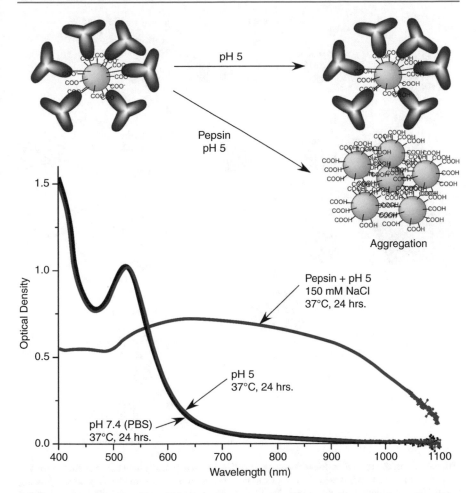

Fig. 9.1 Change in absorption spectra under various conditions. Construct II showed stability in PBS at 37 µC for 24 h (black trace) and also negligible spectral change at pH 5 after 24 h (blue trace). However, at pH 5 and in the presence of pepsin, extensive aggregation was observed (red trace), greatly increasing the absorbance in the near-infrared region (IR-A-region). Reproduced with permission from [5]

9.1.3   Construct III

AuNPs were coated with glutathione, then glutaraldehyde, and anti-EGFR. AuNPs with anti-EGFR covalently bound by Schiff's base were internalized by receptor-mediated endocytosis. Again, the acidic environment of the lysosome resulted in protonation of carboxyl groups, release of antibody, and AuNP aggregation.

All three AuNP constructs remained stable in the blood; the ability to resist aggregation in the blood prior to delivery to the tumor was a critical requirement for success. pH 5 alone caused Construct I but not Construct II and III to

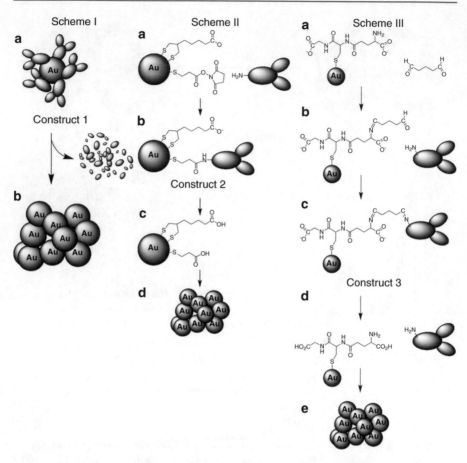

Fig. 9.2 Schemes for tumor delivery and aggregation in endosomes/lysosomes. Scheme 1: AuNPs have anti-tumor antibodies adsorbed (**a**, Construct I) that in the lysosome are degraded, allowing the AuNPs to aggregate (**b**). Scheme II: AuNPs are coated with lipoic acid and dithio(succinimidyl propionate) (DSP) (**a**), covalently coupled to anti-EGFr antibodies (**b**, Construct II), then protonated in the endosome with enzymatic antibody digestion in the lysosome (**c**), leading to aggregation (**d**). Scheme III: AuNPs are coated with glutathione (**a**), reacted with glutaraldehyde (**b**), and then anti-EGFr antibodies (**c**, Construct III) to form Schiff's bases vulnerable to cleavage at endosomal pH (**d**), resulting in protonation of carboxyl groups and along with enzymatic antibody degradation, causing aggregation (**e**). Reproduced with permission from [5]

aggregate—presumably due to the less-stable electrostatic absorption of anti-EGFR to AuNPs used in Construct I vs the covalent attachments used in Constructs II and III.

9.2   Treatments and Results

In vivo testing was performed in athymic nude mice with advanced (100–150 mm³) A431 squamous cell carcinomas growing on their flanks subcutaneously and Constructs II and III. The anti-EGFR AuNP conjugates were injected intravenously via the tail vein and showed preferential tumor localization (Fig. 9.3a). Six hours post-i.v. injections, tumor-to-muscle ratios of gold content (determined by atomic absorptions) was 12.9 ± 1.8 to 1; gentle extraction with NaOH and detergent confirmed that all of the tumoral AuNP was in the aggregated state. Water-filtered infrared A irradiation using the Hydrosun wIRA radiator proved very effective treating of tumors that had accumulated anti-EGFR-AuNP constructs that had been injected i.v. or directly into the tumors. Figure 9.3b shows typical before and after wIRA treatment results (1.5 W/cm², exposed for 1.9 min to the wIRA radiator; short exposure times necessitate higher irradiances) when mice received A, D, No AuNP treatment, B. E, anti-EGFR-AuNP injections directly into the tumors (0.2 g Au/kg in 10 L, and C, F, i.v. injections of anti-EGFR (1.0 g Au/kg). Tumors that received direct injections of Construct II (B, E) or were loaded with Construct II after i.v. injections (C, F) necrosed after wIRA treatment, formed a scab, and healed with no apparent scarring over 2–3 weeks. Untreated tumors progressed. Figure 9.4 shows an experiment

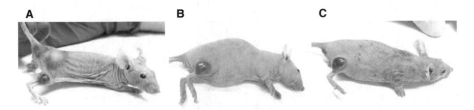

Fig. 9.3a Photographs of mice after intravenous injection of AuNPs. (A) Mouse 1.5 h after tail vein injection of 15 nm AuNPs with adsorbed anti-tumor antibody (Construct I) which localized to the tumor on its leg. (B) Mouse before injection of AuNPs. (C) Mouse in (B) 1.5 h after iv injection of non-targeted 15 nm AuNPs coated with 2 k MW PEG. Reproduced with permission from [5]

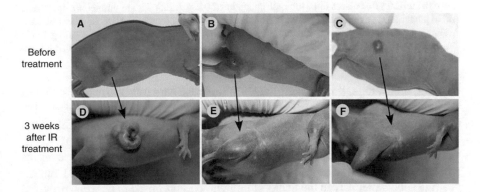

Fig. 9.3b Mice with Tumors before and after IR/AuNP treatment. Top row before treatment, bottom row 3 weeks after wIRA treatment. (A, D) No AuNPs, but exposed to IR. (B, E) Mouse with 10 μL direct intratumoral injection of 15 nm anti-EGFr lipoic acid AuNP preparation (Construct II) and wIRA. (C, F) Mouse with intravenous 15 nm anti-EGFr lipoic acid AuNP preparation and wIRA. There was no residual normal tissue or body impairment with little to no scarring seen with the AuNP-IR-treated animals. wIRA treatment: 1.5 W/cm², 1.9-min exposure time. Reproduced with permission from [5]

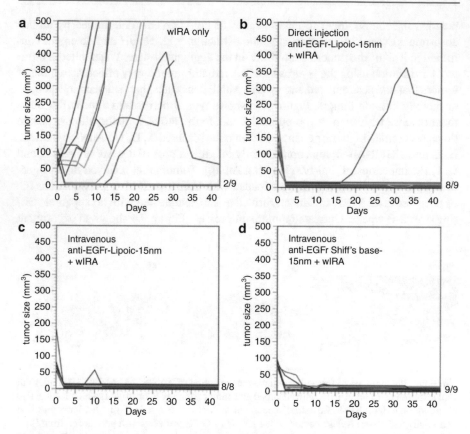

Fig. 9.4 Plots of tumor volume vs. time after wIRA treatments. (**a**) wIRA only, 22% survival (2/9); (**b**) wIRA after direct intra-tumoral injection of 0.2 g Au/kg 15 nm anti-EGFr lipoic acid AuNP preparation (Construct II), 89% tumor ablation (8/9); (**c**) wIRA after i.v. injection of 1.0 g Au/kg Construct II, 100% tumor ablation (8/8); (**d**) wIRA after i.v. injection of 1.5 g Au/kg 15 nm anti-EGFr Schiff's base AuNP preparation (Construct III), 100% tumor ablation (9/9). wIRA treatment: 1.5 W/cm², 1.9-min exposure time. Reproduced with permission from [5]

utilizing, on average, 9 mice per group. Tumors receiving either direct injection of 0.2 g Construct II (Fig. 9.4b) or i.v. injections of 1.0 g Au/kg Construct II (Fig. 9.4c), or i.v. injection of 1.5 g/kg Construct III (Fig. 9.4d) experienced 89%, 89%, and 100% complete ablation, respectively, whereas untreated tumors (Fig. 9.4a) experienced only 22% ablations after wIRA treatment (1.5 W/cm², 1.9 min). These results proved the efficacy of Constructs II and III to cure advanced human A431 tumors growing subcutaneously in the flanks of immune-compromised mice when provided either directly to the tumors or intravenously prior to wIRA therapy using the Hydrosun radiator. A follow-up experiment was performed combining gold nanoparticle-mediated wIRA heating and radiation therapy (RT). The synergy between heat and RT has been well known for many years. In this experiment, the radioresistant mouse SCCVII squamous cell carcinoma was implanted subcutaneously in immune-compromised mice and allowed to progress to an advanced stage (100–150 mm³) before initiating therapy. The SCCVII tumor expresses EGFR. The anti-EGFR conjugated to AuNPs in Construct II bind to EGFR on SCCVII cells. The experimental plan was to intratumorally infuse via convection enhanced delivery (CED) Construct II, the lipoic acid AuNPs. After allowing time for adequate diffusion of the AuNPs and cellular uptake (24 hours), tumors receiving heating were treated with wIRA at 48 °C for 5 min. Those tumors slated for RT were irradiated at the indicated doses within minutes after heating. Table 9.1 shows the different experimental groups and how they were treated. The results, shown in Fig. 9.5, are as follows:

1. wIRA-hyperthermia treatment alone after AuNP administration (48 °C, 5 min, Group B) is not effective at tumor control (1 out of 7 or 14% survived (no tumor after 250 days).
2. RT alone (25 Gy) is also not effective therapeutically; 2/6 or 33% survived.
3. RT (25 Gy) plus wIRA (no prior AuNP) was not effective (0/7 survived). Note that wIRA without prior AuNP does not heat the tumor in the experimental set-up chosen.
4. AuNP infusion followed by 25 Gy RT alone (Group D) was also ineffective (1/8 or 12% surviving). The SCCVII is a radiation-resistant tumor requiring 55 Gy for half-maximal control. However, AuNPs + wIRA irradiation followed by X-ray irradiation was very effective. For the radiation doses used, 15 Gy (Group E), 20 Gy (Group F), and 25 Gy (Group G), survival was 5/7 (71%) in all three groups.

Additional controls (AuNPs only) or wIRA treatment only showed no benefit (0/7 survival). While RT without effective heating slowed tumor growth as would be expected, only the combination of effective heating and RT, even at reduced radiation doses, was effective. At 250 days, there was some loss of muscle mass in treated mice (15–20%), but there was no loss of leg function. Hence, wIRA hyperthermia not only enabled RT to be effective but reduced the dose of RT needed to be effective. This would be very significant therapeutically if translated to the clinic.

Other gold nanostructures (nanoshells, nanorods, nanotubes, nanorings, nanostars, nanocages) have been developed that also convert near-infrared irradiation into heat and are useful for hyperthermia therapy [7, 8]. Gold nanoshells and gold nanorods were nicely described in the introduction to Hainfeld et al. [5] and have been the subject of reviews since then. Gold nanoshells (Nanospectra

Table 9.1 Experimental groups. Reproduced with permission from [6]

Group	AuNPs	NIR	Radiation 15 Gy	Radiation 20 Gy	Radiation 25 Gy	number of mice	Survival (>250 days)
A					√	6	2/6=33%
B	√	√				7	1/7=14%
C		√			√	7	0/7=0%
D	√				√	8	1/8=12%
E	√	√	√			7	5/7=71%
F	√	√		√		7	5/7=71%
G	√	√			√	7	5/7=71%
H	√					7	0/7=0%
I		√				7	0/7=0%

Note: Heating was only observed with AuNPs + NIR (Fig. 9.5)

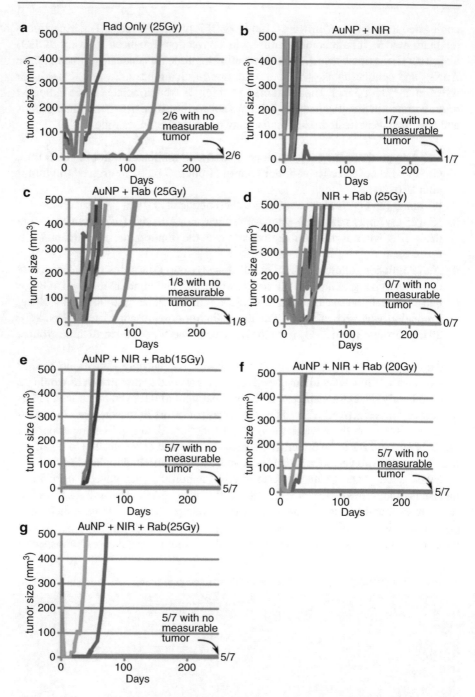

Fig. 9.5 Tumor volume vs. time for various treatments corresponding to Table 9.1 (group **a–g**). Survivors that were tumor-free at 250 days are given at the right of the horizontal axes (e.g., 5/7 meaning 5 out of 7 survived with no measurable tumor). Tumor volumes of individual mice are plotted. Each colored line represents one mouse. Reproduced with permission from [6]

Biosciences, Inc.) are constructed with a ≈ 110 nm silica core and a ≈ 10-nm-thick gold outer layer. Their absorption properties at 800 nm can be tuned by varying core and shell properties. Efficacy in preclinical studies after both direct and i.v. injections was demonstrated in the early 2000s. Gold-silica nanoshells (GSN) have progressed to clinical trials in which laser excited nanoshells in combination with MRI-ultrasound fusion imaging were used to treat 16 patients with low-to-intermediate grade prostate tumors confined to the prostate, when they are curable [9]. On day 1, patients received 7.5 mg/kg i.v. infusion of GSN (4.8 mg/mL), and on day 2, patients received laser illumination under general anesthesia. Follow-up biopsy showed GSN-mediated focal laser ablation was achieved in 15/16 patients without serious complications or deleterious changes in genitourinary function. A noteworthy feature of this technology is the relatively low amount of GSN infused into patients compared to the gold nanoparticle studies. Presumably, GSNs are more efficient at generating heat after infrared absorption, and numerous avenues are being explored to see how GSNs can be used therapeutically to good advantage.

Gold nanorods (GNRs) (≈50–100 nm in length) also adsorb in the NIR range more efficiently than nanoshells. Preclinical experiments performed over 10 years ago demonstrated subcutaneous tumor control; PEG-coated 13 × 47 nm gold nanorods injected i.v. at 20 mg/kg demonstrated control of small subcutaneous tumors on mice when tumors were irradiated 72 h post-injection with NIR. Once again, the low levels of GNRs required for efficacy was notable. Mammary tumors in dogs and cats were treated with NIR and GNRs directly injected into the tumors [10]. A regimen in which the tumors were injected every 2 weeks for 3 weeks with 7.5 nM, 3.75 nM, and 1.88 nM GNR per 100 mm^3 tumor volume used for the first, second, and third injections followed by NIR resulted in complete, durable remissions (>1 year) in all seven of the dogs and cats with spontaneous mammary tumors. A safety study of seven dogs mainly with soft tissue sarcomas with i.v. GNR and NIR treatment was also performed recently [11]. Photothermal therapy with anti EGFR-conjugated GNRs selectively targeted head and neck cancer decreased tumor size with minimal side effects in more recent preclinical experiments. We are not aware of any clinical trial results using the GNRs.

Mouse, cat, and dog trials have shown the gold nanoparticles, gold nanoshells, and the gold nanorods to be safe when administered by direct injection or i.v. They have shown some degree of efficacy for the treatment of diverse collections of tumors including low- and intermediate-risk prostate cancer confined to the prostate, mammary tumors, and soft tissue sarcomas. In most cases, optimized treatment regimens have not been worked out so that it is not known yet how useful this approach can be for superficial tumors of many different origins and some localized deeper tumors. Nor have optimized combination therapy strategies been developed combining heat, radiation, surgery, chemotherapy, and gene-based therapies. As companies raise the millions of dollars needed for the development and testing of these strategies, the clinical potential of nanogold/NIR therapy will become clearer. Hopefully, out of the myriad of nanogold constructs that have been reported on, a small number of most-effective constructs will emerge with the attendant investment and focus needed to have a positive patient impact.

9.3 Conclusion

While treatment of prostate tumors requires a surgically inserted optical fiber and the use of a laser, treatment of superficial tumors with nanogold and NIR could use the wIRA radiator instead of the laser that is used in a large fraction of preclinical studies. The wIRA radiator is portable and relatively inexpensive. If nanogold/NIR therapy is proven to be useful to treat a readily accessible human tumor, the use of the wIRA radiator used might make such therapy accessible to large numbers of patients in low- and middle-income countries that lack access to very high-tech expensive therapies. Foundations with a strong interest in bringing healthcare to low- and middle-income nations might take note of the potential benefits the wIRA radiator has to offer.

References

1. Khlebtsov B, Zharov V, Melnikov A, et al. Optical amplification of photothermal therapy with gold nanoparticles and nanoclusters. Nanotechnology. 2006;17:5167–79.
2. Su KH, Wei QH, Zhang X, et al. Interparticle coupling effects on plasmon resonances of nano-gold particles. Nano Lett. 2003;3:1087–90.
3. Souza GR, Christianson DR, Staquicini FI, et al. Networks of gold nanoparticles and bacteriophage as biological sensors and cell-targeting agents. Proc Natl Acad Sci U S A. 2006;103:1215–20.
4. Nam J, Won N, Jin H, et al. pH-induced aggregation of gold nanoparticles for photothermal cancer. J Am Chem Soc. 2009;131:13639–45.
5. Hainfeld JF, O'Connor MJ, Lin P, et al. Infrared-transparent gold nanoparticles converted by tumors to infrared absorbers cure tumors in mice by photothermal therapy. PLoS. 2014;9:e88414.
6. Hainfeld JF, Lin L, Slatkin DN, et al. Gold nanoparticle hyperthermia reduces radiation dose. Nanomed: Nanotechnol Biol Med. 2014;10:1609–17.
7. Ahmad T, Sarwar R, Iqbal A, et al. Recent advances in combinatorial cancer therapy via multifunctionalized gold nanoparticles. Nanomedicine (Lond). 2020;15:1221–37.
8. Wang JI, Wu X, Shen P, et al. Applications of inorganic nanomaterials in Photothermal therapy based on combinational cancer treatment. Int J Nanomedicine. 2020;15:1903–14.
9. Rastinehad AR, Anastosa H, Wajswola E, et al. Gold nanoshell-localized photothermal ablation of prostate tumors in a clinical pilot device study. Proc Natl Acad Sci U S A. 2019;116:18590–6.
10. Ali MRK, Ibrahim IM, Ali HR, et al. Treatment of natural mammary gland tumors in canines and felines using gold nanorods-assisted plasmonic photothermal therapy to induce tumor apoptosis. Int J Nanomedicine. 2016;11:4849–63.
11. Schuh EM, Portela R, Gardner HL, et al. Safety and efficacy of targeted hyperthermia treatment utilizing gold nanorod therapy in spontaneous canine neoplasia. BMC Vet Res. 2017;13:294.

Mild Hyperthermia Induced by Water-Filtered Infrared A Irradiation: A Potent Strategy to Foster Immune Recognition and Anti-Tumor Immune Responses in Superficial Cancers?

10

G. Multhoff, E. A. Repasky, and Peter Vaupel

10.1 Introduction

Dated back to the 1970s and 1980s, the rationale for the clinical application of hyperthermia (HT) in oncology was to induce direct cytotoxic effects in cancer cells by high, lethal temperatures (tT $\geq$43 °C). However, this concept was partially abandoned after recognizing that, with the heating technologies available at that time, tumor temperatures (tT $\geq$43 °C) could not be reached in all tumors/tumor regions treated in the clinical setting [1]. Using the contactless, thermography-controlled water-filtered infrared A (wIRA) irradiation technique which could heat superficial, large-sized tumors, tissue temperatures in the fever-range (tT = 39–41 °C) or mild hyperthermia levels (tT = 39–43 °C) up to tissue depths of $\approx$25 mm can be reached. The advantages of this novel technique used in the clinical setting in combination with subsequent hypofractionated radiotherapy have been summarized recently [2–4].

Apart from a number of mechanisms of action as an adjuvant to radio- or chemo-therapy, HT also impacts various beneficial effects on anti-tumor immunity. In

G. Multhoff (✉)
Project Group Radiation Immuno-Oncology, Central Institute for Translational Cancer Research, Klinikum rechts der Isar, Technical University München, München, Germany

Department of Radiation Oncology, Klinikum rechts der Isar, Technical University München, München, Germany
e-mail: gabriele.multhoff@tum.de

E. A. Repasky
Department of Immunology, Roswell Park Comprehensive Cancer Center, Buffalo, NY, USA

P. Vaupel
Department of Radiation Oncology, University Medical Cente, University of Freiburg, Freiburg/Breisgau, Germany

© The Author(s) 2022
P. Vaupel (ed.), *Water-filtered Infrared A (wIRA) Irradiation*,
https://doi.org/10.1007/978-3-030-92880-3_10

addition to specific effects exerted on various anti-tumor immune responses also related to the overexpression of heat shock proteins (HSPs), HT-induced increases in tumor blood flow and microvascular permeability, and the impact on local delivery of blood-borne immune cells, antibodies, and cytokines will be discussed in this article. HT-induced increases in tumor blood flow, associated with an improvement of the tumor oxygenation status ("reversal of tumor hypoxia"), will be elucidated, based on the fact that tumor hypoxia, a hallmark of cancer growth, is a potent inhibitor of anti-tumor immune mechanisms.

10.2   Mild Hyperthermia Can Enhance the Delivery of Blood-Borne Anti-Tumor Immunity

Mild hyperthermia (tT = 39–43 °C) can (at least temporarily) increase blood flow in human tumors (for a review, see [5]). In inflammatory, recurrent breast cancer, a frequent medical indication for superficial wIRA-HT, increases in tumor perfusion and hyperemia [i.e., locally increased amount of intravascular blood and O_2-carrying hemoglobin] outlast the time period needed for the subsequent radiation therapy in the thermo-radiotherapy schedule [6]. In addition to radiosensitization, the increase in blood flow may foster the delivery of blood-borne anti-tumor immunity, i.e., the purposeful accumulation of immune cells, antibodies, and cytokines within the heated tumor mass combined with an upregulation of immunogenic cell surface ligands, such as non-classical (e.g., MICA/B) and classical major histocompatibility complex antigen (MHC) molecules [7].

Intratumor trafficking of anti-tumor immune cells, delivery of antibodies, and anti-tumor cytokines may additionally be supported by hyperthermia-induced increases in microvascular permeability which promotes the diapedesis of immune cells and extravasation of anti-tumor cytokines.

10.3   Mild Hyperthermia Can Attenuate Tumor Hypoxia, a Potent Suppressor of Anti-Tumor Immune Reactions

Tumor hypoxia, i.e., the critically reduced oxygenation of cancer cells and of the TME with oxygen tensions <10 mmHg, is one of the hallmarks of cancers [8]. Tumor hypoxia is a consequence of an impaired oxygen supply due to (a) perfusion-limited delivery, (b) diffusion-limited availability, and (c) hypoxemia (i.e., reduced O_2 transport capacity of the blood in anemic patients or HbCO formation in heavy smokers) [9]. Further details of the various pathogeneses, classifications, time frames, spatial and temporal distributions/heterogeneities of hypoxic subvolumes, variability in the extent (severity) of hypoxia, and consequences of tumor hypoxia have been described elsewhere [10, 11].

Apart from driving malignant progression of primary cancers, firstly described by Höckel and Vaupel, [11–13], hypoxia can lead to acquired resistance in radio- and chemotherapy. Furthermore, hypoxia (and/or upregulation of HIF-1α) distinctly impairs immune cells (derived from the TME) exerting effective anti-tumor immune responses (immune hallmark of cancer) [14] while facilitating immunosuppressive cells in terms of their suppressive functions, thus inducing immune tolerance and immune escape (for recent reviews, see [15–19]).

Figure 10.1 schematically illustrates the effects of tumor hypoxia on key immune cell populations. In general, hypoxia negatively impacts the survival and functions of antigen-presenting cells (APCs) and effector cells and decreases the release of effector and proliferative cytokines [e.g., interferon-γ (IFN-γ), interleukin 2 (IL-2)],

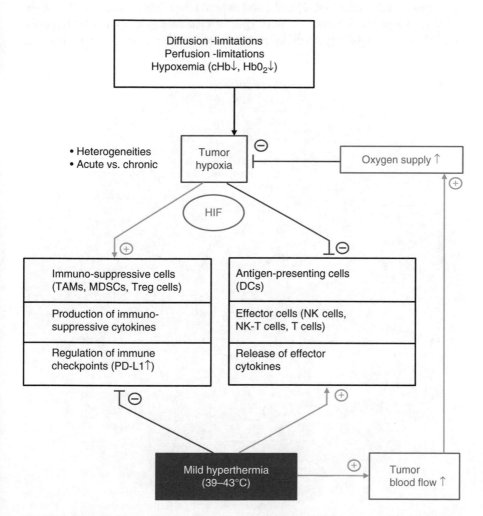

Fig. 10.1 Simplified flow chart describing the supportive impact of tumor hypoxia (with pathogeneses and some characteristics) and HIF-1α on immunosuppressive measures (left), and compromising effects on anti-tumor immunity (right). Mild hyperthermia with tumor temperatures of 39 °C–43 °C can lead to a reversal of tumor hypoxia through improvements in the oxygen supply triggered by increased tumor blood flow upon tissue heating

while supporting immunosuppressive cells and promoting the production of immunosuppressive cytokines (e.g., transforming growth factor-β). Besides these mechanisms, several immune checkpoint molecules are regulated by hypoxia (e.g., PD-L1) and thus contribute to immune evasion. Tumor hypoxia can be reversed by mild hyperthermia (tT = 39–43 °C) via heat-induced increases in tumor blood flow and, in turn, enhanced oxygen supply, as shown in this simplified flowchart.

In more detail, hypoxia (and upregulated, stabilized HIF-1α) dampens antitumor immune responses by (a) reducing the survival as well as the cytolytic and migratory activities of *effector cells* [e.g., CD4+ T helper cells, CD8+ cytotoxic T cells, natural killer-like (NK-T) cells, and natural killer (NK) cells; Fig. 10.2a]; (b) reducing the production and release of *effector cytokines* [e.g., granzyme B, perforin, IFN-γ]; (c) impairing the differentiation and function of *APCs* [e.g., dendritic

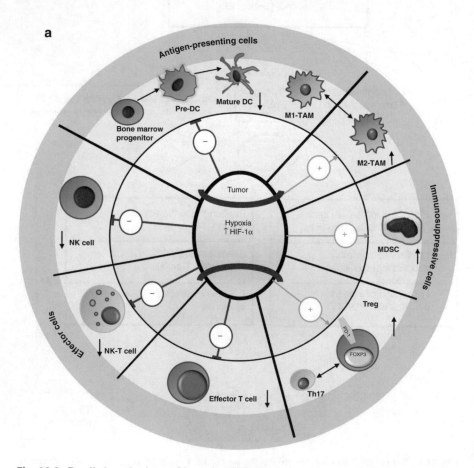

Fig. 10.2 Detailed mechanisms of hypoxia- (HIF-1α-) induced immunosuppression in cancers (**a**), and improved anti-tumor immune responses upon reversal of tumor hypoxia triggered by mild hyperthermia, HT (**b**). Green arrows: activation, red T-bars: inhibition. *TBF* tumor blood flow

b

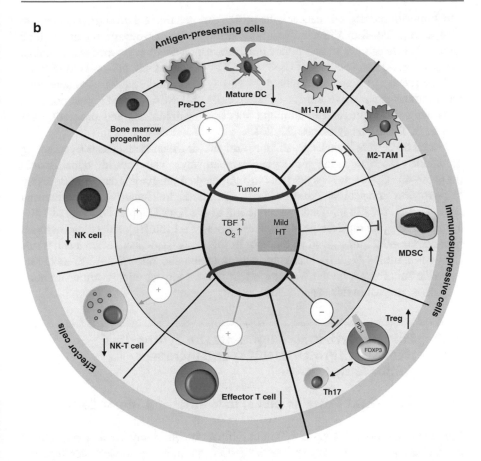

Fig. 10.2 (continued)

cells (DCs), Langerhans cells in the epidermis of the skin]; (d) driving *immunosuppressive cells* [e.g., regulatory T (Treg) cells, myeloid-derived suppressor cells (MDSCs) and tumor-associated M2-macrophages (TAMs)]; (e) increasing the production and release of *immunosuppressive cytokines* (e.g., IL-10); and (f) upregulating of the expression of *immune checkpoint inhibitors* (e.g., PD-L1, [19]).

10.4   Metabolic Reprogramming Impacts Anti-Tumor Immune Responses: Role of Mild Hyperthermia?

Another hallmark of cancer cells is metabolic reprogramming [8]. A major metabolic pathway of this phenotype is aerobic glycolysis (Warburg effect), which is characterized—inter alia—by a high lactate$^-$ and H$^+$ (proton) output/export into the TME [20, 21], finally leading to an extracellular lactate accumulation (up to 40 mM) and tissue acidosis (pH <6.8). Both conditions constitute major inhibitors of anti-tumor immunity, i.e., cancer cells utilize this detrimental microenvironment to escape from anti-tumor immunity. Acidification of the microenvironment and high lactate⁻ levels can thwart anti-tumor immune responses by (a) compromising, e.g., the proliferation and activity of $CD8^+$ and $CD4^+$ T cells, DCs, NK and NK-T cells, and the release of immuno-stimulatory TH-1 type cytokines, and by (b) activating the immuno-suppressive effects of Treg cells, MDSCs, and M2 macrophages, increasing the expression of immune checkpoints inhibitors and promoting the release of TH-2 type cytokines [22, 23].

Based on current knowledge, shaping anti-tumor immune responses by targeting metabolic reprogramming or signaling pathways using mild hyperthermia (tT = 39–43 °C, 60 min) has not been investigated so far. Earlier experiments using fast-growing rat tumor isotransplants exposed to localized hyperthermia (tT = 43.4 °C for 120 min) led to a reduction of the laser Doppler flow rate of 18%, a minimal drop of the average pO_2 values ($\Delta pO_2 = -1$ mmHg), a decrease in mean pH ($\Delta pH = -0.21$ units), and an increase in the mean tissue lactate⁻ concentrations ($\Delta C = +8$ mM) [24, 25]. These findings question the role of mild-to-moderate hyperthermia for 2 h on the Warburg effect and its impact on anti-tumor immune responses, at least in this experimental setting.

10.5   Mild Hyperthermia Augments the Synthesis of Heat Shock Proteins (HSPs) and Increases Tumor Antigenicity

10.5.1 Heat Shock Proteins (HSPs) in Normal and Tumor Cells

Mild hyperthermia (tT = 39–43 °C) in combination with X-ray irradiation increases the formation of reactive oxygen species (ROS), promotes genomic instability, and impairs the DNA double-strand break repair [26]. Moreover, fever-like temperatures interfere with pathways involved in cell cycle regulation and proliferation and can cause protein denaturation and aggregation. Therefore, after exposure of cells to heat generally reduces the synthesis of proteins, apart from that of a special class of proteins, termed heat shock (HSPs) or stress proteins, which consist of at least one ATPase domain and a substrate-binding domain. Apart from thermal stress, their synthesis is also strongly upregulated upon a large variety of different environmental stress factors including changes in oxygen supply, pH, nutrient deficiency, heavy metals, ethanol, radiation (UV, ionizing), cytostatic drugs, hypoxia, and re-oxygenation, etc. [27]. HSPs maintain protein homeostasis, assist protein transport under physiological conditions (e.g., cell proliferation, differentiation, maturation, antigen presentation), and protect cells from lethal damages induced by stress. The biological relevance of HSPs is documented by their ubiquitous distribution, high abundance, and conserved sequence homology in prokaryotic as well as eukaryotic cells.

Normal and tumor cells differ significantly in their proliferative capacity and metabolic demand which is closely related to molecular features of the Warburg effect [21]. Therefore, rapidly proliferating tumor cells generally exhibit a cytosolic overexpression of HSPs which are localized in nearly all subcellular compartments including cytosol, nucleus, endoplasmic reticulum, lysosomes, endosomes, and mitochondria [28]. Following environmental stress including elevated temperatures, hypoxia, chemotherapy, and radiotherapy, the synthesis of all HSPs and especially that of the major stress-inducible Hsp70 is further upregulated to prevent tumor cells from stress-induced lethal damages including protein misfolding, denaturation and aggregation, and transport deficiencies [29, 30]. In contrast to normal cells, viable tumor cells present a number of HSPs, including Hsp70 on their plasma membrane [31, 32] via a tumor-specific glycosphingolipid anchorage [33], and actively release HSPs in lipid micro-vesicles termed exosomes [34].

10.5.2   Role of HSPs in NK and T-Cell-Mediated Immunity

Depending on their intracellular, membrane, or extracellular localization, HSPs fulfill different tasks. High cytosolic and mitochondrial HSPs increase the tumorigenic and metastatic potential of tumor cells and prevent apoptosis, whereas membrane-bound and extracellular HSPs [35, 36] have been identified as potent stimulators of the adaptive and innate anti-cancer immune responses. Following cross-presentation of HSP-chaperoned immunogenic peptides on MHC class I molecules, HSPs support $CD8^+$ cytotoxic T-cell responses [37, 38] with Toll-like, scavenger, and C-type lectin receptors playing pivotal roles in mediating the uptake of HSP-chaperoned peptides [39, 40]. In the absence of immunogenic peptides, Hsp70 stimulates the cytolytic activity of NK cells in a pro-inflammatory (e.g., IL-2, IFN-γ) environment against membrane Hsp70-positive tumor cells. A phase I clinical trial revealed an excellent safety profile of adoptively transferred, ex vivo Hsp70-activated NK cells [41], and favorable clinical responses in a phase II clinical study in patients with advanced NSCLC after radio-chemotherapy [42]. In line with these findings, a mild heat treatment of tumor cells (including chondro-, osteosarcoma, and liposarcoma) cells increases the membrane Hsp70 density on tumor cells and thereby enhances their susceptibility to NK cell-mediated killing [43–45]. In a preclinical colon carcinoma model, the beneficial effects of a unilateral applied hyperthermia could be associated with an increased $CD4^+/CD8^+$ T and NK cell activity in mice with bilateral tumors, which indicates that local heat to one tumor site has the capacity to induce abscopal effects [46, 47]. Moreover, local hyperthermia used in combination with radiotherapy and/or chemotherapy [48–50] enhances the efficacy of both therapeutic concepts and boosts protective anti-cancer immune responses mediated by $CD8^+$ T, NK-T, and NK effector cells.

10.6   Conclusion

Mild hyperthermia (tT = 39–43 °C) increases tumor blood flow and microvascular permeability, the trafficking of blood-borne immune cells, and the delivery of antibodies and cytokines. In addition, HT-related increases in tumor blood flow are also associated with an improvement of the tumor oxygenation status ("reversal of tumor hypoxia") which in turn attenuates hypoxia. The complexity of molecular pathways that coordinate a response to heat is mirrored by diverse cell types that are affected by hyperthermia including DCs, M1 macrophages, effector T, NK-T and NK cells, and immunosuppressive TAMs (M2 macrophages), MDSCs and Treg cells, cytokines, and chemokines (Fig. 10.2b). The majority of data support the hypothesis that temperature shifts in immune cells that may be associated with the application of localized hyperthermia in cancer therapy could promote long-term protection against tumor growth via the recruitment of several mechanisms of the immune system. Furthermore, mechanistic insight into the immune-protective nature of mild hyperthermia has revealed new avenues to exploit the immunostimulatory activities of thermal stress in the context of cancer therapy.

References

1. Streffer C. Hyperthermia and the therapy of malignant tumors. Berlin: Springer; 1987.
2. Vaupel P, Piazena H, Müller W, Notter M. Biophysical and photobiological basics of water-filtered infrared-a hyperthermia of superficial tumors. Int J Hyperthermia. 2018;35:26–36. https://doi.org/10.1080/02656736.2018.1469169.
3. Notter M, Piazena H, Vaupel P. Hypofractionated re-irradiation of large-sized recurrent breast cancer with thermography-controlled, contact-free water-filtered infra-red-A hyperthermia: a retrospective study of 73 patients. Int J Hyperthermia. 2017;33:227–36. https://doi.org/10.1080/02656736.2016.1235731.
4. Notter M, Thomsen AR, Nitsche M, Hermann RM, Wolff HA, Habl G, et al. Combined wIRA-hyperthermia and hypofractionated re-irradiation in the treatment of locally recurrent breast cancer: evaluation of therapeutic outcome based on a novel size classification. Cancers (Basel). 2020;12:606. https://doi.org/10.3390/cancers12030606.
5. Vaupel PW, Kelleher DK. Pathophysiological and vascular characteristics of tumours and their importance for hyperthermia: heterogeneity is the key issue. Int J Hyperthermia. 2010;26:211–23. https://doi.org/10.3109/02656731003596259.
6. Thomsen ARS, Nicolay, N. H. et al. Temperature profiles and oxygenation status in human skin and subcutis upon thermography-controlled wIRA-hyperthermia. Adv. Exp. Med. Biol. 2022; in press.
7. Ostberg JR, Dayanc BE, Yuan M, Oflazoglu E, Repasky EA. Enhancement of natural killer (NK) cell cytotoxicity by fever-range thermal stress is dependent on NKG2D function and is associated with plasma membrane NKG2D clustering and increased expression of MICA on target cells. J Leukoc Biol. 2007;82:1322–31. https://doi.org/10.1189/jlb.1106699.
8. Hanahan D, Weinberg RA. Hallmarks of cancer: the next generation. Cell. 2011;144:646–74. https://doi.org/10.1016/j.cell.2011.02.013.
9. Vaupel P. Tumor microenvironmental physiology and its implications for radiation oncology. Semin Radiat Oncol. 2004;14:198–206.
10. Vaupel P, Mayer A. Hypoxia in cancer: significance and impact on clinical outcome. Cancer Metastasis Rev. 2007;26:225–39. https://doi.org/10.1007/s10555-007-9055-1.
11. Vaupel P, Mayer A, Höckel M. Tumor hypoxia and malignant progression. Methods Enzymol. 2004;381:335–54.
12. Höckel M, Knoop C, Schlenger K, Vorndran B, Baussmann E, Mitze M, et al. Intratumoral pO_2 predicts survival in advanced cancer of the uterine cervix. Radiother Oncol. 1993;26:45–50. https://doi.org/10.1016/0167-8140(93)90025-4.
13. Höckel M, Schlenger K, Aral B, Mitze M, Schäffer U, Vaupel P. Association between tumor hypoxia and malignant progression in advanced cancer of the uterine cervix. Cancer Res. 1996;56:4509–15.

14. Cavallo F, De Giovanni C, Nanni P, Forni G, Lollini PL. 2011: the immune hallmarks of cancer. Cancer Immunol Immunother. 2011;60:319–26. https://doi.org/10.1007/s00262-010-0968-0.
15. Vaupel P, Multhoff G. Accomplices of the hypoxic tumor microenvironment compromising antitumor immunity: adenosine, lactate, acidosis, vascular endothelial growth factor, potassium ions, and phosphatidylserine. Front Immunol. 2017;8:1887. https://doi.org/10.3389/fimmu.2017.01887.
16. Vaupel P, Multhoff G. Hypoxia-/HIF-1α-driven factors of the tumor microenvironment impeding antitumor immune responses and promoting malignant progression. Adv Exp Med Biol. 2018;1072:171–5. https://doi.org/10.1007/978-3-319-91287-5_27.
17. Multhoff G, Vaupel P. Hypoxia compromises anti-cancer immune responses. Adv Exp Med Biol. 2020;1232:131–43. https://doi.org/10.1007/978-3-030-34461-0_18.
18. Chang WH, Lai AG. The hypoxic tumour microenvironment: a safe haven for immunosuppressive cells and a therapeutic barrier to overcome. Cancer Lett. 2020;487:34–44. https://doi.org/10.1016/j.canlet.2020.05.011.
19. Wang B, Zhao Q, Zhang Y, Liu Z, Zheng Z, Liu S, et al. Targeting hypoxia in the tumor microenvironment: a potential strategy to improve cancer immunotherapy. J Exp Clin Cancer Res. 2021;40:24. https://doi.org/10.1186/s13046-020-01820-7.
20. Vaupel P, Schmidberger H, Mayer A. The Warburg effect: essential part of metabolic reprogramming and central contributor to cancer progression. Int J Radiat Biol. 2019;95:912–9. https://doi.org/10.1080/09553002.2019.1589653.
21. Vaupel P, Multhoff G. Revisiting the Warburg effect: historical dogma versus current understanding. J Physiol. 2021;599:1745–57. https://doi.org/10.1113/JP278810.
22. Wegiel B, Vuerich M, Daneshmandi S, Seth P. Metabolic switch in the tumor microenvironment determines immune responses to anti-cancer therapy. Front Oncol. 2018;8:284. https://doi.org/10.3389/fonc.2018.00284.
23. Domblides C, Lartigue L, Faustin B. Control of the antitumor immune response by cancer metabolism. Cell. 2019;8:104. https://doi.org/10.3390/cells8020104.
24. Mayer WK, Stohrer M, Krüger W, Vaupel P. Laser Doppler flux and tissue oxygenation of experimental tumours upon local hyperthermia and/or hyperglycaemia. J Cancer Res Clin Oncol. 1992;118:523–8. https://doi.org/10.1007/BF01225267.
25. Schaefer C, Mayer WK, Krüger W, Vaupel P. Microregional distributions of glucose, lactate, ATP and tissue pH in experimental tumours upon local hyperthermia and/or hyperglycaemia. J Cancer Res Clin Oncol. 1993;119:599–608. https://doi.org/10.1007/BF01372723.
26. Heselich A, Frohns F, Frohns A, Naumann SC, Layer PG. Near-infrared exposure changes cellular responses to ionizing radiation. Photochem Photobiol. 2012;88:135–46. https://doi.org/10.1111/j.1751-1097.2011.01031.x.
27. Radons J, Multhoff G. Immunostimulatory functions of membrane-bound and exported heat shock protein 70. Exerc Immunol Rev. 2005;11:17–33.
28. Schmitt E, Gehrmann M, Brunet M, Multhoff G, Garrido C. Intracellular and extracellular functions of heat shock proteins: repercussions in cancer therapy. J Leukoc Biol. 2007;81:15–27.
29. Gehrmann M, Marienhagen J, Eichholtz-Wirth H, Fritz E, Ellwart J, Jaattela M, et al. Dual function of membrane-bound heat shock protein 70 (Hsp70), Bag-4, and Hsp40: protection against radiation-induced effects and target structure for natural killer cells. Cell Death Differ. 2005;12:38–51.
30. Gehrmann M, Pfister K, Hutzler P, Gastpar R, Margulis B, Multhoff G. Effects of antineoplastic agents on cytoplasmic and membrane-bound heat shock protein 70 (Hsp70) levels. Biol Chem. 2002;383:1715–25.
31. Multhoff G, Botzler C, Wiesnet M, Müller E, Meier T, Wilmanns W, et al. A stress-inducible 72-kDa heat-shock protein (HSP72) is expressed on the surface of human tumor cells, but not on normal cells. Int J Cancer. 1995;61:272–9.
32. Weidle UH, Maisel D, Klostermann S, Schiller C, Weiss EH. Intracellular proteins displayed on the surface of tumor cells as targets for therapeutic intervention with antibody-related agents. Cancer Genomics Proteomics. 2011;8:49–63.

33. Gehrmann M, Liebisch G, Schmitz G, Anderson R, Steinem C, De MA, et al. Tumor-specific Hsp70 plasma membrane localization is enabled by the glycosphingolipid Gb3. PLoS One. 2008;3:e1925.
34. Gastpar R, Gehrmann M, Bausero MA, Asea A, Gross C, Schroeder JA, et al. Heat shock protein 70 surface-positive tumor exosomes stimulate migratory and cytolytic activity of natural killer cells. Cancer Res. 2005;65:5238–47.
35. Todryk SM, Gough MJ, Pockley AG. Facets of heat shock protein 70 show immunotherapeutic potential. Immunology. 2003;110:1–9.
36. Taha EA, Ono K, Eguchi T. Roles of extracellular HSPs as biomarkers in immune surveillance and immune evasion. Int J Mol Sci. 2019;20:4588. https://doi.org/10.3390/ijms20184588.
37. Binder RJ, Han DK, Srivastava PK. CD91: a receptor for heat shock protein gp96. Nat Immunol. 2000;1:151–5.
38. Sondermann H, Becker T, Mayhew M, Wieland F, Hartl FU. Characterization of a receptor for heat shock protein 70 on macrophages and monocytes. Biol Chem. 2000;381:1165–74.
39. Delneste Y, Magistrelli G, Gauchat J, Haeuw J, Aubry J, Nakamura K, et al. Involvement of LOX-1 in dendritic cell-mediated antigen cross-presentation. Immunity. 2002;17:353–62.
40. Zhang Y, Zheng L. Tumor immunotherapy based on tumor-derived heat shock proteins (review). Oncol Lett. 2013;6:1543–9. https://doi.org/10.3892/ol.2013.1616.
41. Krause SW, Gastpar R, Andreesen R, Gross C, Ullrich H, Thonigs G, et al. Treatment of colon and lung cancer patients with ex vivo heat shock protein 70-peptide-activated, autologous natural killer cells: a clinical phase i trial. Clin Cancer Res. 2004;10:3699–707.
42. Multhoff G, Seier S, Stangl S, Sievert W, Shevtsov M, Werner C, et al. Targeted natural killer cell-based adoptive immunotherapy for the treatment of patients with NSCLC after radiochemotherapy: a randomized phase II clinical trial. Clin Cancer Res. 2020;20:5368. https://doi.org/10.1158/1078-0432.CCR-20-1141.
43. Kubista B, Trieb K, Blahovec H, Kotz R, Micksche M. Hyperthermia increases the susceptibility of chondro- and osteosarcoma cells to natural killer cell-mediated lysis. Anticancer Res. 2002;22:789–92.
44. Farjadian S, Norouzian M, Younesi V, Ebrahimpour A, Lotfi R. Hyperthermia increases natural killer cell cytotoxicity against SW-872 liposarcoma cell line. Iran J Immunol. 2013;10:93–102.
45. Dayanc BE, Beachy SH, Ostberg JR, Repasky EA. Dissecting the role of hyperthermia in natural killer cell mediated anti-tumor responses. Int J Hyperthermia. 2008;24:41–56.
46. Li TC, Liu CC, Lee YZ, Hsu YH, Chiang CF, Miaw SC, et al. Combination therapy of pulsed-wave ultrasound hyperthermia and immunostimulant OK-432 enhances systemic antitumor immunity for cancer treatment. Int J Radiat Oncol Biol Phys. 2020;108:140–9. https://doi.org/10.1016/j.ijrobp.2020.04.021.
47. Evans SS, Repasky EA, Fisher DT. Fever and the thermal regulation of immunity: the immune system feels the heat. Nat Rev Immunol. 2015;15:335–49. https://doi.org/10.1038/nri3843.
48. Lee S, Son B, Park G, Kim H, Kang H, Jeon J, et al. Immunogenic effect of hyperthermia on enhancing radiotherapeutic efficacy. Int J Mol Sci. 2018;19:2795. https://doi.org/10.3390/ijms19092795.
49. Issels RD, Lindner LH, von Bergwelt-Baildon M, Lang P, Rischpler C, Diem H, et al. Systemic antitumor effect by regional hyperthermia combined with low-dose chemotherapy and immunologic correlates in an adolescent patient with rhabdomyosarcoma - a case report. Int J Hyperthermia. 2020;37:55–65. https://doi.org/10.1080/02656736.2019.1709666.
50. Multhoff G, Botzler C, Jennen L, Schmidt J, Ellwart J, Issels R. Heat shock protein 72 on tumor cells: a recognition structure for natural killer cells. J Immunol. 1997;158:4341–50.

Part III

Clinical Practice: Psychiatry

Whole-Body Hyperthermia (WBH): Historical Aspects, Current Use, and Future Perspectives

11

S. Heckel-Reusser

Abbreviations

DGHT	Deutsche Gesellschaft für Hyperthermie (German Society for Hyperthermia)
ECG	Electrocardiogram
ESHO	European Society for Hyperthermic Oncology
FRWBH	Fever-range whole-body hyperthermia
HR	Heart rate
IR	Infrared
NIBP	Non-invasive blood pressure
RESP	Respiration
sCMT	systemic cancer multistep therapy
SpO$_2$	Oxyhemoglobin (HbO$_2$) saturation (using peripheral pulse oximetry)
T	Temperature
WBH	Whole-body hyperthermia

11.1 History of Whole-Body Hyperthermia (WBH)

Numerous ancient cultures already knew the beneficial effects of physical heating of the organism, using hot water baths, hot sand, or hot steam. In the seventeenth century, the English physician Sir Thomas Sydenham emphasized: "Fever itself is Nature's instrument," making a claim in the controversial discussion whether fever is just a troublesome symptom to be suppressed or a mechanism of the organism to stimulate self-healing processes. Before the introduction of anti-inflammatory drugs

S. Heckel-Reusser (✉)
Heckel Medizintechnik, Esslingen, Germany
e-mail: heckel@heckel-medizintechnik.de

© The Author(s) 2022
P. Vaupel (ed.), *Water-filtered Infrared A (wIRA) Irradiation*,
https://doi.org/10.1007/978-3-030-92880-3_11

and antibiotics, physicians deliberately triggered infections in patients suffering from incurable life-threatening diseases in order to induce a strong fever reaction. Julius Wagner-Jauregg was awarded the Nobel Prize in Physiology and Medicine in 1927 for the injection of malarial parasites in the treatment of dementia paralytica. He also reported improvements in depressive disorders [1]. An association between febrile response and tumor regression was noted as early as 1866 by Wilhelm Busch, and independently by Friedrich Fehleisen, who observed cancer remission in patients afflicted by severe erysipelas [2]. A similar case report on a complete remission of a sarcoma encouraged the American surgeon W.B. Coley to intravenously inject a mixture consisting of *Streptococcus erysipelas* and *Bacillus prodigiosus*. "Coley's toxins" achieved remissions in refractory progressing malignant diseases. Meanwhile, Coley is acknowledged as the "father of anti-cancer immunotherapy" [3]. Until the 1960s, "active fever therapy" using pyrogenic drugs (e.g., Pyrifer, Pyrexal, Vaccineurin) as well as whole-body hyperthermia, defined as physical warming of the organism, were widely accepted as a medical therapy. "Hot fever baths" were comprehensively described as a treatment for infectious and inflammatory diseases [4, 5]. In 1960, Martin Heckel [6] presented the first whole-body hyperthermia (WBH) device which used near-IR as an alternative to hot water baths. From 1965 onwards, Manfred von Ardenne [7] developed the concept of "systemic cancer multistep therapy" (sCMT), including extreme whole-body hyperthermia. Initially, using a special two-chamber water bath, he later changed to the application of wIRA and developed the first wIRA-WBH device. While interest in hyperthermia in oncology focused more and more on local forms of application, Klaus L. Schmidt [8] published a monograph on "Hyperthermia and Fever" in 1975 which included a comprehensive literature review on the therapeutic application of WBH in infections, allergic, and rheumatic diseases.

11.2   Three Levels of Whole-Body Irradiation (WBH)

WBH, defined as physically induced elevation of body core temperature, ranges from short, mild heat applications that can be performed at home, up to extreme WBH which must be performed in an intensive care unit environment. A classification of WBH into three levels has been published in the Guidelines of the "Deutsche Gesellschaft für Hyperthermie" (German Society for Hyperthermie) [9] (Table 11.1).

Notably, this classification is not applicable for local/regional hyperthermia, where "mild HT" includes temperature elevations from 39 °C to 43 °C. Even in the WBH literature, the term "mild" has frequently been used for temperature elevations that are classified here as moderate, resp. fever range.

Temperature limits between the three WBH levels are given just for orientation since they are subject to individual variations. The initial body core temperatures of patients differ significantly (reference range: 36.0 °C–37.5 °C), and it is not known whether the absolute value of the body core temperature achieved, or the relative

Table 11.1 Three levels of WBH [9]

	Mild WBH		Fever-range (moderate) WBH		Extreme WBH
Target temperature of body core, T (rectal)	<38.5 °C		38.5 °C – 40.5 °C		>40.5 °C
Application time in the specified temperature range	≤30 min	>30 min	≤ 180 min	>180 min	≥ 60 min
Patient stress	Perspiration, no thermoregulatory stress	Perspiration, no thermoregulatory stress	Thermoregulatory stress, non-sedated/lightly sedated	Thermoregulatory stress, lightly/heavily sedated	Thermoregulatory stress, deep intravenous anesthesia
Patient monitoring	Without nursing care	Nursing care or T (axillary) or T (rectal) or T (sublingual) or T (tympanic)	Nursing care under medical supervision Continuous T (rectal/vaginal) ± T (axill/tymp) + HR/SpO_2 ± ECG Periodic ± NIBP ("+" means mandatory, "±" means optional)	Nursing care under medical supervision Continuous T (rectal/vaginal) + T (axill) + HR/SpO_2 + ECG/RESP Periodic + NIBP	Medically supervised treatment Intensive care monitoring
Indications (selection)	Relaxation, wellness	Rehabilitation, physical therapy, rheumatology, orthopedics	Rheumatology, dermatology, oncology, psychiatry, immunology, environmental medicine	Oncology, chronic infections	Oncology, chronic infections

value of the temperature increase compared to the baseline temperature is more important for the therapeutic effect.

11.3 Practical Implementation, Mechanisms of Action, Indications

11.3.1 Mild WBH

During the first phase of WBH, the temperature of the body shell is elevated up to the level of the core temperature which is a temperature increase of several degrees in the extremities (Fig. 11.1). The duration of this phase is individually most heterogeneous, generally ranging between 10 and 20 min, in rare cases even up to 30 min. The same goes for the speed of the following increase in body core temperature. For mild WBH, the heating of the body can be stopped as soon as the patient feels uncomfortable due to the initiation of thermoregulatory stress. The duration of the following heat-retention phase—with activation of the parasympathetic system— ranges from 30 to 120 min. Data on duration–efficacy relationships are currently not

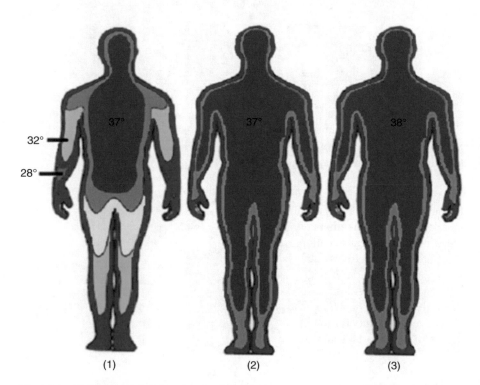

Fig. 11.1 (1) Temperature fields of body shell (skin, extremities) and of body core (with radial and axial temperature gradients in a 20 °C environment, (2) expansion of the core temperature in a 35 °C environment, (3) mild whole-body hyperthermia. Modified from [10]

available. A total treatment duration of 90 min is recommended as this allows for a new assignment of the treatment station every 2 h.

The primary physiological effects of mild WBH are a decrease in the tone of skeletal and smooth musculature, and an increased perfusion in the periphery including the extremities. This might be especially important for bradytrophic tissue which has been damaged by degenerative diseases.

Indications of mild WBH include diseases of the musculoskeletal system (e.g., chronically raised skeletal muscle tone, especially chronic back pain, post-accident care, degenerative osteoarthritis, fibromyalgia (see Chap. 19, this book), arterial hypertension [11]), systemic scleroderma [11], and Raynaud's syndrome [12].

11.3.2 Fever-Range Whole-Body Hyperthermia (FRWBH)

After reaching a core temperature in the fever range, most patients find the treatment exhausting, but nevertheless an "interesting" body experience. The nurse will assist this situation by empathic communication, application of cold cloths on the forehead, and similar procedures. Patients can listen to music and even watch videos for distraction. Interestingly, the development of thermoregulatory stress is not directly correlated to the rise of core temperature and may suddenly increase and decrease in spite of steadily increasing temperature. After reaching the target temperature level, the wIRA radiators can be switched off and the patient be covered by a blanket and remaining in the tent or wrapped into the tent fabric allowing for a half-sitting position (Heckel device) or the intensity of wIRA irradiation is decreased while the patient keeps lying on the net (Iratherm device). During this plateau phase, body core temperature in most patients rises for another 0.2–1 °C without further increase in stress. The duration of this phase is often 60 min, but can be prolonged as long as it is tolerable for the patient.

Clinical protocols of long-duration fever-range WBH (FRWBH, 4–6 hours above 39 °C) require sedation of the patients. These protocols have demonstrated safety and suggested efficacy in combination with chemo- and immunotherapy [13–15]. In the latter cases, "WBH may have the great advantage of allowing treatment of widely disseminated tumors in metastatic patients, with the same HT" [16].

At the end of heat retention, when all insulation or further energy supply is terminated and the thermoregulatory cooling mechanisms are no longer counteracted, most patients feel immediately well and free of stress, even if the temperature has not yet started to decline. The stress is obviously not caused by the increased temperature itself, but by the impeded thermoregulation.

The requirements for monitoring of vital parameters and the staff specifications are listed in Table 11.1 and are comprehensively described in the WBH guidelines of DGHT [9] (Fig. 11.2).

The concept of fever-range WBH (FRWBH) is mainly based on the assessment of elevated body core temperature as an essential trigger for initiating a strongly activated immune response. While in cold-blooded animals, elevation of body core temperature occurs by movement to warmer environments, warm-blooded creatures

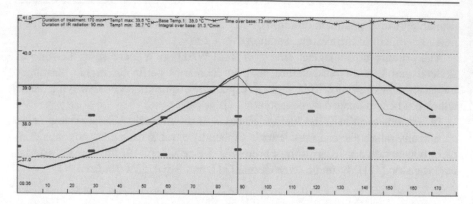

Fig. 11.2 FRWBH treatment, documented in the software Febrodata®, Heckel Medizintechnik (Esslingen, Germany). Blue curve: T rectal, starting at 36.8 °C and reaching 39.4 °C after 90 min. Heat-retention phase (90th to 145th min). Cool-down phase (145th–170th min). Red curve: heart rate (min. 65/minute, max. 120/minute). Pink spots indicate sporadically measured blood pressure (min. 110/78 mmHg, max. 115/82 mmHg)

develop a fever. Even if fever, as a response to infection, cannot be equated with hyperthermia as a physical heating of the body, FRWBH can strongly activate innate and adaptive immune responses. Interestingly, fever temperatures can also promote anti-inflammatory effects in case of chronic inflammation and autoimmune diseases [17]. To simplify, it could be considered as a "reset of the immune system" to overcome chronic pathologic dysfunctions correlating with too high or too low immune activity. Numerous preclinical studies have confirmed the therapeutic potential of controlled increases in body core temperature and have gradually examined the underlying biological mechanisms [18, 19].

Indications for FRWBH include major depression (see Chap. 12, this book), chronic inflammatory diseases of the muscolo-skeletal system such as ankylosing spondylitis and psoriasis arthritis (see Chap. 20, this book), and additive use in oncology (see Chap. 8, this book). FRWBH may increase the efficacy of antibiotic drugs in the treatment of chronic Lyme disease [20] and stimulate anti-bacterial immune responses.

11.3.3 Extreme Whole-Body Hyperthermia (WBH)

Extreme WBH is an intensive care application under deep intravenous anesthesia and requires comprehensive preparation, extensive monitoring of vital parameters, and a careful follow-up directly upon treatment [9, 21]. Risks of side effects are considerably higher than in FRWBH, since the set body core temperature is far beyond the range of fever which is developed in humans regarding immune reactions to common infections. Moreover, specific skills and experience in visual monitoring of the skin and in positioning of the patient are required to minimize the risk of thermal skin damage. Extreme WBH has been used to directly damage malignant cells in the oncological setting and to fight bacteria and viruses in chronic infection. In 1965, M. von Ardenne introduced extreme WBH as a key element of his "systemic cancer multistep therapy (sCMT)," consisting of the three main steps: (a) extreme whole-body hyperthermia (maximum temperature of at least 42 °C), (b) induced hyperglycemia, and (c) respiratory hyperoxemia. Hyperglycemia was applied in order to render cancer cells selectively more heat sensitive, by lowering the pH values in the cancer tissues. In 1974, the concept was extended by including a chemotherapy protocol adapted to the respective tumor entity [7, 22, 23]. Since hyperglycemia may stimulate cancer growth [24], it must be carefully considered whether this growth-promoting effect is fully excluded if applied in the framework of sCMT.

From the mid-1990s until 2005, numerous phase I and II trials with extreme WBH were published, most of them with target temperatures between 41.5 °C and 41.8 °C, combined with chemotherapy. Interest in this therapeutic schedule rapidly declined thereafter. A recently published review presents an excellent overview on these publications, concluding that "as modern oncology offers many less invasive treatment options, it is unlikely WBH will ever find its way in routine clinical care" [25]. On the other side, promising results in the above-mentioned trials may justify further research in this field, and extreme WBH should not completely be excluded as a therapy option for patients not satisfyingly responding to modern standard therapies.

In 2018, Douwes [26] published the concept of "antibiotically augmented thermal eradication of chronic Lyme disease," combining extreme WBH up to 41.6 °C and antibiotics, based on the heat sensitivity of *Borrelia* and the temperature-dependent efficacy of antibiotics [20]. Results in 601 of 809 patients treated in the past 3 years were "very good" or "good" (data presented at the ESHO Annual Meeting, Berlin 2018) [27].

11.4   Contrary Effects of WBH on Blood Flow of Inner Organs and Body Periphery

Regarding the impact of all WBH levels on blood flow, a widespread misunderstanding needs to be addressed. Contrary to general assumptions, WBH does not necessarily increase perfusion in the whole organism. In contrast, the thermoregulatory response on passive heating of the body includes a shift of large blood volumes into the periphery in order to cool the body by increased heat transfer and subsequent heat release to the environment supported by evaporation/perspiration. Consequently, blood flow through inner organs can be decreased. Deja et al. [28] reported a significant decrease in liver perfusion during extreme WBH in approximately 50% of the treatments. In a self-experiment conducted in 2009 (S. Heckel-Reusser), these basic mechanisms were tested during FRWBH. Liver blood flow was measured directly before and immediately after WBH when the rectally measured body core temperature reached 39 °C. In this experiment, liver perfusion immediately after WBH was 70% of the baseline value measured before WBH (personal communication, Dr. J. Gellermann, Charité University Hospital, Berlin). A few weeks later, the same measurements were repeated before injection of a pyrogenic drug (Coley's toxin), and 3 h later, when fever temperature had reached 39 °C. As expected, there was no difference in liver perfusion. By administration of Coley's toxin, the temperature setpoint was shifted to >39 °C and body core temperature thus increased in order to achieve this elevated setpoint. Consequently, thermoregulation did not aim at any cooling of the organism and no blood redistribution from the core to the periphery was observed. In contrast, the perfusion of inner organs might decrease during WBH. This must be taken into account for the timing of medication, e.g., in case of combined thermochemotherapy in the treatment of liver metastasis.

11.5   Currently Applied WBH Techniques

Techniques applied for therapeutic WBH include extracorporeal blood heating, water immersion, 27 MHz short waves, long-wave IR irradiation in a chamber with almost 100% humidity, IR A/B ("near IR"), and wIRA irradiation [29, 30].

In 2010, Jia et al. [29] listed four commercially available medical WBH devices "for high-performance whole-body hyperthermia therapy": ET Space (Energy Technology, Shenzhen, China), IRATHERM1000 (von Ardenne Institute of Applied Medical Research, Dresden, Germany), heckel-HT3000 (Hydrosun Medizintechnik, Müllheim, Germany), and Oncotherm WBH2000 (Oncotherm, Budaörs, Hungary). Currently, only the heckel-HT3000 and IRATHERM1000 (in addition, a slightly modified model IRATHERM800 just for mild WBH) are commercially available. wIRA irradiation penetrates deeply into the subcutis, followed by (mainly) convective transport of the absorbed heat energy to all regions of the body by blood flow. At the same time, heat dissipation to the environment is impeded by a tent tempered with IR-C (heckel-HT3000) or by an insulating blanket (IRATHERM). Both techniques have proven high treatment tolerability and patient compliance. The main features of these two devices and of heckel-HT2000 (which was available until 2006 and is still in use in many clinics) are listed in Table 11.2.

11.6   Contraindications and Side Effects

There are no general contraindications for mild hyperthermia as long as body core temperature is only slightly increased. However, a good general health condition is absolutely required for fever-range and extreme WBH. Contraindications of fever-range WBH depend on the level of temperature increase and are primarily based on cardiovascular stress and the possibility of unwanted activation of inflammatory processes and destabilization of unbalanced hormonal and metabolic constellations. Most important absolute contraindications are cardiac insufficiency (>grade 2), major internal organ insufficiencies, and peripheral artery diseases. Relative contraindications, which must be individually assessed and may require prior treatment,

Table 11.2 Features of three different WBH devices

Products	heckel-HT3000	heckel-HT2000(M)	IRATHERM 1000
WBH levels (intended use)	Mild, fever range, extreme	Mild, fever range	Mild, fever range
Energy input	wIRA from above to the upper part of the body	Diffuse-reflected IR-A-/-B from chest to knees	wIRA from below
wIRA irradiance	Max. 100 mW/cm² to the uncovered skin	Max. 100 mW/cm² to the skin covered by cotton fabric	Max. 140 mW/cm² to the uncovered skin
Prevention of heat dissipation	Tent tempered by IR-C	Tent tempered by IR-A/-B	Insulating blanket from above
Patient positioning	Supine or prone position on a mattress	Possibility of half-sitting position in the heat-retention phase	Supine position on a knotless net
Maintenance of temperature plateau	wIRA switched OFF, tent still lightly tempered or heat-retention package allowing for a half-sitting position		Decreased power of wIRA radiators
Power consumption, total	3000 W	1250 W	5500 W
Rated voltage	230 V		3 phase 230/400 V

include cardiac arrhythmias, acute infections, major lymphedemas, high risk of thrombosis, and erratically progressive diseases (e.g., multiple sclerosis). In case of inflammatory diseases manifesting in exacerbations, such as progressive primary chronic polyarthritis, WBH is generally applied in the subacute phase, based on the concern of an unintended stimulation of acute inflammatory activities. This paradigm may be controversially discussed in view of new findings on direct anti-inflammatory effects of FRWBH, as described by Lee [17].

A most common side effect of fever-range WBH in almost all patients is a feeling of restlessness due to the strain on the central thermoregulatory system. Headache may indicate a minor dehydration.

IR-WBH, and especially wIRA-WBH, decreases the thermal load to the skin surface compared with conductive HT techniques and, thus, can significantly improve treatment tolerability and patient compliance. Paradoxically, this intended effect of energy absorption in deeper skin layers increases the risk of thermal skin damage in areas with circulatory impediments [23]. The technical design and procedure of wIRA-WBH deliberately prevent heat dissipation to the surroundings. At the same time, disturbed blood perfusion can diminish the intended convective heat transfer from the periphery to the core, in rare cases leading to thermal skin damage. The heckel-HT3000 is designed in a way that the area irradiated with wIRA is free of any compression and fully accessible for visual inspection and countermeasures in case of the development of hot spots.

In detail, contraindications and side effects are listed in the WBH guidelines of DGHT [9]. It has to be emphasized that the performance of extreme WBH treatments requires a comprehensive training in experienced centers in order to decrease the rate of side effects, the latter decreasing significantly with experience [31].

11.7   Conclusion and Outlook

Given the growing importance of immunotherapies in oncology, rheumatology, and other indications of chronic inflammation, it is worth considering the concept of WBH. Modern WBH techniques using wIRA have been proven to be safe, feasible, and well tolerated. Nevertheless, there is a general need to enhance the level of evidence by documenting treatment outcome data of routine use and by conducting controlled clinical trials.

References

1. Wagner-Jauregg J. The history of the malaria treatment of general paralysis. 1946. Am J Psychiatry. 1994;151:231–5. https://doi.org/10.1176/ajp.151.6.231.
2. Dobosz P, Dzieciątkowski T. The intriguing history of cancer immunotherapy. Front Immunol. 2019;10:2965. https://doi.org/10.3389/fimmu.2019.02965.
3. Bickels J, Kollender Y, Merinsky O, et al. Coley's toxin: historical perspective. Isr Med Assoc J. 2002;6:471–2.
4. Lampert H. Überwärmung als Heilmittel. Stuttgart: Hippokrates; 1948.

5. Schlenz M. Wie kann man unheilbar scheinende Krankheiten mit Erfolg behandeln? Innsbruck: Inn-Verlag; 1951.
6. Heckel M. Beliebig langdauernde und gezielt dosierbare Erhöhung der Körpertemperatur durch eine Infrarotbestrahlungsanordnung. Strahlentherapie. 1960;111(1):149–53.
7. von Ardenne M. Principles and concept 1993 of the Systemic Cancer Multistep Therapy (sCMT). Extreme whole-body hyperthermia using the infrared-A technique IRATHERM 2000--selective thermosensitisation by hyperglycemia--circulatory back-up by adapted hyperoxemia. Strahlenther Onkol. 1994;170(10):581–9.
8. Schmidt KL. Hyperthermie und Fieber. Stuttgart: Hippokrates; 1987. p. 2.
9. Deutsche Gesellschaft für Hyperthermie (DGHT). Leitlinie zur Ganzkörperhyperthermie - Version 1.0. Forum Hyperthermie. 2018;1:5–24.
10. Aschoff J, Wever R. Kern und Schale im Wärmehaushalt des Menschen. Naturwissenschaften. 1958;45(20):477–85.
11. Meffert H, Scherf HP, Meffert B. Milde Infrarot-A-Hyperthermie: Auswirkungen von Serienbestrahlungen mit wassergefilterter Infrarotstrahlung auf Gesunde und Kranke mit arterieller Hypertonie bzw. systemischer Sklerodermie. Akt Dermatol. 1993;19:142–8.
12. Förster J, Fleischanderl S, Wittstock S, et al. Letter to the editor: infrared-mediated hyperthermia is effective in the treatment of scleroderma-associated Raynaud's phenomenon. J Investig Dermatol. 2005;6:1313–6.
13. Kraybill WG, Olenki T, Evans SS, et al. A phase I study of fever-range whole body hyperthermia (FR-WBH) in patients with advanced solid tumours: correlation with mouse models. Int J Hyperthermia. 2002;18(3):253–66.
14. Bull JM, Scott GL, Strebel FR, et al. Fever-range whole-body thermal therapy combined with cisplatin, gemcitabine, and daily interferon-alpha: a description of a phase I-II protocol. Int J Hyperthermia. 2008;24(8):649–62.
15. Kleef R, Nagy R, Baierl A, et al. Low-dose Ipilimumab plus Nivolumab combined with IL-2 and hyperthermia in cancer patients with advanced disease: exploratory findings of a case series of 131 stage IV cancers - a retrospective study of a single institution. Cancer Immunol Immunother. 2021;70:1393–403.
16. Hall EJ, Giaccia AJ. Hyperthermia. In: Radiobiology for the radiologist. 8th ed. Philadelphia: Wolters Kluwer; 2019.
17. Lee CT, Kokolus KM, Leigh ND, et al. Defining immunological impact and therapeutic benefit of mild heating in a murine model of arthritis. PLoS One. 2015;10:e0120327.
18. Evans SS, Repasky EA, Fisher DT. Fever and the thermal regulation of immunity: the immune system feels the heat. Nat Rev Immunol. 2015;15(6):335–49.
19. Repasky EA, Evans SS, Dewhirst MW. Temperature matters! And why it should matter to tumor immunologists. Cancer Immunol Res. 2013;1(4):210–6.
20. Reisinger E, Wendelin I, Gasser R, et al. Antibiotics and increased temperature against Borrelia burgdorferi in vitro. Scand J Infect Dis. 1996;2:155–7.
21. Hildebrandt B, Hegewisch-Becker S, Kerner T, et al. Current status of radiant whole-body hyperthermia at temperatures >41.5°C and practical guidelines for the treatment of adults. The German 'Interdisciplinary working group on Hyperthermia'. Int J Hyperthermia. 2005;21(2):169–83.
22. von Ardenne A, Wehner H. Extreme whole-body hyperthermia with water-filtered infrared-A radiation. In: Baronzio GF, Hager ED, editors. Hyperthermia in cancer treatment: a primer. Boston: Springer; 2006. p. 237–46.
23. Wehner H, von Ardenne A, Kaltofen S. Whole-body hyperthermia with water-filtered infrared radiation: technical-physical aspects and clinical experiences. Int J Hyperthermia. 2001;17(1):19–30.
24. Koobotse MO, Schmidt D, Holly JMP, et al. Glucose concentration in cell culture medium influences the BRCA1-mediated regulation of the lipogenic action of IGF-I in breast cancer cells. Int J Mol Sci. 2020;21(22):8674.
25. Lassche G, Crezee J, van Herpen CML. Whole-body hyperthermia in combination with systemic therapy in advanced solid malignancies. Crit Rev Oncol Hematol. 2019;139:67–74.

26. Douwes F. Komplextherapie der chronischen Borreliose (Lyme disease) - Ein neuer Therapieansatz: die Antibiotika augmentierte Thermoeradikation (AAT). OM & Ernährung. 2018;164:F10.
27. Douwes F. The successful antibiotic augmented thermal eradication of chronic lyme disease. Paper presented at the 32nd ESHO Meeting, Berlin, 16–19 May 2018.
28. Deja M, Ahlers O, Macguill M, et al. Changes in hepatic blood flow during whole body hyperthermia. Int J Hyperthermia. 2010;26(2):95–100.
29. Jia D, Liu J. Current devices for high-performance whole-body hyperthermia therapy. Expert Rev Med Devices. 2010;7(3):407–23.
30. Rowe-Horwege RW. Hyperthermia, systemic. In: Webster JG, editor. Encyclopedia of medical devices and instrumentation. 2nd ed. New York: John Wiley & Sons; 2006. p. 42–62.
31. Wust P, Riess H, Hildebrandt B, et al. Feasibility and analysis of thermal parameters for the whole-body-hyperthermia system IRATHERM-2000. Int J Hyperthermia. 2000;16(4):325–39.

Whole-Body Hyperthermia (WBH) in Psychiatry

12

A. Knobel, K. Hanusch, N. Auen, F. Rübener, S. Fischer, C. Borzim, A. Heinz, and M. Schäfer

Abbreviations

5-HT	5-Hydroxytryptamine/serotonin
CES-D	Center for Epidemiologic Studies Depression Scale
FMS	Fibromyalgia syndrome
HAMD	Hamilton Rating Scale for Depression
MDD	Major depressive disorder
MINI	Mini-International Neuropsychiatric Interview
SD	Standard deviation
SE	Standard error
SSRI	Selective serotonin reuptake inhibitor
TRP	Transient receptor potential
TRPA1	Transient receptor potential cation channel subfamily A member 1
TRPV1	Transient receptor potential cation channel subfamily V member 1
WBH	Whole-body hyperthermia

A. Knobel (✉) · C. Borzim · A. Heinz
Department of Psychiatry and Psychotherapy, Charité Campus Mitte, Charité University Medicine Berlin, Berlin, Germany
e-mail: astrid.knobel@charite.de

K. Hanusch
Department of Health Professions, Berne University of Applied Sciences, Berne, Switzerland

N. Auen · F. Rübener · M. Schäfer
Department of Psychiatry, Psychotherapy, Psychosomatic and Addiction Medicine, Evangelische Kliniken Essen-Mitte, Essen, Germany

S. Fischer
Clinical Psychology and Psychotherapy, Institute of Psychology, University of Zurich, Zurich, Switzerland

© The Author(s) 2022
P. Vaupel (ed.), *Water-filtered Infrared A (wIRA) Irradiation*,
https://doi.org/10.1007/978-3-030-92880-3_12

12.1   Hyperthermia, Fever, and Mental Health

Depressive disorders have significant medical, social, and economic impact [1]. On the one hand, a significant proportion of individuals with mental illness do not have access to specific treatment, and on the other, those who seek help are frequently interested in more natural therapies. A recent critical assessment of conventional pharmacological treatments for depressive episodes has indicated that approximately 30% of patients with depressive episodes do not respond to conventional antidepressant medication or develop side effects [2]. Effective new treatments are therefore urgently needed in psychiatry.

Early written records by Galen of Pergamon (personal physician of Marcus Aurelius, approximately 129–201 B.C.) described the application of therapeutical heat in form of hot baths for the treatment of melancholia. In the early nineteenth century, it was assumed that an impulse to the autonomous nerve system could lead to alterations in the metabolic system, relaxation, and better sleep. In the first half of the twentieth century, "malaria fever cure" was first used by Wagner-Jauregg and Rosenblum for patients with psychiatric symptoms related to syphilis and later for non-syphilitic psychoses. In addition, warm full baths, hot wet packs, and other forms of hydrotherapy have been used to treat agitation, before being replaced by pharmacotherapy [3, 4].

12.2   Whole-Body Hyperthermia (WBH)
for Psychiatric Symptoms

Beneficial effects of WBH on mood and quality of life have repeatedly been observed during and after treatment in various fields of medicine, including rheumatology, orthopedics, and oncology. The significant improvement in depressive symptoms induced by WBH in patients with cancer has been correlated with increases in plasma β-endorphin levels [5].

Recently, WBH has received renewed attention in the context of treating mental health issues, with several studies investigating potential effects and clinical applications, especially for patients with depressive symptoms. Most importantly, a randomized, double-blind, and sham-controlled trial delivered by Janssen and colleagues [6] has reported a significant, rapid, and partially lasting reduction of depressive symptoms in non-medicated patients with major depressive disorder (MDD) following a single session of wIRA-WBH using a Heckel-HT3000™ (Hydrosun Medizintechnik, Müllheim, Germany). In 17 out of 34 patients, body core temperature was increased to 38.5 °C (active treatment condition, within 107 min, followed by a heat-retention phase of 60 min, during which the patients achieved a mean maximal body core temperature of 38.9 °C, i.e., a mean increase of 1.9 °C). Depressive symptoms which were assessed 1, 2, 4, and 6 weeks after WBH using the Hamilton Rating Scale for Depression (HAMD) were significantly reduced (4 points on HAMD scale) from week 2 to week 6 after treatment, when compared to sham treatment (see Table 12.1).

Table 12.1 HAMD scores during follow-up after wIRA-WBH vs. Sham intervention (modified from [6])

	HAMD mean score (SD) WBH	HAMD mean score (SD) Sham
Baseline	20.71 (4.87)	22.75 (4.42)
Week 1 (post-intervention)	14.80 (5.40)	20.86 (3.33)
Week 2	12.67 (6.78)	18.71 (3.17)
Week 4	12.93 (4.92)	17.79 (4.06)
Week 6	12.40 (5.45)	17.21 (4.78)

A preceding open clinical trial by the same group [7] was based on findings which demonstrated that WBH and the selective serotonin reuptake inhibitor citalopram independently increased body temperature and acted synergistically to induce antidepressant-like behavioral responses in a rat model of depression [8]. Hanusch et al. [7] have reported that a single session of mild-intensity WBH, using a Heckel-HT2000™ near-infrared WBH device to increase body temperature (average maximum body core temperature 38.4 °C, i.e., an increase of 1.2 °C; mean session time 127 min) resulted in a rapid and sustained reduction in depressive symptoms (CES-D score before treatment: mean = 29.9 [SD 10.6], 5 days after treatment: mean = 19.2 [SD 12.3], t = 5.53, df = 15, $p < 0.001$, effect size = 1.13) in 16 patients with MDD, with WBH-induced reductions in the mean circadian body core temperature correlating with reduced CES-D scores 5 days after treatment. Interestingly, they observed no significant treatment response in patients treated with selective serotonin reuptake inhibitor (SSRI).

A quasi-experimental, observational study of fibromyalgia by Romeyke et al. [9] found that the integration of WBH into a multi-modal inpatient pain therapy regime appeared to improve depressive symptoms ($p = 0.055$, comparing multi-modal therapies with and without WBH; patients in both groups numerically improved from admission to discharge). This study used a Heckel-HT2000™ device targeting a body core temperature of 38.5 °C for 50 min (followed by 60 min rest) with an average of 4.9 sessions per patient. However, it should be noted that the 103 subjects included in this study were suffering from severely progressive forms of fibromyalgia syndrome with a high degree of chronicity and multiple comorbidities and had received multiple therapies including psychotherapy.

Studies have also assessed the effects of WBH using hot baths instead of IR-heating. A communication by Schaper [10] described the antidepressant effects (HAMD-17) of weekly hyperthermic baths ($n = 4$ to 13, depending on the length of their in-patient stay with an average maximum body core temperature of 38.4 °C and an increase of 1.7 °C) in 20 patients with unipolar depression or bipolar disorder. Statistically significant reductions in depression were seen after the second session and during the second week of treatment. Gödl and Glied [11] also reported on results from a study involving weekly WBH treatments of 10 patients in hot tubs for 6–8 weeks with an average maximum body core temperature of 39.3 °C and an average increase of 2.3 °C. At the end of the treatment phase, 50% of all included subjects were below the cutoff for a diagnosis of depression. However, baseline HAMD scores were not obtained, since heart rate variability was chosen as the main outcome measure. In another study involving 17 patients with confirmed depressive disorder (ICD-10: F32/F33), WBH in hot tubs (twice a week for 4 weeks) significantly reduced depression (HAMD) after four interventions compared with patients in the sham condition. In this study, water was heated to 40.2 °C, and participants spent, on average, 22.6 min in the tub, followed by 33.2 min rest [12].

Taken together, these studies indicate that WBH treatment is generally well tolerated with reported side effects *during* treatment being tachycardia, restlessness, and agitation, as well as emotions such as anger, sadness, or insufficiency. *After* treatment, participants often exhibited short and complete remitting symptoms such as headaches, nausea, ringing in ears, insomnia, vertigo, reduced libido, or areas of hypesthesia in extremities [13].

12.3   Mechanisms of Action of WBH

Depressive disorders are characterized by an altered mineralocorticoid receptor (MR) response, often increased cortisol levels, as well as serotonergic alterations including a down-regulation of $5\text{-}HT_{1A}$ receptors, and increased binding of $5\text{-}HT_{2A}$ receptors in the hippocampus [14, 15]. It is also known that serotonergic ($5\text{-}HT_{1A}$) receptor function and SSRI administration influence temperature and hormone responses [16]. Hyperthermic interventions may modify the release of serotonin in the raphe nuclei via functional transient receptor potential (TRP) channels (see Fig. 12.1). Transient receptor potential ankyrin 1 ($TRPA_1$) and vanilloid 1 ($TRPV_1$) receptors are implicated in the sensation of pain, temperature, inflammation, and cough. $TRPA_1$ is activated by temperatures below 17 °C, $TRPV_1$ (capsaicin receptor) by temperatures above 43 °C. $TRPA_1$ and $TRPV_1$ are often co-expressed in neurons. Consequently, the formation of functional $TRPA_1$-$TRPV_1$ tetramers imparts unique activation profiles, presumably altering the release of serotonin [17].

In summary, WBH may activate warm-sensitive afferent thermosensory pathways and affect mood-regulating neural activity in the midbrain, including nuclei

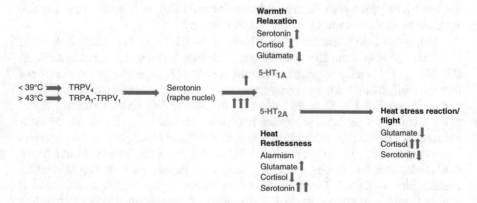

Fig. 12.1 Assumed mechanisms of action of WBH (according to Hanusch, unpublished)

implicated in serotonergic neurotransmission, and thereby elicit antidepressant-like effects as well as thermoregulatory cooling (reduced circadian body temperatures).

The immune hypothesis of depression describes a connection between a chronic subclinical stimulation of the immune system and the development of depression and other mood disorders [18]. There is evidence that at least in subgroups of patients with clinical depression, levels of pro-inflammatory cytokines are elevated during negative mood states and that treatment responses may be related to immune changes, including a decrease in pro-inflammatory markers. Levels of C-Reactive Protein (CRP), IL-1, IL-6, and TNF-α have consistently been reported to be increased in depressed patients [19, 20]. WBH activates or modulates the immune system in a reproducible manner [13], and therapeutic hyperthermia and fever have been associated with a variety of immunological reactions which can be exploited for the treatment of cancer, but which might also have positive therapeutic effects in clinical depression, and the course of at least some forms of depression that are characterized by a chronic subclinical activation of pro-inflammatory cytokines [21].

12.4   Current Research

Three randomized, double-blind, and (sham-) controlled clinical studies are currently being conducted by our groups in Berlin and Essen (Germany). Studies are based on the hypothesis that WBH is a fast-acting non-medical stimulation treatment against depressive symptoms which is well tolerated and improves quality of life. Overall, we are focusing on generating safety and tolerability data and attempting to confirm if WBH improves depressive symptoms and whether antidepressants influence treatment response and possible side effects. We are also monitoring immune parameters in the serum of patients to detect (subclinical) immune activation and possible changes after WBH and their potential correlations to clinical response.

12.4.1 Patients and Methods

In contrast to Janssen et al. [6], our new studies include patients with and without psychopharmacological treatment. The study protocol in Essen compares two different patient groups with depression. The diagnosis of MDD (as an inclusion/exclusion criterion) is undertaken using the MINI interview in version 7.0.2, and the severity of the current state of depression is determined using the Hamilton Depression Scale (HAMD-17). The first group of patients consists of patients with mild or moderate depression (HAMD-17 Score ≥ 17) who are treatment naïve or do not currently receive any antidepressant medication. The other group includes patients with moderate-to-severe depression who are non- or only partial responders to standard pharmacological treatment according to current S3 guidelines for unipolar depression [22]. In each subgroup, patients are randomized to either a treated group receiving two treatments with WBH in 2 weeks, or an untreated group as controls. For inclusion, patients have to present in a good physical status and have to be free of conditions resulting in an immune-suppressed state at the time of participation. Exclusion criteria are other severe psychiatric comorbidities, relevant somatic disorders, acute suicidality, and prior treatment with WBH. All patients are examined and rated by an experienced psychiatrist who confirms diagnosis and estimates the severity of depression. Response, safety, and efficacy are assessed using expert-rated clinical scales for depression, as well as self-rating instruments (Beck Depression Inventory, Multidimensional Fatigue Inventory, Perceived Stress Scale, Short-Form-Health Survey). To verify the presence of short-term effects of WBH, we distributed a questionnaire that had to be completed within 3 days after treatment. Clinical outcome variables were assessed at weeks 1, 3, and 6 by an experienced psychiatrist who is blinded to the treatment group of the patients. Blood samples were taken at the time of inclusion, at weeks 1, 3, 6, and 12 and stored frozen until the measurement of specific biomarkers (e.g., TNF-α, sICAM-1, hsCRP, IL-6). For the second patient group who have previously received pharmacological treatment, changes in medication or acute pharmaceutical interventions were allowed as clinically required in both the treated and untreated control groups. Any alteration or influence on the participant by medication was recorded in the study protocol. Determining the primary study endpoint after 6 weeks was selected to enable effects to be compared with those reported in the study of Janssen et al. [6].

In contrast to the Janssen study [6], patients received two applications of WBH in the first 2 weeks of the trial. During wIRA-WBH (Heckel HT-3000™ device), the body core temperature was raised to 38.5 °C (peak temperature), followed by 1 h of heat congestion. This process was monitored and vital signs such as blood pressure, heart rate, blood oxyhemoglobin (HbO_2) saturation, and body core temperature were recorded. One treatment of WBH is considered complete when the participant's vital parameters return to a normal state. Control subjects in the control group had the option to receive WBH after their 6-week observation period.

12.4.2 Preliminary Results and Clinical Experience

According to our experience, close support and care is crucial for a successful WBH session in order to provide the patient with a sense of safety and empowerment. For a successful implementation of the procedure, it was also necessary to inform participants of the opportunity to interrupt the process of hyperthermia at any stage. We especially recognized that some patients require mental or emotional support when approaching a core temperature of 38.5 °C. Finally, because thirst was often experienced by participants undergoing WBH, drinking water at room temperature should be offered. Treatment responses regarding negative mood and further symptoms of depression are currently being examined.

Preliminary results regarding safety and tolerability are currently available for 34 participants treated in Essen (16 participants were treatment naïve, 18 participants were non- or partly-responders). WBH was well tolerated (physically and psychologically) in most psychiatric patients with or without antidepressant treatment. To

Table 12.2 Differences in reaching the body core temperature of 38.5 °C between patients with and without antidepressants (*SD* standard deviation, *SE* standard error)

	Treatment group	No. of treatments	Average time (min)	SD	SE
Time to reach 38.5 °C	Not medicated	16	67.1	22.9	5.7
	+ antidepressants	12	83.2	20.5	5.9

date, the dropout rate, independent of treatment group, has been approximately 20%. In patients who received an antidepressant treatment (moderate-to-severe depression), the overall dropout rate was 22% compared with 19% in the group of treatment naïve patients (mild-to-moderate depression). For individuals with moderate-to-severe depression, the dropout rate for the treated and control groups has been 11%. The dropout rate for treatment naïve patients with mild-to-moderate depression has been 12% in the control group and 6% in the group treated with WBH. We have also analyzed the average time necessary to reach a body core temperature of 38.5 °C. Overall, a slight difference was observed between the two treatment groups. Medication prolonged time to reach the core temperature of 38.5 °C (see Table 12.2).

Risk factors for discontinuation of WBH sessions have also been analyzed. Of the patients with moderate-to-severe depression receiving antidepressant treatment, 33% discontinued WBH treatment, compared with only 11% of the patients with mild and moderate depression.

No serious side effects of wIRA-WBH that would have required further treatment have been observed. Side effects that have been noted are related to the physiological body cooling mechanisms and the activation of the sympathetic stress system. For example, almost all patients experienced a drop in systolic and diastolic blood pressure resulting in an increase in heart rate which continued until the end of the warm-up period. Some participants described cardiac palpitations, headache, increase in respiratory rate, or restlessness. Overall, the risk for adverse effects during WBH was increased in individuals having somatic comorbidities (e.g., bronchial asthma).

12.5   Outlook to Future Research

In summary, accumulating evidence from new, randomized, and controlled clinical trials using water-filtered Infrared A (wIRA-) heating shows this to be a well-tolerated and effective approach for treating depressive symptoms, with even a single session being able to improve depressive symptoms [6, 7]. Due to small sample sizes and a lack of suitable control groups in some studies, more randomized, controlled studies with higher numbers of patients are necessary. As implemented in our current studies in Essen and Berlin, well-designed sham conditions should allow participants to experience heat without increasing body core temperature above 38.0 °C. To reflect a realistic clinical population and allow transfer of study results to clinical practice, it is necessary to allow and control for antidepressant medication, since most patients in the psychiatric setting receive multi-modal therapies due to the severity and chronicity of symptoms. Evidence, albeit limited, indicates that a gradual increase in ambient temperature aimed at delivering a body core temperature between 38 °C and 39 °C followed by 60 min rest while maintaining the temperature is the most effective [13]. Treatment can be repeated in defined time intervals. Defining subtypes of depressive disorders that are most responsive to WBH may be important for better predicting who should be offered a hyperthermia treatment. In this context, examining underlying mechanisms of action is of prime importance. Since endocrine alterations are a frequent finding in major depressive disorder [23–26], future research to investigate whether hormones, such as cortisol, oxytocin, and triiodothyronine/thyroxine (T3/T4), can serve as predictors and indicators of treatment outcomes is warranted. Similarly, as immune effects may play an important role in major depressive disorder, there is a need for studies investigating inflammatory markers such as TNF-α, interleukins, or cell adhesion molecules before and after hyperthermia treatments [27, 28]. Finally, the molecular underpinnings of major depressive disorders are only beginning to be understood, and it would be highly important to unravel which (epi-)genetic signatures are linked with better treatment outcomes and whether at least some of these could be changed by WBH.

In conclusion, wIRA-WBH holds great promise as a treatment for depressive disorders given the findings listed above, especially given its good tolerability. Hopefully, further studies will help to establish recommended applications of WBH, e.g., for patients declining antidepressant medication, as a complimentary treatment for patients that do not, or insufficiently respond to standard therapies, or as a "door opener" enabling patients to engage in other therapies such as psychotherapy, exercising, or medication. At this point, WBH may be considered for individual patients unresponsive to standard therapies providing fully informed consent ("single patient use"). It may be particularly helpful for patients with high psychological strain and unresponsiveness to well-established therapies or those suffering from comorbidities known to respond to hyperthermia, after careful consideration of possible risks.

References

1. Otte C, Gold SM, Penninx BW, et al. Major depressive disorder. Nat Rev Dis Primers. 2016;2:1–20.
2. Cipriani A, Furukawa TA, Salanti G, et al. Comparative efficacy and acceptability of 21 antidepressant drugs for the acute treatment of adults with major depressive disorder (MDD): a systematic review and network meta-analysis. Lancet. 2018;391:1357–66.
3. Hanusch KU, Janssen C. Die passive Ganzkörperhyperthermie in der Psychiatrie- Eine historische Analyse. Naturheilkunde. 2013;2:40–3.
4. Woesner M. What is old is new again: the use of whole-body hyperthermia for depression recalls the medicinal uses of hyperthermia, fever therapy, and hydrotherapy. Curr Neurbiol. 2019;10(2):56–66.
5. Koltyn KF, Robins HI, Schmitt CL, et al. Changes in mood state following whole-body hyperthermia. Int J Hyperthermia. 1992;8:305–7.

6. Janssen CW, Lowry CA, Mehl MR, et al. Whole-body hyperthermia for the treatment of major depressive disorder: a randomized clinical trial. JAMA Psychiatry. 2016;73:789–95.

7. Hanusch KU, Janssen CH, Billheimer D, et al. Whole-body hyperthermia for the treatment of major depression: associations with thermoregulatory cooling. Am J Psychiatry. 2013;170:802–4.

8. Hale MW, Raison CL, Lowry CA. Integrative physiology of depression and antidepressant drug action: implications for serotonergic mechanisms of action and novel therapeutic strategies for treatment of depression. Pharmacol Ther. 2013;137:108–18.

9. Romeyke T, Stummer H. Multi- modal pain therapy of fibromyalgia syndrome with integration of systemic whole-body hyperthermia- effects on pain intensity and mental state: a non-randomised controlled study. J Musculoskeletal Pain. 2014;22:341–55.

10. Schaper L. Wiederholte Hyperthermiebehandlung durch Überwärmungsbäder bei Patienten mit depressiven Störungen: Effekte auf die Interleukin-6 sowie auf die mittlere Körpertemperatur und den psychopathologischen Befund, Albert-Ludwig-Universität Freiburg im Breisgau. Dissertation; 1995.

11. Gödl R, Glied N. Veränderungen der autonomen Regulation durch Überwärmungsbadtherapie bei Patienten mit depressiven Störungen. Universtätsbibliothek (Dissertation): Karl-Franzens-Universität Graz; 2000.

12. Naumann J, Grebe J, Kaifel S, et al. Effects of hyperthermic baths on depression, sleep and heart rate variability in patients with depressive disorder: a randomised clinical pilot trial. BMC Complement Altern Med. 2017;17:172.

13. Hanusch KU, Janssen CW. The impact of whole-body hyperthermia interventions on mood and depression- are we ready for recommendations for clinical application? Int J Hyperthermia. 2019;36(1):572–80.

14. Heinz A. New understanding of mental disorders. In: Computational models for dimensional psychiatry. Boston: MIT Press; 2017.

15. Young EA, Lopez JF, Murphy-Weinberg V, et al. Mineralocorticoid receptor function in major depression. Arch Gen Psychiatry. 2003;60(1):24–8.

16. Lerer B, Gelfin Y, Gorfine M, et al. 5-HT1A receptor function in normal subjects on clinical doses of fluoxetine: blunted temperature and hormone responses to ipsapirone challenge. Neuropsychopharmacology. 1999;20(6):628–39.

17. Sadofsky LR, Sreekrishna KT, Lin Y, et al. Unique responses are observed in transient receptor potential ankyrin 1 and vanilloid 1 (TRPA1 and TRPV1) co-expressing cells. Cell. 2014;3(2):616–26.

18. Capuron L, Miller AH. Immune system to brain signaling: neuropsychopharmacological implications. Pharmacol Ther. 2011;130(2):226–38.

19. Howren MB, Lamkin DM, Suls J. Associations of depression with C-reactive protein, IL-1, and IL-6: a meta-analysis. Psychosom Med. 2009;71(2):171–86.

20. Dowlati Y, Herrmann N, Swardfager W, et al. A meta-analysis of cytokines in major depression. Biol Psychiatry. 2010;67(5):446–57.

21. Wohleb ES, Franklin T, Iwata M, et al. Integrating neuroimmune systems in the neurobiology of depression. Nat Rev Neurosci. 2016;17(8):497–511.

22. Schneider F, Härter M, Schorr S. Leitlinie/Nationale VersorgungsLeitlinie Unipolare Depression. Berlin: Springer; 2017.

23. Reimold M, Knobel A, Rapp MA, et al. Central serotonin transporter levels are associated with stress hormone response and anxiety. Psychopharmacology (Berl). 2011;213(2–3):563–72.

24. Stetler C, Miller GE. Depression and hypothalamic-pituitary-adrenal activation: quantitative summary of four decades of research. Psychosom Med. 2011;73:114–26.

25. Engel S, Laufer S, Knaevelsrud C, et al. The endogenous oxytocin system in depressive disorders: a systematic review and meta-analysis. Psychoneuroendocrinology. 2018;101:138–49.

26. Fountoulakis KN, Kantartzis S, Siamouli M, et al. Peripheral thyroid dysfunction in depression. World J Biol Psychiatry. 2006;7(3):131–7.

27. Raison CL, Janssen CW, Lowry CA. Hyperthermia for major depressive disorder? JAMA Psychiatry. 2016;73(10):1096–7.

28. Schaefer M, Sarkar S, Schwarz M, et al. Soluble cell adhesion molecule sICAM-1 in patients with unipolar or bipolar affective disorders. Neuropsychobiology. 2016;74:8–14.

Part IV

Clinical Practice: Neonatology

Mode of Action, Efficacy, and Safety of Radiant Warmers in Neonatology

13

D. Singer

13.1 Risk of Hypothermia in Term and Preterm Neonates

Human neonates are at heightened risk of hypothermia. However, contrary to what is often believed, their propensity to cool down is not, or not merely, due to an "immaturity" of thermoregulation. In fact, at least term neonates are well adapted to their small body size by their comparatively high specific (i.e., weight-related) metabolic rate and by the ability to produce extra heat in their brown adipose tissue. Nevertheless, as a result of their relatively large surface-to-volume ratio and the steeply increasing heat loss with decreasing ambient temperatures, their maximal thermogenic capabilities are already attained at temperatures which are still deemed to be comfortable by adults. Moreover, the "invisibility" of non-shivering thermogenesis often leads to an underestimation of the thermal stress experienced by neonates with subsequent neglect of thermal care. The risk of hypothermia is even more pronounced in preterm neonates due to their smaller body size in conjunction with a true "immaturity" of the thermoregulatory effector systems (lack of both white and brown adipose tissue, slow increase in basal metabolic rate up to a level appropriate for body size, elevated permeability of skin resulting in higher evaporative water and heat losses) [1–4].

The adverse effects of cold are primarily caused by the combination of diminished peripheral perfusion (to decrease heat loss) and elevated metabolic rate (to increase heat production). The imbalance of oxygen supply and demand results in a metabolic acidosis that triggers pulmonary vasoconstriction and leads to a "vicious cycle" of hypoxia. The indirect effects of counter-regulation are potentiated by the direct effects of cold, especially by the impairment of blood coagulation which contributes to the increased risk of brain hemorrhage in hypothermic preterm

D. Singer (✉)
Division of Neonatology and Pediatric Critical Care Medicine, University Medical Center Eppendorf, Hamburg, Germany
e-mail: dsinger@uke.de

© The Author(s) 2022
P. Vaupel (ed.), *Water-filtered Infrared A (wIRA) Irradiation*,
https://doi.org/10.1007/978-3-030-92880-3_13

neonates. Altogether, unintentional (accidental) hypothermia is known to increase morbidity and mortality in term and even more so in preterm neonates [1, 5, 6]. This contrasts with therapeutic (induced) hypothermia which has long been used in cardiac surgery to prevent brain damage during extracorporeal circulation and has now been established as a neuroprotective treatment for posthypoxic states in both adults (cardiac arrest) and neonates (perinatal asphyxia) [7, 8]. However, the undisputable beneficial effects of a cold-induced reduction in metabolic rate are only attained if thermoregulation is pharmacologically suppressed and are thus completely different from the potentially life-threatening *sequelae* of accidental hypothermia to be prevented by appropriate thermal care.

13.1.1 Methods of Thermal Care in Neonatology

To avoid unintentional cooling in term and preterm babies, extensive precautions to prevent and, where inevitable, replace heat losses are mandatory in clinical neonatology. In delivery rooms and on neonatal wards, thermal care is basically provided by either radiant warmers or incubators [2, 3, 9, 10]. In the latter, thermal protection comes from circulating warm air (heat convection) and, even more importantly, from high saturations of water vapor to reduce evaporation from the newborn's body surface. In radiant warmers, heat is supplied/replaced by infrared irradiation. Since radiant heat elicits evaporation on the body surface, part of its warming effect is instantaneously counteracted by heat losses so that, when directly compared, heat radiators are slightly less effective in supplying heat than humidified incubators. If, however, evaporation is inhibited (e.g., by plastic sheets used to cover the babies), radiant warmers and incubators are equivalent in their thermo-protective effects [10, 11].

Despite their heating power, radiant warmers are often insufficient to compensate for the huge heat losses occurring in extremely low birthweight neonates during delivery room care. This could theoretically be counteracted by a corresponding increase in radiant power density (irradiance). However, conventional radiant warmers have one major drawback which limits their practical use: The low-energy, longwave infrared (IR-B and IR-C) radiation they emit has a relatively low depth of penetration. The accumulation of heat within the outer skin layers not only causes some thermal discomfort in the caregivers, but also leads to a dependency of the newborn's heat uptake on its peripheral circulation [4, 12, 13]. If skin perfusion were to be greatly reduced (e.g., under conditions of circulatory shock), or if the irradiance were to be further increased, a local overheating would inevitably result. In fact, severe cases of burns have been observed after resuscitation of asphyctic neonates under conventional IR radiators [14].

13.1.2 Aim of the Studies Reported

In view of the aforementioned limitations of conventional radiant warmers, the technology of water-filtered heat radiators [12], which emit a modified IR-A spectrum and should combine an enhanced depth effect with less surface overheating, has attracted some interest in neonatal care [13]. Several studies which have tested the potential benefits of water-filtered IR-A (wIRA) irradiation in neonates will be summarized in this contribution. Briefly, these studies can be subdivided into physical investigations, conducted to elucidate the particular mode of action of wIRA in comparison with conventional IR irradiation in agar phantoms, and clinical observations that have been performed to test the efficacy and safety of either type of heat radiators in human term and preterm neonates under common hospital conditions.

13.2   Materials and Methods

13.2.1 Physical Investigations

Most of the physical investigations were carried out on agar phantoms like those used in radiotherapy [12, 13, 15, 16]. Since these are mainly composed of water and allow direct evaporation from the surface, they have thermal properties somewhat similar to human tissues, and, more specifically, to preterm neonates. The phantoms were exposed to either conventional radiant warmers from different suppliers (DR = Dräger, H&L = Heinen & Löwenstein; F&P = Fisher & Paykel) or to the water-filtered infrared-A (wIRA) radiator manufactured by Hydrosun. The radiation power density (irradiance) was uniformly adjusted to 30 mW/cm^2 and the duration of irradiation amounted to 60 min. Temperature measurements were performed using customary temperature probes placed within the core and on the surface of the phantoms. Alternatively, surface temperatures were assessed by infrared thermometry. In addition to the phantom studies, a number of thermographic measurements were carried out on the skin of healthy adult volunteers.

13.2.2 Clinical Observations

Clinical observations were performed on term and preterm neonates who were exposed to conventional IR or to wIRA irradiation as an alternative or supplementary source of heat. They were all in typical clinical settings in which an extra heat loss could be anticipated (primary care in the delivery room, incubator care in the intensive care unit, physical examinations on the neonatal ward). Body core and/or surface temperatures were alternatively measured by customary rectal thermometers, single spot infrared thermometers, or infrared thermography (Nikon LAIRD-S270). Since the latter often yields rather qualitative results, extra effort was undertaken to quantify the thermographic records. To this end, a grid of measuring points was laid over the body. By calculating the arithmetic means of closely adjacent measuring points, a total of four regional temperatures (of head, trunk, arm, and leg) was obtained which were then weighted according to the relative contribution of the respective regions to the total body surface area. In this way, a mean body surface temperature was determined (Fig. 13.1).

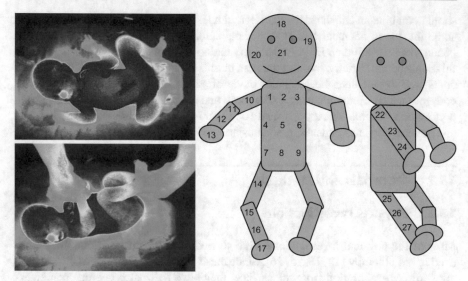

$$Tm_{Surface} = (Tm_{Head} \times 0.2) + (Tm_{Trunk} \times 0.3) + (Tm_{Arm} \times 0.2) + (Tm_{Leg} \times 0.3)$$
$$Tm_{Head} = (18 + 19 + 20 + 21) / 4 \text{ (e.g.)}$$

Fig. 13.1 Thermographic observations comparing the effects of water-filtered IR-A (wIRA) and conventional IR irradiation on human neonates during routine examinations. To quantify the results, a grid of measuring points was laid over the thermographic pictures. Regional temperatures (e.g., head temperature) were calculated as arithmetic means of several measuring points. The mean body surface temperature was determined as the weighted mean of regional temperatures (according to the contribution of the respective regions to the total body surface area)

13.3   Results and Discussion

13.3.1 Physical Investigations

The physical measurements on agar phantoms revealed a surprisingly clear difference in the effects of wIRA in comparison with conventional IR irradiation: Whereas with conventional radiators, the surface temperatures at the end of the 60-min irradiation period clearly exceeded the core temperatures, the wIRA radiator resulted not only in an improved central warming, but also in a markedly diminished superficial overheating with the surface temperature being even lower than the core temperature (Fig. 13.2). The central warming effect was uniformly augmented when plastic sheets were used to attenuate evaporation. However, whereas under conventional IR radiators this related to an excessive increase in surface temperatures, the surface temperature in the wIRA-exposed phantoms did not reach higher levels than under conventional irradiation without plastic sheets (Fig. 13.3). From the time course of the heating process, it became evident that the central warming is preceded by a superficial accumulation of heat in conventional IR irradiation, with the heat transfer occurring by "secondary" conduction (in living beings, also by

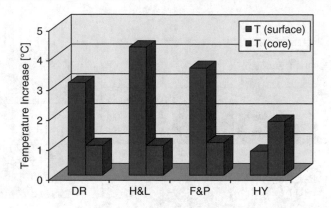

Fig. 13.2 Surface and core temperatures of agar phantoms after 60-min exposure to different types of IR irradiation (30 mW/cm², means of $n = 3$, each): Whereas conventional radiant warmers (Dräger [DR], Heinen & Löwenstein [H&L], or Fisher & Paykel [F&P]) all lead to a much higher increase in surface than core temperatures, the wIRA radiator (Hydrosun [HY]) results in a predominant, and more pronounced increase in body core temperature with markedly reduced surface warming

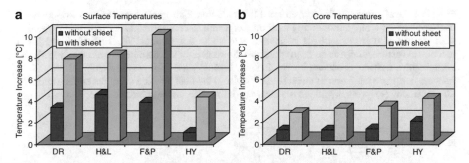

Fig. 13.3 Effects of plastic sheets on surface (**a**) and core (**b**) warming under different types of IR irradiation (60 min, 30 mW/cm², mean of $n = 3$, each): With the use of a plastic sheet, the increase in core temperature is more pronounced with all types of irradiation. However, whereas this is associated with an excessive increase in surface temperature for conventional radiators (DR, H&L, F&P), the surface temperature for wIRA irradiation (HY) is not higher than for conventional IR irradiation without a plastic sheet

convection) from the surface to the core (Fig. 13.4). In contrast, the heat seems to be primarily deposited in deeper "tissue" layers under wIRA irradiation, with the warming of the surface being due to a back-diffusion of heat rather than to a direct local effect. Therefore, a comparatively low gradient between the (higher) core and the lower (surface) temperature is established (Fig. 13.5). In both cases, a leveling of the surface temperature increase can be observed which indicates a new equilibrium between radiative heat uptake and evaporative heat loss, and thus disappears when evaporation is prevented by plastic sheets.

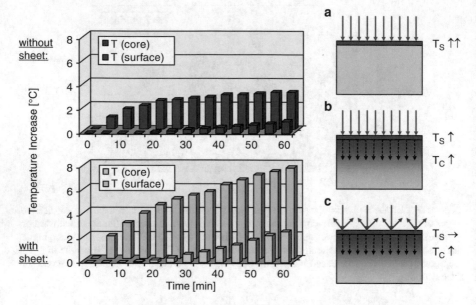

Fig. 13.4 Heat transfer under conventional IR irradiation: The graphs represent the time course of core and surface temperature during a 60-min exposure to conventional IR irradiation without or with the use of plastic sheets. It is obvious that under conventional IR irradiation, a primary increase in surface temperature T_S (**a**) precedes the secondary increase in core temperature T_C (**b**), with the heat transfer occurring by conduction. With the use of a plastic sheet, not only is the increase in surface temperature much steeper, but also the final leveling off of the surface temperature is missing (**c**), probably due to the lacking cooling effect of evaporative water loss

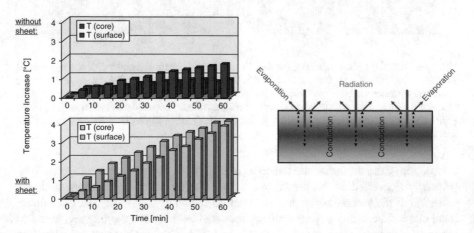

Fig. 13.5 Heat transfer under wIRA irradiation: The graphs represent the time course of core and surface temperature during a 60-min exposure to wIRA irradiation without or with the use of plastic sheets. In contrast to conventional IR irradiation (see Fig. 13.4), the increase in core temperature precedes superficial warming, which thus appears to be due to the back-diffusion of heat from deeper "tissue" layers. Using of a plastic sheet results in a largely homogeneous warming of outer and inner parts of the phantom

Incidentally, in parallel to the weaker surface heating effect, the induction of evaporation was also seen to be less pronounced in wIRA irradiation. This was found in complementary studies on either agar phantoms or pieces of meat which both exhibited an approx. 20–30% smaller loss of water at equal duration of wIRA exposure compared to conventional IR irradiation.

To further complement the physical investigations, a number of thermographic measurements were carried out in adult volunteers exposed to a 20-min irradiation with conventional "baby warmers" in comparison with the wIRA radiator. Remarkably, with the conventional radiant warmers, an almost painful elevation of skin temperature by approx. 5 °C was attained at the end of the observation period, whereas the skin temperature only rose by approx. 2.5 °C with the wIRA radiator (at equal irradiances).

13.3.2 Clinical Observations

Clinical observations were focused on the changes in body surface temperature or on the maintenance of core temperature in term and preterm neonates subjected to either type of IR irradiation.

With regard to the *body surface temperature*, a thermographic study was performed on neonates who underwent routine examinations at a room temperature of 25 °C (i.e., without extra heat sources), under a conventional radiant heater (Weyer Ceramotherm 2000) or with the aid of a wIRA radiator (Hydrosun). At "pure" room temperature, a marked decrease in the mean body surface temperature occurred, reflecting the peripheral vasoconstriction of thermoregulating newborns. This could be prevented using radiant warmers, with the mean body surface temperature being slightly, but significantly higher in the conventional than in the wIRA group (Fig. 13.6). Although this result was biased by a slightly longer duration of examinations in the conventional IR than in the wIRA group, the study has once more demonstrated that the two types of IR irradiation differ in their surface effects. Incidentally, it has also shown that the calculation of a mean body surface temperature using a mathematical weighting algorithm is a valuable method for quantifying thermographic records.

With respect to *body core temperatures*, it was found that the use of two additional wIRA radiators as supplementary sources of heat did not alter the rectal temperature at the end of delivery room care, but still resulted in a smaller decrease in body temperature during the subsequent transport to the neonatal intensive care unit (Fig. 13.7). This implies that the heat deposits built up by wIRA irradiation in the depth of tissues exert a preventive effect against cooling, whereas the warming effect of conventional radiant warmers terminates as soon as the newborns are removed from the heat source.

In addition to these results, it has been shown that wIRA irradiation exhibits a lower absorption and better transmission rate through incubator walls so that the risk of heat-induced material damage is lower, and the thermoprotective effect of

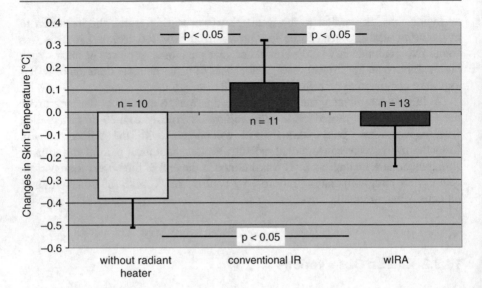

Fig. 13.6 Mean body surface temperature changes in term neonates subjected to routine clinical examinations without (room temperature, 25 °C) or with either conventional (Weyer) or wIRA radiators (Hydrosun; 15 mW/cm² in both cases). At room temperature, a marked decrease in the mean surface temperature is to be observed as an effect of peripheral vasoconstriction. This is prevented by heat radiators, with the mean body surface temperature for conventional IR irradiation being slightly but significantly higher than for wIRA irradiation

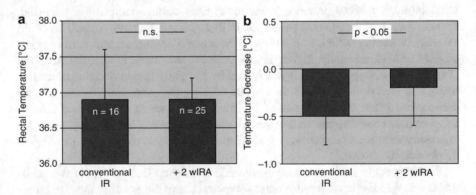

Fig. 13.7 Effective rectal temperature in preterm neonates after primary care in the delivery room (**a**), as compared with the temperature drop occurring during the subsequent incubator transport to the neonatal intensive care unit (**b**): Whereas the use of two wIRA radiators (in addition to the conventional radiant heater) did not lead to a measurable increase in rectal temperature at the end of delivery room care, the drop in temperature during the transport was significantly lower than after conventional IR irradiation alone. Apparently, the heat deposits built-up by wIRA irradiation in deeper tissue layers exert a preventive effect in terms of less subsequent cooling

wIRA radiators used as a "back-up" to incubator care is superior to that obtained with conventional infrared "lamps" (Hanau Sollux 750) [13].

13.4   Current Practice and Unresolved Issues

Based on these and other results, wIRA radiators have been introduced on many neonatal wards over the past few years where they are currently used as a supplementary source of heat for use during procedures which bear a risk of cooling (primary care in the delivery room, intensive care procedures with opened incubator doors). The possibility of supplying extra heat without an increased risk of superficial burns has greatly promoted the acceptance of this novel technology.

In contrast to the short-term use of wIRA radiators, their long-term use in neonatal care (as a continuous source of heat) has, however, so far been limited by two issues:

First, concerns have been raised that near-infrared irradiation might cause retinal damage due to its ability to penetrate the posterior chamber of the eye [17, 18]. However, no IR-related injury to the newborn eye has ever been reported [19], and computational models show that even when using a wIRA radiator at short distances, the respective irradiations would remain below critical limits [20]. Furthermore, animal studies on the use of wIRA irradiation as an adjunctive treatment for chlamydial eye infections found no evidence of retinal damage [21, 22], whereas conversely, near-infrared exposure has been shown to reverse age-related visual impairment [23, 24]. Thus, although further studies are needed on the potential impact of IR irradiation on the developing eye [25], there is currently no evidence of any adverse wIRA effects that would outweigh the risk of superficial burns induced by conventional radiant warmers.

Second, the cylindrical shape of currently used wIRA radiators results in a defined beam which differs from the rectangular irradiation area of ceramic or steel tube heaters designed to be mounted over diaper changing tables. Here, further research is necessary to examine whether the natural filtering effect of water might not be imitated by artificial materials, thus enabling a flatter design of radiant warmers without loss of the specific wIRA properties.

13.5   Summary and Conclusions

In summary, a series of physical investigations on agar phantoms and adult volunteers, as well as several clinical observations on term and preterm babies, have shown that wIRA irradiation has surprisingly different thermal effects as compared to conventional radiant warmers used in neonatal care. Due to its specific physical properties, resulting in an "enhanced depth effect with less surface overheating," it is especially suited as a supplementary source of heat under conditions where extra heat losses need to be replaced without an increased risk of burns. Provided some minor technical and biomedical issues are satisfactorily addressed, wIRA irradiation appears to have further potential for the thermal care of term and preterm neonates.

Acknowledgments The majority of the results presented in this chapter were obtained by Meike Schröder (Dr. med. Thesis, Göttingen 2000), Christina Aumann (Dr. med. Thesis, Göttingen 2001), Verena Löwe (Dr. med. Thesis, Würzburg 2009), and Ulrike Benninghoff, Dr. med. (Würzburg), within the context of their doctoral or postdoctoral work, respectively. Many thanks to all the undergraduate and graduate collaborators and to the nursing staff of the involved neonatal wards and intensive care units for their enthusiasm and efforts. The expert technical assistance of Ms. B. Hallmann, Göttingen, and Ms. E. Maurer, Würzburg, in the physical investigations and part of the clinical observations is gratefully acknowledged. This project had been initiated and funded by a grant from the Dr. med. h.c. Erwin Braun Stiftung, Basel, Switzerland.

References

1. Gekle M, Singer D. Wärmehaushalt und Temperaturregulation. In: Pape H-C, Kurtz A, Silbernagl S, editors. Physiologie. Stuttgart: Thieme; 2019. p. 570–87.
2. Okken A, Koch J, editors. Thermoregulation of sick and low birth weight neonates: temperature control, temperature monitoring, thermal environment. Berlin: Springer; 1995.
3. Agren J. The thermal environment of the intensive care nursery. In: Martin RJ, Fanaroff AA, Walsh MC, editors. Fanaroff & Martin's neonatal-perinatal medicine: diseases of the fetus and infant. 10th ed. Philadelphia: Elsevier Saunders; 2015. p. 502–12.
4. Singer D, van der Meer F, Perez A. What is the right temperature for a neonate? In: Herting E, Kiess W, editors. Innovations and frontiers in neonatology. Basel: Karger; 2020. p. 95–111.
5. Wilson E, Maier RF, Norman M, Effective Perinatal Intensive Care in Europe [EPICE] Research Group, et al. Admission hypothermia in very preterm infants and neonatal mortality and morbidity. J Pediatr. 2016;175:61–7.
6. Laptook AR, Bell EF, Shankaran S, NICHD (Neonatal Research Network), et al. Admission temperature and associated mortality and morbidity among moderately and extremely preterm infants. J Pediatr. 2018;192:53–59.e2.
7. Jacobs SE, Berg M, Hunt R, et al. Cooling for newborns with hypoxic ischaemic encephalopathy. Cochrane Database Syst Rev. 2013;2013(1):CD003311.
8. Wassink G, Davidson JO, Dhillon SK, et al. Therapeutic hypothermia in neonatal hypoxic-ischemic encephalopathy. Curr Neurol Neurosci Rep. 2019;19(2):2.
9. Flenady VJ, Woodgate PG. Radiant warmers versus incubators for regulating body temperature in newborn infants. Cochrane Database Syst Rev. 2003;4:CD000435.
10. McCall EM, Alderdice F, Halliday HL, et al. Interventions to prevent hypothermia at birth in preterm and/or low birth weight infants. Cochrane Database Syst Rev. 2018;2(2):CD004210.
11. Li S, Guo P, Zou Q, et al. Efficacy and safety of plastic wrap for prevention of hypothermia after birth and during NICU in preterm infants: a systematic review and meta-analysis. PLoS One. 2016;11(6):e0156960.
12. Vaupel P, Krüger W, editors. Wärmetherapie mit wassergefilterter Infrarot-A-Strahlung, Grundlagen und Anwendungsmöglichkeiten. 2nd ed. Stuttgart: Hippokrates; 1995.
13. Singer D, Schröder M, Harms K. Vorteile der wassergefilterten gegenüber herkömmlicher Infrarot-Strahlung in der Neonatologie. Z Geburtsh Neonatol. 2000;204:85–92.
14. Simonsen K, Graem N, Rothman LP, Degn H. Iatrogenic radiant heat burns in severely asphyxic newborns. Acta Paediatr. 1995;84:1438–40.
15. Ishida T, Kato H. Muscle equivalent agar phantom for 13.56 MHz RF-induced hyperthermia. Shimane. J Med Sci. 1980;4:134–40.
16. Visser AG, Deurloo IKK, Levendag PC, et al. An interstitial hyperthermia system at 27 MHz. Int J Hyperthermia. 1989;5:265–76.

17. Okuno T. Thermal effect of visible light and infra-red radiation (i.r.-A, i.r.-B and i.r.-C) on the eye: a study of infra-red cataract based on a model. Ann Occup Hyg. 1994;38:351–9.
18. International Electrotechnical Commission. International standard. Medical electrical equipment—part 2–21: particular requirements for the basic safety and essential performance of infant radiant warmers (IEC 60601–2-21). 3rd ed. Geneva: IEC; 2020.
19. Baumgart S, Knauth A, Casey FX, Quinn GE. Infrared eye injury not due to radiant warmer use in premature neonates. Am J Dis Child. 1993;147:565–9.
20. Piazena H. Ergebnisbericht zur Risikoanalyse gemäß DIN EN 62471 bei Anwendung eines Bestrahlungsgerätes zur lR-Hauttherapie des Typs hydrosun 750 mit BTE 595. Berlin: Persönl. Mittlg; 2017.
21. Rahn C, Marti H, Frohns A, et al. Water-filtered infrared A reduces chlamydial infectivity in vitro without causing ex vivo eye damage in pig and mouse models. J Photochem Photobiol B. 2016;165:340–50.
22. Kuratli J, Pesch T, Marti H, et al. Water filtered infrared A and visible light (wIRA/VIS) irradiation reduces *Chlamydia trachomatis* infectivity independent of targeted cytokine inhibition. Front Microbiol. 2018;9:2757.
23. Nelidova D, Morikawa RK, Cowan CS, et al. Restoring light sensitivity using tunable near-infrared sensors. Science. 2020;368(6495):1108–13.
24. Shinhmar H, Grewal M, Sivaprasad S, et al. Optically improved mitochondrial function redeems aged human visual decline. J Gerontol A Biol Sci Med Sci. 2020;75:e49–52.
25. Söderberg PG. Optical radiation and the eyes with special emphasis on children. Prog Biophys Mol Biol. 2011;107:389–92.

Part V

Clinical Practice: Dermatology

Water-Filtered Infrared A Irradiation in Wound Treatment

14

U. Lange, I. Aykara, and P. Klemm

14.1 Introduction

Water-filtered Infrared A (wIRA) irradiation is a special form of heat radiation which has high tissue penetration while delivering a low thermal load to the skin surface. wIRA increases tissue temperature, blood flow, oxygen partial pressure, and HbO_2 saturation in the treated tissue and may induce further non-thermal cellular effects. The range of applications is correspondingly large due to pain reduction, inhibition of inflammation and exudation, increase in local defense against infection, and regenerative properties. Therefore, wIRA is used to improve the healing of acute and chronic wounds. Even in non-critical wounds, wIRA accelerates the undisturbed "normal" wound healing and attenuates pain. The available evidence for wIRA in acute and chronic wounds is presented.

14.2 Historical Notes

At the Congress of the International Society on Oxygen Transport to Tissue (ISOTT) in Mainz, Germany, the successful effect of the therapeutic combination of hyperbaric oxygenation and local wIRA on chronic ulcers of the lower leg was presented for the first time by Hoffmann [1]. The concept of treating acute surgical wounds with wIRA was subsequently implemented in a randomized clinical trial, the results from which were published in 2006 [2].

U. Lange (✉) · I. Aykara · P. Klemm
Department of Rheumatology, Clinical Immunology, Osteology and Physical Medicine,
Justus-Liebig-University Giessen, Campus Kerckhoff, Bad Nauheim, Germany
e-mail: u.lange@kerckhoff-klinik.de

© The Author(s) 2022
P. Vaupel (ed.), *Water-filtered Infrared A (wIRA) Irradiation*,
https://doi.org/10.1007/978-3-030-92880-3_14

14.3 Basic Concepts and Mode of Action of wIRA

wIRA is a special form of infrared radiation in the range of 780–1400 nm. The water filter reduces radiation components within the infrared A, as well as most parts of the infrared B and C range, which are associated with undesired thermal side effects of the skin surface. Compared to conventional halogen radiators without water filtering (e.g., "red light lamps"), which emit approximately 50–80% of their radiation in the undesired, skin-damaging infrared B and C range, less than 0.5% of this potentially damaging irradiation is delivered with wIRA radiators. As a special form of infrared irradiation (thermal radiation), wIRA exhibits a high tissue penetration and significantly increased energy input alongside low thermal loads to the skin surface. A distinction is made between thermal (associated with heat energy transfer), temperature-independent (occurring without relevant temperature change), temperature-dependent (occurring with temperature change), and non-thermal (without relevant heat energy transfer) effects [3, 4].

The tissue temperature is increased by ≈ 6 °C superficially and by ≈ 2.7 °C at a tissue depth of 2 cm, the oxygen partial pressure is increased by 30% at 2 cm tissue depth, and the tissue perfusion is increased eightfold superficially with a lasting effect up to 5 cm tissue depth [3, 4].

It is well known that pain reduction elicited by wIRA results from both thermal and non-thermal effects. The increased blood flow better eliminates accumulated metabolites (including pain mediators, lactate, bacterial toxins), and metabolism is activated by the elevated tissue temperature (improved metabolism of accumulated substances and regeneration).

Non-thermal effects include direct effects on cells and cellular structures and substances, possibly also on pain receptors (nociceptors). It is known that wIRA causes significant muscle relaxation and associated reduction in pain, an improvement in the quality of life, and reduces the risk of local infections by increasing blood HbO_2 saturation and the tissue oxygen partial pressure [3, 4]. Irradiation with visible light (VIS) and wIRA presumably act in conjunction with endogenous protoporphyrin IX (or protoporphyrin IX from bacteria) and have a similar effect to mild photodynamic therapy by promoting cell regeneration and wound healing (old or pre-damaged cells are apoptotic and replaced by new cells) and having an antibacterial effect (photodynamic inactivation of bacteria) [3, 4]. The essential part of the antibacterial and antiviral effect is probably based on an improvement of the endogenous defense by increasing temperature, tissue perfusion, and oxygen partial pressure, as well as the associated provision of energy-rich substrates and oxygen (thermal wIRA effect). Presumably, this is combined with non-thermal wIRA effects on immunocompetent cells, resulting in an immunomodulatory effect and improved local immune defense [3, 4]. The limitation of wound inflammation is comparable to the pain reduction described above, i.e., via thermal as well as non-thermal effects. A reduction in wound secretion by wIRA may be explained by non-thermal, direct effects on cells [3, 4].

14.4   Clinical Application Aspects

wIRA is a non-contact, easy-to-use, and non-painful method which has good depth effects and establishes a prolonged heat depot. Further advantages of wIRA are maintenance of the blood circulation, hygienically clean application (compared to fango/mud), use in different body positions without fixation (compared to wraps), the possibility of combining with exercise, and adequate dose adaption by varying the irradiation time and distance. The irradiation distance should be chosen so that the irradiance is perceived as comfortable (subjective comfort distance usually between 35 and 80 cm). In patients with limited sensory perception (e.g., patients with diabetic polyneuropathy), impaired ability to respond, inadequately perfused tissue, cold tissues, or subcutaneous tissue (e.g., along the tibia ridge), a lower irradiation intensity (irradiance) should be used by increasing the radiator-patient distance.

The application of wIRA to wounds is by no means limited to wound-healing disorders. The "normal" unimpeded wound-healing process can also benefit from wIRA. In this setting, an accelerated and less painful wound healing with a good cosmetic result has been described.

Irradiation of the uncovered skin/wound is carried out vertically, for at least 60 min/day (some longer application times are possible, e.g., 2–6 h/day). The recommendation is to treat more frequently and longer with lower irradiances than shorter with higher irradiances until wound healing is completed. The wIRA irradiance for wounds is recommended to be 70 mW/cm². Wounds with reduced thermal tolerance of the irradiated tissue should be treated with 35 mW/cm². Based on extensive findings from many years of clinical experience, the use of wIRA with adequate irradiances can be considered to be safe [3–5].

14.5   wIRA for the Treatment of Acute and Chronic Wounds

Wound healing is a highly energy-consuming process, and energy production in the tissue depends on an adequate supply of oxygen and energy-rich substrates. Tissue temperature, perfusion, and oxygen partial pressure are therefore crucial factors, all of which are increased by wIRA.

Based on the current data, it can be concluded that wIRA accelerates the healing of acute and chronic wounds, including infected wounds, via thermal and temperature-dependent, non-thermal, and temperature-independent effects, as well as normal wound-healing processes. In this context, wIRA has pain-reducing (with reduced need for analgesics), anti-inflammatory, infection-reducing, wound secretion-reducing, and regeneration-promoting effects (reviewed in [3, 4]). In total, there have been seven prospective clinical studies (overview and details in [3, 4]) which demonstrate good wound healing with wIRA at the highest level of evidence (evidence level 1a/1b), six of which were randomized controlled trials.

14.5.1 Acute Wounds

14.5.1.1   Acute Abdominal Surgical Wounds

The effects of wIRA in acute wounds have been investigated in a prospective, randomized, controlled, double-blind study in 111 patients after abdominal surgery [2]. For this, wIRA was applied twice daily for 20 min (starting on the second postoperative day). In addition to a highly significant reduction in pain in the wIRA group compared to the control group (visible light, VIS) (acute pain reduction at 230 irradiations: 18.5 vs. 0 on a visual analog scale (VAS) of 0–100, $p < 0.000001$), a reduction in pain medication (52–59% less pain medication versus the control groups with VIS or peridural catheter analgesia only, $p = 0.00002/p = 0.00037$) was demonstrated. Upon irradiation with wIRA, the partial pressure of oxygen increased by 32% and the temperature by 2.7 °C in the 2 cm depth tissue, whereas no changes were recorded in the control group (42 vs. 30 mmHg, $p < 0.000001$; 38.9 vs. 36.4 °C, $p < 0.000001$). The surgeon's assessment of overall wound healing on a VAS scale of 0–100 was also significantly better in the group treated with wIRA (79 vs. 46.8 for the control, $p < 0.000001$), and the cosmetic result was comparable (84.5 vs. 76.5, $p < 0.0002$). Although not significant, there was a positive trend in favor of a lower rate of wound infections in the wIRA group ((3 of 46 (7%) vs. 7 of 49 (15%), $p = 0.21$)), including subsequent infections after discharge. Interestingly, there was a discernible trend toward a shorter postoperative inpatient stay in the wIRA group (9 vs. 11 days, $p = 0.02$). A key finding of this study was that postoperative irradiation with wIRA alone can also improve the normal wound-healing process.

14.5.1.2   Burn Wounds

A prospective, randomized, controlled, double-blind study investigated the effect of wIRA in 45 severely burn injured children (overview and details in [3, 4, 6]). Daily wIRA irradiation was applied for 30 min from day 1 of the burn injury. Irradiation with wIRA significantly increased the rate of wound area reduction and epithelialization (90% wound area reduction after 9 vs. 13 days, $p = 0.00001$) compared to control (VIS only). After 5 days, the physician decided whether surgical debridement of necrotic tissue was indicated or whether conservative therapy could be continued. Surgery was performed on 11 of 21 patients in the wIRA group and 14 of 24 in the control group. Furthermore, the wIRA group showed better results in the overall surgical assessment of the wound and with regard to the assessment of the irradiation effect versus the control (not significant, but tending to show better effects up to 3 months after the burn injury). However, a difference in *stratum corneum* formation between the 4 treatment arms was verified by laser scanning microscopy, especially for days 5–7. The fastest formation of the *stratum corneum* was seen in wounds treated with wIRA and dexpanthenol ointment, followed by wIRA alone. Analysis of wound bacterial counts performed every 2 days showed that wIRA and the combination of wIRA with dexpanthenol ointment prevented colonization with physiological skin bacteria by day 5 versus the other two treatment arms. Among other effects, bacterial colonization was more distinctively suppressed upon wIRA than following treatment with wIRA and dexpanthenol ointment.

14.5.1.3   Experimental Wounds

In this prospective randomized controlled trial, 4 experimental superficial wounds (each 5 mm in diameter) were induced in each of 12 subjects (overview and details in [3, 4]). Subsequently, 4 different therapies were applied for 10 days: (1) no treatment, (2) wIRA only with 30 min of irradiation daily, (3) dexpanthenol ointment only once daily, and (4) wIRA and dexpanthenol ointment once daily.

It was found that wound healing was very good from a clinical point of view with all four types of treatment. There were only small differences between these treatment options, with small advantages for the combination wIRA and dexpanthenol ointment and only for dexpanthenol ointment in terms of relative wound area changes.

14.5.1.4   Other Aspects and Perspectives in Acute Wounds

Reviews report on further positive effects of wIRA after endoprosthetic treatment of knee and hip joints [4, 6]. During the rehabilitation process, wIRA irradiation rapidly enhances the resorption of wound seroma and wound hematoma, which was objectively demonstrated clinically and sonographically. Pain relief was demonstrated in parallel.

Successful treatment with wIRA has been documented after urological surgery, with rapid wound healing and resorption of recurrent wound seroma. wIRA has also been shown to have a positive effect on wound healing after cesarean surgery. An amelioration of postoperative pain has also been successfully observed after thoracotomy.

14.5.2   Chronic Wounds

It is well known that the wound center is often hypoxic and relatively hypothermic and that this combination is unfavorable for wound healing. As optimal wound healing requires an adequate supply of energy-rich substrates and oxygen to the tissue, temperature, oxygen partial pressure, and blood flow are indispensable central factors in wound healing. Since wIRA irradiation increases temperature, tissue perfusion, and the tissue oxygen partial pressure, the wound healing is improved by wIRA application. The clinically beneficial effect is based, among other things, on an improved energy supply (increase in metabolic status) and oxygen supply [3, 4].

14.5.2.1   Chronic Venous Stasis Leg Ulcers

wIRA irradiation has positive effects on wound healing in three prospective, randomized, controlled clinical studies in patients with chronic venous stasis leg ulcers (overview and details in [3, 4]).

A Swiss study has shown significantly faster wound healing and a significantly lower need for analgesics in 40 patients with 3×30 min of wIRA irradiation over 6 weeks versus the control. Wound closure was objectifiable in the wIRA group after 14 days and in the control after 42 days ($p < 0.000005$). After 42 days, 19 of 20 (95%) of the wIRA group and 9 of 20 (45%) of the control showed completed wound healing ($p < 0.001$).

A Norwegian-Danish study [7] prospectively analyzed the effect of wound healing in 10 patients with thermographic follow-up. In 7 patients, the therapy resulted in complete or almost complete healing of the therapy-refractory chronic lower leg ulcers and in 2 other patients in a significant reduction of the ulcer size. In addition, pain relief with a substantially reduced need for analgesics was demonstrated. The thermographic picture typically showed a hyperthermic ulcer border, hypothermic wound center, and temperature differences up to 4.5 °C before the start of therapy, which normalized in the course of treatment. Of special interest are the results in a study participant, who had an ulcer on one leg treated with wIRA, and another ulcer on the other leg treated with VIS as control. There was a clear difference in favor of wIRA. Furthermore, a significant improvement in the effect of irradiation (reported by patient and examiner), assessment of wound healing (by the examiner), the cosmetic result (by patient and examiner), and an improved quality of life was demonstrated for the wIRA group (using a visual analogue scale).

In another prospective, randomized, controlled, blinded study involving 51 patients with non-healing chronic venous leg ulcers [8], there was a trend toward faster wound healing, better healing tendency, granulation, reduced exudation, and diminished wound coatings by combining compression treatment, wound cleaning and non-adhesive wound pad, and 30 min of wIRA irradiation (5 × 30 min per week for 9 weeks) versus control (VIS only).

A lower wound infection rate was observed after a single preoperative irradiation with wIRA (evidence level 1b). Wound infections occurred in 5.1% (9 of 178 patients) in the intervention group and in 12.1% (22 of 182 patients) in the control group ($p < 0.02$). A wound infection during postoperative days 9–30 was noted in 1.7% (3 of 178) of the irradiation group versus 7.7% (14 of 182) of the control group [9].

14.5.2.2   Other Indications

Indications for improved wound healing upon wIRA irradiation have been described in case reports for arterial-venous ulcers or arterial ulcers (at low irradiance), ulcers due to external pressure, i.e., decubitus ulcers (preventive and therapeutic with reduction of the wound area and better granulation of the wound area), diabetic foot (preventive and therapeutic, with thermographic proof of effect), healing of fistulas (in dentistry), and for improved absorption of topically applied substances on wounds (overview in [3, 4]).

14.5.3   Variable Irradiations Used in Different Studies

All studies listed above differed significantly in the wIRA application time. The latter ranged from 9 to 40 min/day, with one exception not exceeding 30 min/day. Interestingly, one study [5] recommended a significantly longer application time of up to 60 min/day, although this was also increased to up to 2–6 h/day. It was found that longer daily irradiations were associated with better effects on wound healing. Thus, more frequent and prolonged irradiations at low irradiances are preferable over shorter application times at higher irradiances.

It is possible that the therapeutic effects in the studies conducted can be further improved by longer irradiation times and this possibility should be considered in future studies.

14.5.4 Conclusions and Perspectives

Based on the data presented, the positive effects of wIRA-irradiation in wound treatment can be summarized as follows:

- wIRA is a useful therapeutic option recommended for the treatment of acute and chronic wounds. wIRA can provide significant pain relief with substantially reduced need for analgesics;
- wound exudation and inflammation are reduced;
- wound healing, clinical outcome, and cosmetic result are improved;
- wIRA application is reasonable before and after surgical procedures;
- wIRA is a positive adjunct to pre- or postoperative routine administration of antibiotics (under certain conditions, wIRA may even replace antibiotics, although this has not yet been evaluated);
- for chronic ulcers of the lower legs, wIRA is a positive adjunct to common therapies for wounds of various etiologies;
- wIRA can be used to improve the absorption of topically applied substances.

Furthermore, some perspectives for the implementation of wIRA-irradiation in wound-related indications have only been described in smaller studies or casuistics:

- preoperative wIRA (e.g., over 1–2 weeks) for preconditioning sites for removal and transplantation of skin grafts, transplants, and split-skin grafts;
- postoperative wIRA to promote wound healing and reduce pain, exudation, inflammation, and infection at the mentioned locations;
- wIRA as non-invasive alternative to the punction of wound seromas and wound hematomas, and to wound revisions;
- wIRA for prophylaxis and therapy of decubitus ulcers.

In conclusion, wIRA-irradiation offers a valuable therapeutic option in the overall therapy concept for the treatment of acute, chronic, infected, and burn wounds.

References

1. Hoffmann G. Improvement of wound healing in chronic ulcers by hyperbaric oxygenation and by water-filtered ultrared a induced localized hyperthermia. Adv Exp Med Biol. 1994;345:181–8.
2. Hartel M, Hoffmann G, Wente MN, et al. Randomized clinical trial of the influence of local water-filtered infrared a irradiation on wound healing after abdominal surgery. Br J Surg. 2006;93(8):952–60.

3. Hoffmann G. Wassergefiltertes Infrarot A in Chirurgie, Dermatologie, Sportmedizin und weiteren Bereichen. In: Krause R, Stange R, editors. Lichttherapie. Berlin, Heidelberg, New York: Springer; 2012. p. 25–54.
4. Hoffmann G. Clinical applications of water-filtered infrared-A (wIRA) – a review. Phys Med Rehab Kurort. 2017;27:265–74.
5. Winkel R, Hoffmann G, Hoffmann R. Wassergefiltertes Infrarot A (wIRA) hilft Wunden heilen. Chirurg. 2014;85(11):980–92.
6. Hartel M, Illing P, Mercer JB, et al. Therapy of acute wounds with water-filtered infrared-A (wIRA) (review). GMS Krankenhaushyg Interdiszip. 2007;2:DOC53.
7. Mercer JB, Nielsen SP, Hoffmann G. Improvement of wound healing by water-filtered infrared-A (wIRA) in patients with chronic venous stasis ulcers of the lower legs including evaluation using infrared thermography. GMS Ger Med Sci. 2008;6:Doc11.
8. Schumann H, Calow T, Weckesser S, et al. Water-filtered infrared A for the treatment of chronic venous statis ulcers of the lower legs at home: a randomized controlled blinded study. Br J Dermatol. 2011;165:541–51.
9. Künzli BM, Liebl F, Nuhn P, et al. Impact of preoperative local water-filtered infrared A irradiation on postoperative wound healing: a randomized patient- and observer-blinded controlled clinical trial. Ann Surg. 2013;258(6):887–94.

Clinical Application of wIRA Irradiation in Burn Wounds

15

A. S. Bingoel, S. Strauss, and P. M. Vogt

15.1 Introduction

The treatment of thermal injuries is challenging and is an area of significant, clinical need. Early operative interventions which reduce the burden of skin necrosis and the related morbidity are favored by most patients [1]. In some patients, early necrosectomy is not possible due to compromised general condition, whereas in others, burn wounds need more postoperative care. For these cases, conservative treatment options are on the rise to provide an ideal environment for wound healing, preoperatively as well as postoperatively.

In this context, the therapeutic potential of water-filtrated infrared-A irradiation (wIRA irradiation) in different surgical disciplines is well known [2, 3]. We use wIRA irradiation as additional therapy for burns, scalds, and chemically induced injuries as well as for treating patients with severe skin reactions such as toxic epidermal necrolysis (TEN) on a daily basis. This chapter provides an overview of our experience treating various thermal wound types with wIRA irradiation.

15.2 Pathophysiology of Thermal Injuries

Thermal injuries can derive from heat, hot fluids or steam, chemical irritants, electrical trauma, or cold. Severe skin reactions such as toxic epidermal necrolysis (TEN) can also be included in this framework. The skin, which consists of the epidermis and dermis, is affected by heat. An increased skin temperature of up to

A. S. Bingoel (✉) · S. Strauss · P. M. Vogt
Department of Plastic, Aesthetic, Hand and Reconstructive Surgery, Burn Center, Hannover Medical School, Hannover, Germany
e-mail: bingoel.alperen@mh-hannover.de; Vogt.Peter@mh-hannover.de

© The Author(s) 2022
P. Vaupel (ed.), *Water-filtered Infrared A (wIRA) Irradiation*,
https://doi.org/10.1007/978-3-030-92880-3_15

52 °C can be tolerated for a short period due to evaporation. However, if the temperature exceeds 69 °C for more than 1 s, cells of the skin are irreversibly damaged, with necrosis, with epidermolysis being the consequence [4]. A concept originally presented by Jackson in 1953 is still valid for the explanation of burn wound stages [5]. The center of a thermal wound shows a coagulation-related necrosis, whereas encircled areas present stasis with a mixture of vital and dead cells, constricted vessels, and ischemia. This area can be affected both positively and negatively and is at high risk of becoming necrotic if not treated meticulously. The outer, third zone shows a red appearance due to vasodilatation and is primarily not in danger of necrosis.

15.2.1 First-Degree Burns

First-degree burns appear as an erythema and are painful. There is no blistering, and the redness is caused by vasodilatation. A common trigger is a prolonged exposure to sunlight which damages the epidermis.

15.2.2 Second-Degree Burns

Second-degree burns are divided into superficial partial-thickness and deep partial-thickness burns, both associated with blistering of the skin due to epidermolysis and damage of several areas of the dermis. Whereas superficial partial-thickness burns primarily comprise vital dermis and are very painful, deep partial-thickness burns are characterized by a more injured dermis with a prolonged re-capillarization and less pain (Fig. 15.1).

Fig. 15.1 Hand with both superficial and deep partial-thickness burn wounds

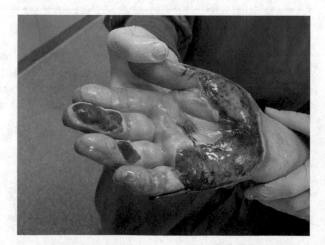

Fig. 15.2 Hand with
third-degree burn wounds

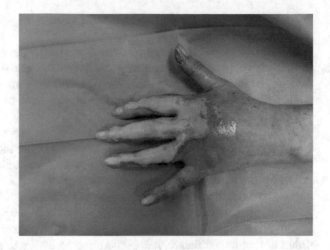

15.2.3 Third-Degree Burns

In third-degree burns, all skin layers are harmed and necrosis can extend to the muscles. There is no blistering, and wounds have a yellowish leather-like appearance (Fig. 15.2) which have to be treated surgically.

15.3   wIRA Irradiation in Thermal Injuries

15.3.1 Effects of wIRA Irradiation on the Skin

Several effects of wIRA irradiation on the skin have been reported [3]. These include the following reactions:

- increase in tissue temperature;
- improvement of tissue perfusion (blood flow); and
- increase in tissue oxygen partial pressure.

Blood flow and oxygen partial pressure in wounds are key features for a successful healing process. Cell proliferation and synthesis of proteins require energy that greatly depends to a major extent on the presence of oxygen [6]. Hypoxic conditions additionally decrease the capability of leukocytes to kill bacteria [7]. These problems are mostly linked to a compromised microcirculation [8]. Microcirculatory disturbances negatively affect wound healing because all above-mentioned key factors are decisively dependent on adequate tissue perfusion.

Reduced inflammatory reactions via modulation of the immune system have also been described. A reduced bacterial colonization in infectious wounds is noticeable in the clinical setting and evidence suggests that wIRA irradiation impairs bacterial colonization [9, 10].

15.3.2 wIRA Application in Thermal Wounds

Although first-degree burns can be treated with wIRA irradiation, such patients are most likely outpatients and are not necessarily hospitalized. wIRA irradiation therefore is primarily used for treating hospitalized patients with second- and third-degree thermal injuries, patients with frostbites, and in particular patients with infectious thermal wounds.

Patients with *superficial partial-thickness burns* are treated with topical polyhexanide ointment and wIRA irradiation 2–4 days after injuries. In these cases, we see quick-drying wounds with a fast-progressing re-epithelialization of the skin. After the onset of epithelialization, dexpanthenol-containing fatty ointments are applied to the skin after wIRA irradiation to further support wound healing [11].

The approach in *deep partial-thickness burns* is slightly different but can have an impact on the dimension of surgical procedures. In patients with poor general condition or multiorgan failure, it is sometimes necessary to postpone surgical procedures in order to stabilize patients with complex treatments on intensive care burn units. In these patients, we intend to preserve the perfusion of wound regions, not fully damaged according to Zone II [5], so that less extensive necrosectomies are necessary, and the risk for bacterial infections is reduced.

If patients are in good clinical condition and surgery can be performed safely, wIRA irradiation is applied preoperatively with the same intention as mentioned above. Postoperatively, wIRA is used for re-epithelialization of split-thickness skin graft donor sites [12].

Due to the capability of the wIRA irradiation to penetrate skin (and other materials), we also started to irradiate tie-over-bolsters in order to support the healing process of split-thickness grafts in the first 5 days after transplantation.

Although third-degree burns are usually dry and do not require wIRA irradiation, it can be used for the adjacent regions with minor degree burns.

The protocol used in this study administers 3–4 irradiation sessions for 30 min/day each, with the distance between the wIRA-radiator exit and targeted body region being set at 30 to 40 cm. Postoperatively, radiators are used for areas that were transplanted with split-thickness skin grafts. After removal of tie-over bolsters, irradiation is applied 3–4 times per day for 20–30 min each session. Treated grafts show a faster epithelialization of the fenestrated spots.

Frostbites are rare and primarily seen in homeless persons in regions with cold winters or in extreme athletes. Cell damage arises due to protein denaturation, dehydration, or formation of ice crystals. Endothelial damage might still continue even if the impact of cold can be stopped due to reperfusion injury (Fig. 15.3). Late ischemia with vasoconstriction and thrombosis impairs microcirculation with consecutive necrosis. Among other therapies, we also apply wIRA irradiation in these patients, albeit with mixed results.

In this context, other severe skin diseases such as toxic epidermal necrolysis are also treated. Here, large wound areas often require extended logistics and medical armamentarium of a specialized burn unit. Initial results appear promising; however, the rarity of these skin diseases impedes systemic analyses.

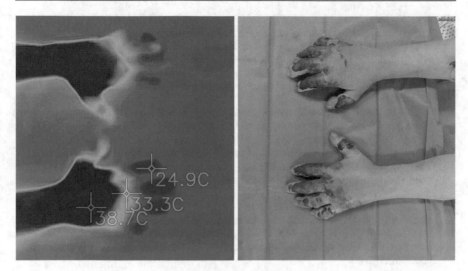

Fig. 15.3 Right: severe frostbites of the fingers. Left: Documentation with FLIR ONE thermography showing the colder parts

Although we have not yet been able to determine any significant reduction in the requirement for pain medication, as postulated earlier [13, 14], most patients report an enjoyable and comfortable warmth and a pleasant sense of relaxation during the application of wIRA.

15.4   Outlook to Further Research

Our preliminary in vitro data also show that wIRA irradiation induces the migration of adipose-derived stromal cells (ASCs). In scratch assays simulating wounds in a cell monolayer, ASCs lead to a faster wound closure after wIRA application compared to untreated or heat-treated controls. Further research is needed to understand the molecular mechanisms that are induced or mitigated/inhibited by wIRA irradiation.

References

1. Ong YS, Samuel M, Song C. Meta-analysis of early excision of burns. Burns. 2006;32(2):145–50.
2. Winkel R, Hoffmann G, Hoffmann R. Water-filtered infrared-A (wIRA) promotes wound healing. Chirurg. 2014;85(11):980–92.
3. Hoffmann G, Hartel M, Mercer JB. Heat for wounds - water-filtered infrared-A (wIRA) for wound healing - a review. Ger Med Sci. 2016;14:Doc08.
4. Herndon DN. Total burn care. 5th ed. Amsterdam: Elsevier; 2017.
5. Jackson DM. The diagnosis of the depth of burning. Br J Surg. 1953;40(164):588–96.
6. Schreml S, Szeimies RM, Prantl L, et al. Oxygen in acute and chronic wound healing. Br J Dermatol. 2010;163(2):257–68.

7. Allen DB, Maguire JJ, Mahdavian M, et al. Wound hypoxia and acidosis limit neutrophil bacterial killing mechanisms. Arch Surg. 1997;132(9):991–6.
8. Sorg H, Tilkorn DJ, Mirastschijski U, et al. Panta rhei: neovascularization, angiogenesis and nutritive perfusion in wound healing. Eur Surg Res. 2018;59(3–4):232–41.
9. Daeschlein G, Alborova J, Patzelt A, et al. Kinetics of physiological skin flora in a suction blister wound model on healthy subjects after treatment with water-filtered infrared-A radiation. Skin Pharmacol Physiol. 2012;25(2):73–7.
10. Kuratli J, Borel N. Perspective: water-filtered infrared-A-radiation (wIRA) - novel treatment options for chlamydial infections? Front Microbiol. 2019;10:1053.
11. Gorski J, Proksch E, Baron JM, et al. Dexpanthenol in wound healing after medical and cosmetic interventions (Postprocedure wound healing). Pharmaceuticals (Basel). 2020;13:7.
12. Aljasir A, Pierson T, Hoffmann G, Menke H. Management of donor site infections in split-thickness skin graft with water-filtered infrared-A (wIRA). GMS Interdiscip Plast Reconstr Surg DGPW. 2018;7:Doc03.
13. von Felbert V, Schumann H, Mercer JB, et al. Therapy of chronic wounds with water-filtered infrared-A (wIRA). GMS Krankenhhyg Interdiszip. 2008;2(2):Doc52.
14. Hartel M, Hoffmann G, Wente MN, et al. Randomized clinical trial of the influence of local water-filtered infrared A irradiation on wound healing after abdominal surgery. Br J Surg. 2006;93(8):952–60.

Influence of wIRA Irradiation on Wound Healing: Focus on the Dermis

16

N. Zöller and S. Kippenberger

Abbreviations

Bcl-2	B-cell lymphoma 2
LLLT	Low-level-light therapy
MMP 1	Matrix metalloproteinase 1
NIR	Near infrared
P1NP	N-terminal domain of procollagen type1
TGF-β1	Transforming growth factor β1
wIRA	Water-filtered infrared-A

16.1 Introduction

"Wound healing" describes a complex process which consists of tissue homeostasis, inflammation, proliferation, and scar-remodelling [1]. Development of chronic wounds, chronic inflammation, and aberrant scarring are the consequences of an imbalanced cell proliferation, cytokine secretion, and extracellular matrix synthesis and degradation. There are two types of aberrant scarring: *hypertrophic scars* and *keloid scars*. In contrast to hypertrophic scarring, keloid development is considered to have a genetic background, and scarring is not limited to the initial defect area. Physical restrictions, stigmatization, and chronic wounds are only some aspects that have a high impact on patients´ lives. Although a broad variety of treatment regimens, such as conservative approaches (e.g., compression therapy), invasive approaches (e.g., cryotherapy, surgical procedures, and laser ablation), and

N. Zöller (✉) · S. Kippenberger
Department of Dermatology, Venereology and Allergology, University Hospital Frankfurt,
Goethe University, Frankfurt/Main, Germany
e-mail: Nadja.Zoeller@kgu.de

© The Author(s) 2022
P. Vaupel (ed.), *Water-filtered Infrared A (wIRA) Irradiation*,
https://doi.org/10.1007/978-3-030-92880-3_16

combination therapies using pharmacological agents (e.g., glucocorticoids, chemotherapeutics and immunomodulators) are used, a high recurrence rate of keloids is observed [2]. Consequently, there remains a great need to develop alternative therapeutic options.

One of these options is the application of water-filtered infrared-A (wIRA) irradiation which is considered by the European Society for Hyperthermic Oncology (ESHO) to be an 'external non-contacting IR heating system'. wIRA is known for its high tissue penetration, reaching the subcutis without inducing harmful increases in skin surface temperature or pain. Clinical, pre-clinical, and in vitro studies have demonstrated its capacity to (a) influence cell metabolism, angiogenesis, thermoregulation, local blood flow, oxygen partial pressures, pain management, bacterial colonisation, total wound infection, and to (b) shorten healing time of acute and chronic wounds [1]. These aspects, together with a potential influence on collagen synthesis, support wIRA as being a promising therapeutic approach to treat hypertrophic scars, in particular keloids. In this study, we have compartmentalised and investigated the thermal and spectral components of wIRA separately and in combination with water bath heating.

16.2   Methods and Results

Aberrant scarring, sometimes solely initiated by micro-fissures, is characterised by an imbalanced wound healing. The treatment of aberrant scarring often results in secondary wounds, for example, after injection or surgical removal of scar tissue and might, therefore, trigger a recurrence. We have been interested in how wIRA irradiation may influence different aspects of aberrant scars, such as cell proliferation, migration, metabolic activity, and the synthesis and degradation of extracellular matrix proteins, specifically collagen type I. Our studies have focussed on investigating the influence of the spectral and thermal components of wIRA irradiation. Therefore, cells were either kept light-protected or were irradiated with 360 J/ cm^2 (780 nm–1400 nm; 106 mW/cm^2) using a wIRA radiator (Hydrosun® 750, Hydrosun Medizintechnik, Müllheim, Germany) equipped with an optical filter eliminating wavelengths <780 nm, for 56–120 min. During irradiation, samples were kept in a temperature-controlled water bath at 37–46 °C (Fig. 16.1).

16.2.1 Morphological Changes and Metabolic Activity

When considering potential new treatment regimens, investigations on cellular morphology, viability, and cytotoxicity are prerequisites. The rhomboid morphology of normal and keloid fibroblasts was not altered neither by the spectral component of wIRA nor by water bath heating up to 44 °C (Fig. 16.1). Independent of the fibroblast origin, the rhomboid cell shape changed to a more spherical shape after light-protected exposure to 46 °C. Fibroblast cells treated with the spectral component of wIRA at 46 °C were significantly less spherical. The lack of spherical cell

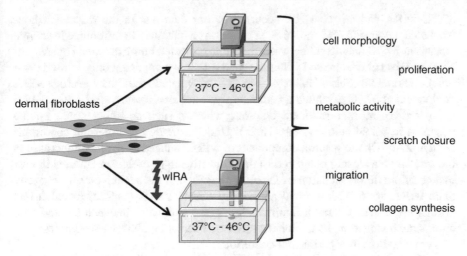

Fig. 16.1 Experimental setup and analysed parameters

morphology in the co-treated cultures might be associated with reverse pro-apoptotic effects, for example, by upregulating Bcl-2 (data not shown). The spectral wIRA component might antagonize mitochondrial membrane destabilisation, cytochrome C release, and consequently downregulate anoikis, a cell adhesion-dependent associated programmed cell death which is known to be induced (a) intrinsically through mitochondrial membrane permeabilization, as well as (b) extrinsically via death receptor signalling.

A moderate, exclusively temperature-dependent reduction of the metabolic activity without inducing cytotoxic effects was observed in all fibroblasts. Comparable effects have been observed after application of pulsed or prolonged hyperthermia by laser or convective heat [3, 4]. Therefore, it is unlikely that the in vitro observed reduced metabolic activity is clinically relevant.

16.2.2 Wound Closure

In normal fibroblast cultures, treatment is conducted with the spectral component of wIRA at 37 °C stimulated proliferation, as indicated by an increased incorporation of a thymidine analogue during mitosis, and an increase in the binucleate index, cytokinesis, and total cell number. Photo-documentation of the respective scratch closure additionally showed that the induced scratch closed faster in the wIRA at 37 °C exposed cultures compared to sham-irradiated cultures. These results indicated that the spectral component of wIRA promoted proliferation and migration without inducing pro-inflammatory cytokines and had only a moderate effect on the production of reactive oxygen species (ROS) [5]. Thereafter, we investigated whether scratch closure for normal and keloid fibroblasts differed. In a previous study we observed that wIRA differentially influenced normal and keloid fibroblasts under hyperthermic conditions [6]. Scratch closure in cultures exposed to

37 °C wIRA and 46 °C wIRA occurred earlier than that in the respective non-irradiated cultures (37 °C and 46 °C). There was a quantitative difference in scratch closure at 37 °C and 46 °C between the light-protected/non-irradiated (open symbols) and the cultures treated with the spectral wIRA-component only (closed symbols). Normal fibroblast cultures (Fig. 16.2a) treated with the spectral wIRA component at 37 °C exhibited a significantly faster area closure after 6 h and 12 h compared to the non-irradiated cultures, whereas such an effect could not be observed in keloid cultures (Fig. 16.2b). Under extreme hyperthermia conditions (wIRA at 46 °C), the spectral component of wIRA induced a significant increase in the scratch area closure compared to the respective light-protected cultures in normal or keloid fibroblast cultures. Direct comparison of the scratch closure capacity upon wIRA at 46 °C in normal and keloid fibroblasts (Fig. 16.2c) revealed that normal fibroblasts covered a significantly larger scratch area between 6 h and 36 h after scratch induction than keloid fibroblasts. Thereafter, almost the complete area was covered in both experimental conditions.

In the studies presented, wound-healing velocity was likewise influenced after treatment with the spectral component of wIRA under hyperthermic (40–46 °C) and normothermic conditions (37 °C). It has previously been reported that irradiation with different irradiances (doses) of low-intensity red light (dominant wavelength 628 nm) upregulates genes involved in proliferation [7]. Another indicator supporting wIRA treatment is that under various thermal conditions, wavelengths of the NIR spectrum and LLLT influence mitochondrial mass, mitochondrial membrane

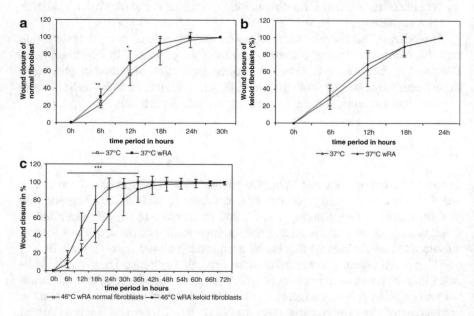

Fig. 16.2 Scratch closure of normal and keloid fibroblasts depending on wIRA-irradiation. Quantitative analysis of the wound closure of normal fibroblasts (**a**) and keloid fibroblasts (**b**). Comparison of scratch closure of normal (cross) and keloid (dot) fibroblasts after wIRA irradiation at 46 °C (**c**). * $p \leq 0.05$, ** $p \leq 0.01$ compared to non-irradiated control cultures (**a, b**) *** $p \leq 0.001$ compared to irradiated normal fibroblast cultures (**c**)

potential, and moderate ROS-induction, all of which are likely responsible for pro-liferation and the induction of migration [5, 8].

16.2.3 Extracellular Matrix Synthesis

As described above, the thermal component of the wIRA irradiation was eliminated and all applied thermal stimuli were exclusively administered using a temperature-controlled water bath. This enabled the influence of the spectral component of wIRA irradiation to be separated from its thermal component. As described in Sect. 16.2.2 that normal fibroblasts close an artificial wound faster than keloid fibroblasts after treatment with the spectral component of wIRA, it is also important to validate the synthesis of the extracellular matrix, which is closely balanced under physiolog-ical conditions. Monitoring collagen synthesis is an important criterion for develop-ing a possible keloid therapy. As a consequence, we assessed the dependence of collagen type I synthesis in normal and keloid fibroblast on the spectral and/or the thermal components of wIRA [6]. As depicted in Fig. 16.3, keloid fibroblasts (black columns) can be clearly distinguished from normal fibroblasts (white columns) due to higher collagen synthesis. Whereas collagen type I synthesis of normal fibro-blasts was neither influenced by the spectral component of wIRA nor by increasing the water-bath temperature during treatment from 37 °C up to 44 °C; a distinct decrease of the collagen type I concentration was observed in keloid fibroblast cul-tures that had been treated at 44 °C. At the latter temperature, there was no difference between the hyperthermia treatment (44 °C) and the co-treatment (wIRA

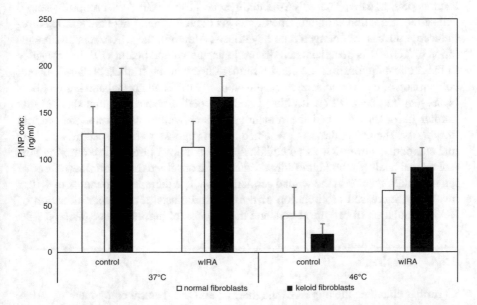

Fig. 16.3 Comparison of collagen type I synthesis of normal and keloid fibroblasts

at 44 °C). Increasing the water-bath temperature to 46 °C significantly reduced collagen type-I synthesis in normal and keloid fibroblasts (Fig. 16.3). The relative reduction of collagen type I synthesis of keloid fibroblasts after treatment at 46 °C was four times higher than the observed reduction in normal fibroblasts. Collagen type I synthesis in cells exposed to wIRA at 46 °C was partially reconstituted. The restored collagen type I synthesis remained proportionally lower than the collagen type I synthesis of the normal fibroblasts under these conditions.

Further investigations focussing on transforming growth factor-β1 (TGF-β1), a well-known promoter of collagen synthesis, revealed a temperature-related reduction of TGF-β1 secretion in normal and in keloid fibroblasts. In keloid fibroblasts, this temperature-induced reduction in secretion was completely restored in cultures exposed to wIRA at 46 °C. In our studies, we observed neither a temperature nor a spectral wIRA component-related effect on the secretion of the matrix metalloproteinase-1 (MMP-1).

16.3 Conclusions

The rationale for the treatment of hypertrophic scars/keloids is (a) to increase the catabolism of extracellular matrix proteins and their de novo synthesis and (b) to inhibit cells, especially fibroblasts, that are responsible for their synthesis in order to regain a physiological equilibrium. The results presented indicate that applying moderate to extreme hyperthermia with wIRA qualifies as a potential approach due to its capacity to inhibit TGF-β1 secretion. This in turn influences signal transduction pathways which impact migration, proliferation, and collagen type I synthesis, such as p38, MAPK. The wIRA-related rescue of the TGF-β1 secretion in keloid cells after incubation at high temperatures is not able to neutralize the temperature-induced reduction of collagen type I synthesis. Although the wIRA-related upregulation of TGF-β1 is beneficial and desirable during wound healing [9], its relevance in the clinical application in keloid treatment needs to be further validated. Direct comparison of the wound/scratch closure capacity between normal and keloid fibroblasts that had been wIRA irradiated under hyperthermic conditions showed that normal fibroblasts reduced the remaining scratch/wound area faster than keloid fibroblasts. Therefore, the data presented herein suggest both the spectral and thermal components of wIRA as potential adjuvant therapy options for promoting normal wound healing after keloid surgery due to the observed differential responses of the fibroblast species in the wound scratch assay. The therapeutic benefits of wIRA involve an increased proliferation of normal fibroblasts, a moderate induction of ROS, stimulation of cell migration, and the low risk of thermal tissue damage.

16.4 Outlook

To further elucidate the impact of the thermal and the spectral component of wIRA as an anti-fibrotic therapy regimen, it is advisable to employ more complex systems such as tissue cultured skin equivalents [10], which might be adapted to represent scar tissue to monitor extracellular matrix structure and morphological and biochemical properties of the cells. Additionally, ex vivo explants and long-term analysis of the above-described treatment regimen are planned in order to further discriminate between the relevant factors in normal and diseased cells. Considering a broad experience concerning the development of phytochemically based photodynamic treatment regimens, we are currently investigating the influence of photosensitizers in combination with wIRA irradiation on benign keloid fibroblasts, other neoblastic cells, and their normal counterparts. These studies are focussing on the signalling pathways that are involved in proliferation, migration, apoptosis, anoikis, cell cycle progress, and autophagy.

Acknowledgments Dr. Anke König, Dr. Gabi Reichenbach, Anne Jeute, and Svenja Missalla contributed to the results described in this article.

References

1. Velnar T, Bailey T, Smrkolj V. The wound healing process: an overview of the cellular and molecular mechanisms. J Int Med Res. 2009;37(5):1528–42. https://doi.org/10.1177/147323000903700531.
2. Danielsen PL, Rea SM, Wood FM, et al. Verapamil is less effective than triamcinolone for prevention of keloid scar recurrence after excision in a randomized controlled trial. Acta Derm Venereol. 2016;96(6):774–8. https://doi.org/10.2340/00015555-2384.
3. Dams SD, de Liefde-van BM, Nuijs AM, et al. Pulsed heat shocks enhance procollagen type I and procollagen type III expression in human dermal fibroblasts. Skin Res Technol. 2010;16(3):354–64. https://doi.org/10.1111/j.1600-0846.2010.00441.x.
4. Kalamida D, Karagounis IV, Mitrakas A, et al. Fever-range hyperthermia vs. hypothermia effect on cancer cell viability, proliferation and HSP90 expression. PLoS One. 2015;10:e0116021. https://doi.org/10.1371/journal.pone.0116021.
5. König A, Missalla S, Valesky EM, et al. Effect of near-infrared photobiomodulation therapy in a cellular wound healing model. Photodermatol Photoimmunol Photomed. 2018;34(4):279–83. https://doi.org/10.1111/phpp.12390.
6. Zöller N, König A, Butting M, et al. Water-filtered near-infrared influences collagen synthesis of keloid-fibroblasts in contrast to normal foreskin fibroblasts. J Photochem Photobiol B. 2016;163:194–202. https://doi.org/10.1016/j.jphotobiol.2016.08.020.
7. Zhang Y, Song S, Fong CC, et al. cDNA microarray analysis of gene expression profiles in human fibroblast cells irradiated with red light. J Invest Dermatol. 2003;120(5):849–57. https://doi.org/10.1046/j.1523-1747.2003.12133.x.
8. Shingyochi Y, Kanazawa S, Tajima S, et al. Low-level carbon dioxide laser promotes fibroblast proliferation and migration through activation of Akt, ERK, and JNK. PLoS One. 2017;12(1):e0168937. https://doi.org/10.1371/journal.pone.0168937.
9. Danno K, Mori N, Toda K, et al. Near-infrared irradiation stimulates cutaneous wound repair: laboratory experiments on possible mechanisms. Photodermatol Photoimmunol Photomed. 2001;17(6):261–5. https://doi.org/10.1034/j.1600-0781.2001.170603.x.
10. Zöller NN, Kippenberger S, Thaçi D, et al. Evaluation of beneficial and adverse effects of glucocorticoids on a newly developed full-thickness skin model. Toxicol In Vitro. 2008;22(3):747–59. https://doi.org/10.1016/j.tiv.2007.11.022.

Water-Filtered Infrared A Irradiation: From Observations in Clinical Studies to Complex In Vitro Models

17

C. Wiegand, J. Tittelbach, U. -C. Hipler, and P. Elsner

17.1 Clinical Effectiveness of wIRA in the Treatment of Warts

Water-filtered infrared-A (wIRA) irradiation is characterized by deep-reaching thermal effects with comparatively low level of heat-induced pain on the skin surface using typical irradiances (60–120 mW/cm^2) [1, 2]. wIRA has been successfully employed in a broad range of areas including physiotherapy, sports medicine, internal medicine, pediatrics, as adjuvant therapy in radiation oncology, as well as in the treatment of chronic and acute wounds [3], and also for antimicrobial treatment ± photodynamic therapy (aPDT) [4, 5]. Previous studies have reported PDT to be efficient in warts [6, 7].

Warts are a common skin condition with an overall prevalence of 2.4–12.9% which are caused by the human papillomavirus (HPV) [8, 9]. Warts seriously impair quality of life due to possible functional impairment, pain, and unsightly appearance. As well as having a physical impact, the concern that warts might spread and/ or lead to infections in other people has a negative psychological impact [9]. Although warts most commonly involve hands and feet, they can affect other areas of the skin including anogenital regions where they can manifest as sexually transmitted infections [8, 9]. Additional manifestations of HPV-associated diseases include several genital or upper respiratory/digestive malignancies such as cervical, vaginal, vulvar, penile, anal, and oropharyngeal cancers [8], the latter of which have been in the focus of most investigators in the HPV field [8]. In contrast, Fuchs et al. [4] have concentrated on the therapy of common warts (*verrucae vulgares*) and reported on the first prospective randomized controlled blind trial of PDT and wIRA in the treatment of recalcitrant common hand and foot warts. Although different therapeutic regimens for common warts have been described earlier, there is a lack of a single striking treatment strategy with high efficacy and little side-effects.

C. Wiegand (✉) · J. Tittelbach · U. -C. Hipler · P. Elsner
Department of Dermatology, University Hospital Jena, Jena, Germany
e-mail: C.Wiegand@med.uni-jena.de

© The Author(s) 2022
P. Vaupel (ed.), *Water-filtered Infrared A (wIRA) Irradiation*,
https://doi.org/10.1007/978-3-030-92880-3_17

Standard therapies such as cryotherapy or electrosurgery are invasive, cause burns, blisters, local irritation, itching, bleeding, infection, ulcers, and scarring, and/or are painful, because of which they are traumatizing for patients, especially for young children [4]. Although applying local hyperthermia (44 °C/30 min) has been successfully used for treating common and facial warts, side effects include burning sensations, blister formation, and subsequent hyperpigmentation [10]. No such side effects have been reported using a wIRA radiator (type 501; Hydrosun®, Müllhein, Germany) [4], most probably because IR-A components, which would typically cause unwanted thermal stress and a stinging and burning sensation in the skin by interactions with water molecules, are reduced by a water filter [11]. A combination of wIRA and 5-ALA based PDT has been used for treating actinic keratosis and basal cell carcinoma [5] and some patients with HPV-induced palmar and plantar warts [4]. PDT involves the excitation of a photosensitizer with VIS of 380–780 nm and the subsequent interaction of this with cellular lipids and proteins, either without oxygen (photooxidative reaction type I) or with oxygen (photooxidative reaction type II) [12]. 5-ALA is endogenously transformed into the photosensitizer, protoporphyrin IX by proliferating cells in the skin [6, 12]. The study by Fuchs et al. [4] showed that wIRA irradiation, either with or without 5-ALA-based PDT, significantly reduced recalcitrant foot and hand warts. Furthermore, wIRA distinctly increased the percentage of cleared warts compared to patients receiving the standard treatment scheme (including keratolysis and curettage as pre-treatment and retinoic acid ointment as post-treatment) alone, as well as completely curing some patients. Importantly, no scars or skin side effects were observed, and patients reported no disturbance of function after treatment [4]. Both, thermal and non-thermal effects may explain the wIRA effect. The increase in tissue temperature directly inactivates the thermolabile human papillomaviruses. Indeed, temperature rises above 42 °C have been shown to induce changes in the apolipoprotein B mRNA-editing catalytic polypeptide (APOBEC) 3 proteins, which are potent viral DNA mutators and feature broad antiviral activity [13]. wIRA hyperthermia might also indirectly activate tissue metabolism and may have immunomodulatory effects such as improving the local immune competence of the patient. Non-thermal effects of infrared radiation such as direct stimulation of cells [14], induction of cell growth towards infrared sources [15], and influences on cellular components, such as cytochrome c [16], have also been reported.

17.2   In Vivo and In Vitro Antibacterial Effects of wIRA

The emergence of antibiotic-resistant gram-positive and gram-negative bacteria is considered a global health problem due to the diminishing availability of antibiotics to treat these infections. Nonchemical treatments for infectious diseases using strategies such as local wIRA hyperthermia are being explored [17], as various bacterial species display thermo-sensitivity [18]. The effectiveness of wIRA treatment on infections with *Chlamydia pecorum* and *Chlamydia trachomatis* has been demonstrated in vitro using animal and human cell culture models [17]. Heat treatment has further been proven to be beneficial for *Leishmania*-induced skin lesions and *Mycobacterium ulcerans* (reviewed in [17]). wIRA irradiation in antimicrobial photodynamic therapy (aPDT) combined with toluidine blue as photosensitizer has been reported to be successful against the oral bacteria associated with the development of periodontitis, *Streptococcus mutans,* and *Enterococcus faecalis* [19]. Another wIRA study investigating the effect of PDT using the photosensitizer chlorine e6 on periodontal pathogens and subgingival biofilms in situ has demonstrated a distinct reduction of bacteria and oral biofilms [20]. Furthermore, wIRA irradiation alone has been shown to have beneficial effects on wound infections after abdominal surgery [21].

17.3   Treatment of Wounds and Wound Infections with wIRA

Several physical procedures are currently promoted as an "enhancer" of the treatment of wound infections, including cold atmospheric plasma, electrostimulation, laser therapy and extracorporeal shock wave therapy, and wIRA irradiation [22]. It is important that a distinction is made as to whether the antimicrobial effect is through killing bacteria and/or achieved by promotion of wound healing. Elimination of bacteria in the infected wound can support favorable outcomes, as is seen with a classic antibiosis [22]. A possible, endogenous PDT-like effect has been discussed for wIRA, since VIS and wIRA irradiation could interact with endogenous protoporphyrin IX or protoporphyrin IX of bacteria, and therefore could additionally support wound healing by evoking antibacterial effects [1]. However, direct antimicrobial effects by wIRA on non-thermosensitive bacteria have not yet been reported [23]. Hence, it is more likely that wIRA exerts its beneficial effects in wound infections by promoting the factors that are decisive for healing (e.g., tissue perfusion) and combating germs (e.g., increase in phagocytosis) in the wound environment [22]. Indeed, it has been reported that wIRA irradiation leads to an increase in local temperature [21, 24], in tissue blood flow [24] and in oxygen partial pressure [21]. These effects substantially support the healing process, especially in chronic wounds which are typically ischemic, hypoxic, and hypothermic [25]. wIRA also has non-thermal effects which are based on direct stimulation of cells and cellular structures by IR-irradiation. These effects comprise stimulation of wound repair [26], cell protection events [27], target-oriented growth of neurons [15], and possible effects on pain receptors [21]. Consequently, inflammation, pain, and the required dose of pain medication are reduced [2]. Overall, wIRA irradiation has a positive impact on wound healing, shortens the time to complete wound closure, and thereby can curtail hospitalization [23].

17.4   Investigation of wIRA Effects Using In Vitro Models

Wound healing is a complex process which involves different epidermal and dermal cell types, as well as leukocytes, all of which are coordinated by cytokines and growth factors. The primary focus is on fibroblasts, as they are involved in the production of extracellular matrix, and thus rebuild new tissue in the wound area [26], and keratinocytes which participate in the inflammatory reaction and ultimately close the injured area by epithelization [28]. Given the positive effects on wound healing by VIS-therapy (visible light-therapy), it is of interest to investigate the effects of VIS-therapy on cell viability and cell proliferation during wound healing, and also on cell migration. Zöller et al. [29] have treated foreskin and keloid fibroblasts with convective heat and/or wIRA to assess the potential of these as treatments for keloids and hypertrophic scars. They found a temperature-dependent induction of a spherical cell shape, a reduction of collagen type-I synthesis, and decreased TGF-β1 secretion in the fibroblasts. Although wIRA irradiation had no influence on MMP-1, it restored original cell morphology in foreskin fibroblasts and collagen type-I synthesis, and TGF-β1 secretion in keloid fibroblasts [29]. Knels et al. [30] evaluated wIRA for the treatment of oxidative stress in cells which is found in elderly or diabetic patients. For this, they exposed fibroblast cultures to glyoxal to induce glycation of proteins and lipids to mimic oxidative stress and determined their rescue from apoptotic cell death by wIRA. They found that wIRA irradiation diminished the effects of glyoxal-induced stress, such as ROS-production, translocation of phosphatidylserine, and DNA-fragmentation, which are considered main events of cell apoptosis, while being well tolerated by the cultured fibroblasts [30]. Wound healing is mostly investigated in vitro based on the direct measurement of cell migration and regeneration of the cell layer after mechanical damage to confluent cell layers (scratch wound assay) [31] (Fig.17.1). Cells that have been successfully used in this assay include HaCaT keratinocyte cells, primary epidermal keratinocytes, and primary dermal fibroblasts. Preliminary studies into wIRA effects on wound closure in vitro have shown distinct differences in responses of a wounded HaCaT keratinocyte monolayer after a 10-min treatment compared to the untreated control and heat treatment alone (Fig. 17.1). Cell migration started earlier in wIRA-irradiated cells (Fig. 17.1, middle column) in contrast to untreated cells (Fig. 17.1, left column), whereas heating cells for 10 min in order to induce the same temperature rise in the cells as induced by the wIRA irradiation delayed the healing process (Fig. 17.1, right column). Although, cellular processes induced and mediators involved remain to be elucidated, it is apparent that the observed clinical benefits of wIRA on wound healing can be investigated in vitro using adequate models and experimental settings, thereby allowing further clarification of the underlying biological effects. Several researchers have stressed that temperature changes need to be strictly controlled in vitro in order to distinguish between thermal and non-thermal effects of wIRA [32, 33]. In contrast to skin models or patient's skin in vivo, in cell culture models there is only one cell monolayer and the protective epidermis or temperature control by blood circulation is missing [31, 32]. To evaluate exclusively non-thermal effects of wIRA irradiation, it is necessary to keep the temperature constant during the experiment [32, 33]. Accordingly, Jung et al. [34] tested the effects of wIRA on the generation of reactive oxygen species (ROS) in human dermal fibroblasts. They showed that ROS formation is heat-dependent and not induced by the irradiation alone as long as the temperature was kept constant. Temperature measurements were performed directly on the cell layers with

Fig. 17.1 Regeneration of the cell layer in the scratch wound assay with human HaCaT keratinocytes (1) untreated, (2) irradiated with wIRA for 10 min and (3) exposed to comparable temperatures heating (without wIRA irradiation). Images were obtained using the JuLI™ Br Live Cell Analyzer (Peqlab, Erlangen, Germany)

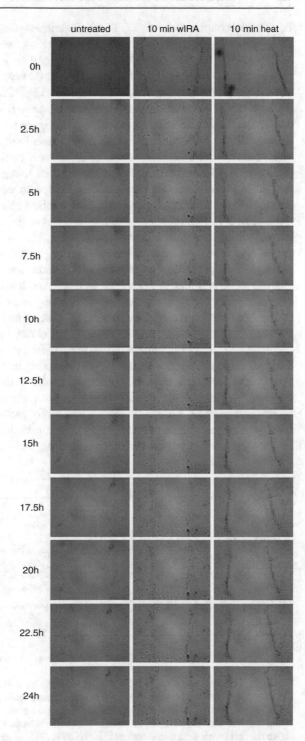

thin thermocouples (type K, TC Direct, Mönchengladbach, Germany) to establish an in vivo like experimental set-up. For the wIRA treatment in the wound healing assays, cell dishes were exposed to different experimental conditions (Fig. 17.2a–c). The results were compared to the temperature curve during a local wIRA irradiation for 10 min on the forearm of a volunteer (Fig. 17.2d). A temperature rise from 34 °C to 42 °C at a skin depth of 1 mm was observed. The cells on the heating plate experienced a drastic increase in temperature since the surface of the plate is additionally heated by wIRA irradiation. In contrast, the temperature in the water bath with constant water exchange could be effectively controlled during the wIRA irradiation [33]. The increase in temperature when using a water bath without water exchange was comparable to the locally treated forearm of the volunteer, thereby confirming in vitro experiments on wound healing effects under in vivo-like conditions. However, in this experimental set-up, it is imperative to include control experiments which simulate increases in temperature to distinguish between effects caused by the wIRA treatment and pure warming of the sample, as they might occur during a clinical application of infrared A irradiation. In this way, it is possible to analyze more complex systems such as tissue models consisting of different layers of different cell types. In these samples, warming due to wIRA absorption cannot be avoided or reliably excluded by cooling [32]. Such an experimental regime is a prerequisite for morphological investigations in 3D cell cultures to ensure close simulation of the in vivo conditions. It is known that cell behavior in 2D systems is different from that in their natural 3D environment in vivo. For instance, fibroblasts very quickly reach confluence in monolayers due to the high proliferation rate, and they show a biosynthetic capacity that does not correspond to the situation in vivo. In 3D collagen gels, fibroblasts show a lower biosynthetic activity and have a regulated growth and degree of differentiation that imitates the in vivo situation. Thus, 3D cell cultures represent an intermediate between 2D monolayer cultures and

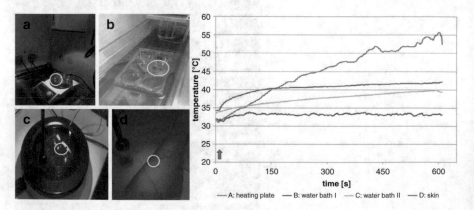

Fig. 17.2 Experimental set-ups for wIRA application on cell layers in vitro: (**a**) with the cell dishes either placed on a heating plate, (**b**) in water bath I with a slow water exchange, and (**c**) in water bath II without water exchange. Results were compared to the local wIRA irradiation for 10 min on the forearm of a volunteer (**d**). Temperature measurements were performed directly above the cell layers with thin thermocouples (type K, TC Direct, Mönchengladbach, Germany)

pre-clinical animal models and are already a viable alternative to animal experiments in some areas of application. Full (3D) skin models are used to test the cytotoxic effects of substances or treatments, as well as their influence on the cellular behavior. Reconstructed human epidermis (RHE) models are often utilized for this purpose and misleadingly referred to as skin models. Although these RHE models show a 3D structure of the epidermis of keratinocytes, they lack a dermal component, and therefore a corresponding interaction with local fibroblasts. 3D skin models consisting of a collagen matrix populated with primary human fibroblasts as the dermis and a completely differentiated epidermis made of primary human keratinocytes are also referred to as "full skin models." Preliminary experiments have shown that wIRA treatment has no negative effects on the morphology in a 3D skin model (Fig. 17.3). In the epidermis, the undifferentiated basal keratinocytes express the keratins 5 (ck5) and 14 (ck14), whereas the cells in the upper epidermis switch to the expression of the keratin pair 1/10 (ck10) specific for differentiation [35]. Keratins are the main structural proteins in epithelial cells, in which they form a cytoplasmic network of 10–12 nm thick intermediate filaments [36]. Markers for the terminal differentiation of the keratinocytes to corneocytes (horn cells) of the stratum corneum are involucrin (IVL), a soluble precursor protein of the horny cell layer, and filaggrin (FLG), the aggregation protein of the keratin filaments in the horny cell layer [37, 38]. Changes in the composition and expression of such structural proteins have been associated with various skin diseases. Fibroblasts in the dermis can be detected by staining the cytoskeletal protein vimentin (VIM), a type-III intermediate filament protein. The detection of proliferating cells is possible using the marker Ki67 [39].

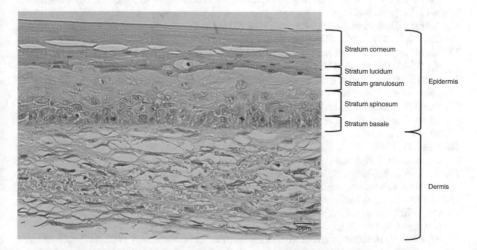

Fig. 17.3 The 3D skin model shows the normal dermis structure as well as differentiated epidermal layers after wIRA irradiation for 10 min. No negative effects on dermal or epidermal components by wIRA irradiation were noted

References

1. von Felbert V, Schumann H, Mercer JB, et al. Therapy of chronic wounds with water-filtered infrared-A (wIRA). GMS Krankenhhyg Interdiszip. 2008;2(2):Doc52.
2. Hartel M, Illing P, Mercer JB, et al. Therapy of acute wounds with water-filtered infrared-A (wIRA). GMS Krankenhhyg Interdiszip. 2007;2(2):Doc53.
3. Hoffmann G. Klinische Anwendungen von wassergefiltertem Infrarot A (wIRA) – eine Übersicht. Phys Med Rehab Kuror. 2017;27:265–74.
4. Fuchs SM, Fluhr JW, Bankova L, et al. Photodynamic therapy (PDT) and waterfiltered infrared a (wIRA) in patients with recalcitrant common hand and foot warts. Ger Med Sci. 2004;2:Doc08.
5. Foss P. Einsatz eines patentierten, wassergefilterten Infrarot-A Strahlers (Hydrosun) zur photodynamischen Therapie aktinischer Dyskeratosen der Gesichts- und Kopfhaut. Z naturheilkundl Onkologie krit Komplementärmed. 2003;6(11):26–8.
6. Fabbrocini G, Di Costanzo MP, Riccardo AM, et al. Photodynamic therapy with topical delta-aminolaevulinic acid for the treatment of plantar warts. J Photochem Photobiol B. 2001;61(1–2):30–4.
7. Stender IM, Na R, Fogh H, et al. Photodynamic therapy with 5-aminolaevulinic acid or placebo for recalcitrant foot and hand warts: randomised double-blind trial. Lancet. 2000;355(9208):963–6.
8. Piguet V. Heat-induced editing of HPV genes to clear mucocutaneous warts? J Invest Dermatol. 2017;137(4):796–7.
9. Kyriakis K, Pagana G, Michailides C, et al. Lifetime prevalence fluctuations of common and plane viral warts. J Eur Acad Dermatol Venereol. 2007;21(2):260–2.
10. Hu L, Qi R, Hong Y, et al. One stone, two birds: managing multiple common warts on hands and face by local hyperthermia. Dermatol Ther. 2015;28(1):32–5.
11. Winkel R, Hoffmann G, Hoffmann R. Wassergefiltertes Infrarot A (wIRA) hilft Wunden heilen. Chirurg. 2014;85(11):980–92.
12. Wolf P. Photodynamic therapy in dermatology: state of the art. J Eur Acad Dermatol Venereol. 2001;15(6):508–9.
13. Yang Y, Wang H, Zhang X, et al. Heat increases the editing efficiency of human papillomavirus E2 gene by inducing upregulation of APOBEC3A and 3G. J Invest Dermatol. 2017;137(4):810–8.
14. Albrecht-Buehler G. Surface extensions of 3T3 cells towards distant infrared light sources. J Cell Biol. 1991;114(3):493–502.
15. Ehrlicher A, Betz T, Stuhrmann B, et al. Guiding neuronal growth with light. Proc Natl Acad Sci USA. 2002;99(25):16024–8.
16. Karu T. Primary and secondary mechanisms of action of visible to near-IR radiation on cells. J Photochem Photobiol B. 1999;49(1):1–17.
17. Borel N, Sauer-Durand AM, Hartel M, et al. wIRA: hyperthermia as a treatment option for intracellular bacteria, with special focus on Chlamydiae and mycobacteria. Int J Hyperthermia. 2020;37(1):373–83.
18. Gazel D, Yılmaz M. Are infectious diseases and microbiology new fields for thermal therapy research? Int J Hyperthermia. 2018;34(7):918–24.
19. Al-Ahmad A, Tennert C, Karygianni L, et al. Antimicrobial photodynamic therapy using visible light plus water-filtered infrared-A (wIRA). J Med Microbiol. 2013;62(Pt 3):467–73.
20. Al-Ahmad A, Walankiewicz A, Hellwig E, et al. Photoinactivation using visible light plus water-iltered infrared-A (Vis+wIRA) and chlorine e6 (Ce6) eradicates planktonic periodontal pathogens and subgingival biofilms. Front Microbiol. 2016;7:1900.
21. Hartel M, Hoffmann G, Wente MN, et al. Randomized clinical trial of the influence of local water-filtered infrared A irradiation on wound healing after abdominal surgery. Br J Surg. 2006;93(8):952–60.

22. Daeschlein G, Lutze S, Arnold A, et al. Stellenwert moderner physikalischer Behandlungsverfahren bei infizierten und kolonisierten Wunden in der Dermatologie. Hautarzt. 2014;65(11):949–59.

23. Daeschlein G, Alborova J, Patzelt A, et al. Kinetics of physiological skin flora in a suction blister wound model on healthy subjects after treatment with water-filtered infrared-A radiation. Skin Pharmacol Physiol. 2012;25(2):73–7.

24. Mercer JB, Nielsen SP, Hoffmann G. Improvement of wound healing by water-filtered infrared-A (wIRA) in patients with chronic venous stasis ulcers of the lower legs including evaluation using infrared thermography. Ger. Med Sci. 2008;6:Doc11.

25. Schreml S, Szeimies RM, Prantl L, et al. Oxygen in acute and chronic wound healing. Br J Dermatol. 2010;163(2):257–68.

26. Danno K, Mori N, Toda K, et al. Near-infrared irradiation stimulates cutaneous wound repair: laboratory experiments on possible mechanisms. Photodermatol Photoimmunol Photomed. 2001;17(6):261–5.

27. Applegate LA, Scaletta C, Panizzon R, et al. Induction of the putative protective protein ferritin by infrared radiation: implications in skin repair. Int J Mol Med. 2000;5(3):247–51.

28. Suter MM, Schulze K, Bergman W, et al. The keratinocyte in epidermal renewal and defence. Vet Dermatol. 2009;20(5–6):515–32.

29. Zöller N, König A, Butting M, et al. Water-filtered near-infrared influences collagen synthesis of keloid-fibroblasts in contrast to normal foreskin fibroblasts. J Photochem Photobiol B. 2016;163:194–202.

30. Knels L, Valtink M, Piazena H, et al. Effects of narrow-band IR-A and of water-filtered infrared A on fibroblasts. Photochem Photobiol. 2016;92(3):475–87.

31. Büth H, Buttigieg PL, Ostafe R, et al. Cathepsin B is essential for regeneration of scratch-wounded normal human epidermal keratinocytes. Eur J Cell Biol. 2007;86(11–12):747–61.

32. Jung T, Grune T. Experimental basis for discriminating between thermal and athermal effects of water-filtered infrared A irradiation. Ann N Y Acad Sci. 2012;1259:33–8.

33. Jung T, Höhn A, Lau AM, et al. An experimental setup for the measurement of nonthermal effects during water-filtered infrared A-irradiation of mammalian cell cultures. Photochem Photobiol. 2012;88(2):371–80.

34. Jung T, Höhn A, Piazena H, et al. Effects of water-filtered infrared A irradiation on human fibroblasts. Free Radic Biol Med. 2010;48(1):153–60.

35. Uitto J, Richard G, McGrath JA. Diseases of epidermal keratins and their linker proteins. Exp Cell Res. 2007;313:1995–2009.

36. Gu LH, Coulombe PA. Keratin function in skin epithelia: a broadening palette with surprising shades. Curr Opin Cell Biol. 2007;19:13–23.

37. Kezic S, Jakasa I. Filaggrin and skin barrier function. Curr Probl Dermatol. 2016;49:1–7.

38. Proksch E, Brandner JM, Jensen JM. The skin: an indispensable barrier. Exp Dermatol. 2008;17:1063–72.

39. Bacchi CE, Gown AM. Detection of cell proliferation in tissue sections. Braz J Med Biol Res. 1993;26:677–87.

Water-Filtered Infrared A Irradiation in Clinical Dermatology

18

P. Jauker, P. Wolf, and A. Tanew

Abbreviations

GvHD	Graft-versus-host disease
IR	Infrared irradiation
LS	Localized scleroderma
MMP	Matrix metalloproteinase
PDT	Photodynamic therapy
PUVA	Psoralen and ultraviolet A
RCT	Randomized controlled trial
RP	Raynaud's phenomenon
SS	Systemic sclerosis
TGF-β	transforming growth factor beta
UV	Ultraviolet irradiation

18.1 Biological Effects of wIRA in Human Skin

Water-filtered infrared-A irradiation (wIRA) is a safe and promising therapeutic modality in dermatology with a number of potential indications. wIRA irradiation can effectively heat the skin and subcutis up to a depth of approx. 2.5 cm with a low thermal load on the skin surface while delivering an effective energy level to deeper tissue layers (see Chap. 3, Fig. 3.5). These properties render wIRA a suitable therapy for dermatologic conditions involving deeper parts of the skin with little risk of associated adverse effects [1, 2].

P. Jauker · A. Tanew (✉)
Department of Dermatology, Medical University of Vienna, Vienna, Austria

P. Wolf
Department of Dermatology and Venereology, Medical University of Graz, Graz, Austria

© The Author(s) 2022
P. Vaupel (ed.), *Water-filtered Infrared A (wIRA) Irradiation*,
https://doi.org/10.1007/978-3-030-92880-3_18

The effects of wIRA on the skin are mediated through heat-dependent and heat-independent mechanisms. Heat-dependent effects result from a rise in tissue temperature (up to 8–9 °C on the surface and about 4.5 °C in a depth of 2 cm) [see Chap. 5, Fig. 5.5], up to ten-fold increases in skin blood flow [3] and an elevated oxygen partial pressure (ΔpO_2 = 25–30 mmHg in a tissue depth of about 2 cm) [see Chap. 5, Fig. 5.5]. These mechanisms enhance the blood flow and increase the supply of oxygen and energy substrates to cells and accelerate the ability of damaged tissue to regenerate and heal [1–6].

The photon energy of wIRA (particularly wavelengths between 780–1000 nm) can also be absorbed by endogenous photosensitizers (particularly porphyrins) which in turn initiate photochemical processes that directly affect cells and cellular structures (e.g., cell protrusions, influence on cytochrome c oxidase and neurostimulation). Some of these biological effects correspond to a mild photodynamic effect and lead to further cell regeneration and tissue healing.

Through all these processes, wIRA reduces pain, improves wound healing, reduces hypersecretion of wounds and exerts antifibrotic and immunomodulatory effects [1, 7–10]. Thus, wIRA has been used as a treatment option for different skin conditions.

18.2 wIRA Treating Dermatological Disorders

18.2.1 Wounds

The effects of wIRA have been investigated in various types of wounds. Numerous studies show that wIRA irradiation promotes the healing of chronic wounds, predominantly venous ulcers, as well as acute wounds (surgical wounds or burns) [10–12].

Venous ulcers are very common in dermatological care and may pose a considerable therapeutic challenge, since healing is often notoriously slow. These ulcers are mostly located on the medial malleolar region. They are caused by impaired venous blood return towards the heart. Insufficient venous valves and/or insufficient contraction of the calf muscles (*calf muscle pump*) result in decreased blood flow, venous reflux and ambulatory venous hypertension. This, in turn, leads to an inadequate tissue perfusion with a decreased supply of oxygen and nutrients, as well as an inadequate removal of metabolites. Chronic hypoxia and hypothermia also impede host defense mechanisms against secondary microbial infection and compromise the healing process such that minimal trauma can lead to chronic wounds that often require long-term management. Treatment includes stage-dependent, wound care, compression, surgical removal of necrotic tissue and insufficient veins, and also infection control. Quality of life is significantly decreased in patients suffering from chronic venous ulcers.

wIRA counteracts several of the functional aberrations underlying the pathophysiology of venous ulcers. wIRA can improve the local wound microenvironment by increasing the temperature, the perfusion, and thus the oxygen supply in the affected tissue. wIRA also reduces wound hypersecretion and inflammation and enhances fluid absorption and thus reduces edema formation. A reduction in pain, which may already be noted during the first wIRA treatment, increases mobility and reduces the need for painkillers. Together, this accelerates healing and shortens the duration of hospitalisation [10–12].

In a prospective trial, Mercer et al. [13] reported on the response of 10 patients with venous stasis ulcers who were treated two to three times weekly with wIRA. Each irradiation lasted 30 min and the maximum treatment period was two months. Of the 10 patients, 7 experienced complete healing of their ulcers and another 2 achieved a distinct reduction in ulcer size. wIRA also reduced pain and the intake of painkillers. Thermographic imaging at baseline showed a hyperthermic ulcer rim and a hypothermic ulcer base that normalized during wIRA treatment.

The largest randomized controlled trial (RCT) in patients with chronic venous stasis ulcers included 51 patients, all receiving basic treatment with compression, wound cleansing and non-adhesive wound dressings [14]. Of these 51 patients, 25 received 5 weekly treatments for 30 min with a wIRA radiator, whereas the other 26 patients were irradiated with visible light (VIS) only. Treatment was given for a maximum of 9 weeks. In the event of earlier complete wound healing, treatment was continued for at least another week. In comparison with VIS alone, wIRA therapy resulted in a significantly greater reduction of the ulcer area (-151 cm^2 vs. -49 cm^2). A greater proportion of patients experienced complete ulcer healing (20% vs. 12%), improved granulation and increased epithelialisation of the ulcer rim, less wound exudation, and also an immediate relief of pain in about 25% of the patients. The irradiations were mostly carried out as a home treatment using a loan device and were reported by the patients as easy to perform. Taken together, this trial provided sound evidence that wIRA can be a useful addition to the therapeutic armamentarium for patients with chronic venous ulcers [14].

The results of all prospective trials that have used wIRA irradiation in different types of wounds (chronic venous stasis ulcers, infected and colonized wounds, surgical wounds and burns) have been reviewed [10]. The duration and frequency of irradiation in these studies have varied between 20 min twice daily and 30 min twice weekly. The numerous effects of wIRA on wounds that were observed in these studies are summarized in Table 18.1.

In summary, wIRA appears to be an effective adjuvant treatment for chronic and acute wounds and may also accelerate wound healing in the perioperative setting [11, 16, 17]. Of note, wIRA treatment is virtually devoid of side effects and is well accepted by the patients. The usual treatment protocol employs three 30-min irradiations per week. Whether more frequent irradiations (up to six daily sessions of 30 min) [11] might further enhance the therapeutic efficacy remains to be substantiated. Home treatment with wIRA is feasible and easy to handle and can be offered to patients on a case-by-case basis. Future studies are required to delineate the optimum treatment protocol and to establish standardized criteria for the use of wIRA in wound management.

Table 18.1 Reported wIRA effects on wounds (modified from [15])

Immediate pain reduction during irradiation
Decreased intake of pain medication
Higher tissue temperature associated with higher oxygen partial pressures during irradiation
Decreased wound exudation
Reduction of inflammation
Accelerated wound healing (formation of granulation tissue and re-epithelialisation)
Lower rate of secondary wound infections
Improved cosmetic outcome
Reduced length of hospitalization

18.2.2 Sclerotic Skin Diseases

Sclerotic skin diseases can be categorized into systemic and localized forms that differ in etiology, pathophysiology, clinical presentation, associated extracutaneous organ involvement, therapy and prognosis. Systemic sclerotic diseases comprise systemic sclerosis (limited and diffuse form), scleromyxedema, scleroderma and nephrogenic systemic fibrosis [18, 19]. Cutaneous and internal organ fibrosis can, however, also occur in chronic graft versus host disease (GVHD), particularly after allogeneic bone marrow transplantation [20].

Systemic sclerosis (SS) is characterized by multiple skin changes (diffuse progressive induration of the skin, sclerodactyly, joint contractures, microstomia, pigmentary changes, telangiectasias, calcinosis cutis and pterygium inversum unguis) and involvement of internal organs, particularly the gastrointestinal tract, kidneys and lungs. In addition to sclerosis and inflammation, vascular abnormalities resulting in impaired tissue perfusion and lowered tissue temperature are also found in systemic sclerosis. Up to 90% of patients with SS suffer from Raynaud's phenomenon (RP) which is characterized by intermittent arteriolar vasospasm of the digits, most often triggered by cold temperature or stress. Prolonged ischemia in Raynaud's phenomenon can lead to ulceration and necrosis of the digits.

Localized scleroderma (LS), also known as morphea, has recently been reclassified into five main types: limited, generalized, linear (including LS en coup de sabre), or mixed LS and eosinophilic fasciitis (Shulman syndrome) [18, 19]. LS differs from systemic sclerosis, in that the sclerosing process is confined to the skin and does not involve other organs. It is characterized by chronic inflammation in the dermal and subcutaneous compartment of the skin and excessive accumulation of collagen. Clinically, LS manifests with single, multiple or generalized sclerotic plaque(s). Depending on the type of LS, the sclerotic process might also affect the joints and result in restricted joint motility. In contrast to SS, no vascular abnormalities are found in LS.

Common therapies for sclerotic skin disorders include immunosuppressive agents like methotrexate, cyclosporine, systemic corticosteroids and azathioprine. Phototherapies, particularly UVA-1 and psoralen plus UVA (PUVA) photochemotherapy are also effective treatments for these conditions. In addition to anti-inflammatory effects, both UVA-1 and PUVA have been shown to significantly upregulate the expression of matrix metalloproteinase-1 (MMP-1; collagenase) in cultured fibroblasts and sclerotic tissue which is essential for degrading accumulated collagen deposits.

In a pioneering study on 58 patients with systemic sclerosis, Foerster et al. [21] made use of the transdermal heating of wIRA and investigated its effect on scleroderma-associated RP. Ten irradiations with wIRA not only significantly attenuated cold response and reduction of subjectively felt RP severity but also decreased the modified Rodnan skin score (a validated score to measure overall skin sclerosis) and scleroderma-associated arthralgia.

Based on demonstrating beneficial effects of wIRA in a child with linear scleroderma [22] and in a small case series of three patents with morphea [23], von Felbert et al. [24] treated ten patients with localized scleroderma (aged 6–62 years) who had not responded to previous conventional therapies. wIRA irradiations of 20–30 min duration were administered two to five times weekly for a maximum of 18–48 sessions, depending on the intermediate therapeutic outcome. Marked improvements (reduction of erythema and sclerosis and diminished pruritus and discomfort) were observed in 7 of the 10 patients, with durometry confirming a decrease in skin sclerosis in 3 patients. Of note, none of the responding patients relapsed during a follow-up period of 1–7.5 years, pointing towards a sustained therapeutic effect of wIRA in patients with LS. No side effects of wIRA were reported.

The mechanisms via which wIRA affects sclerotic tissue remain to be elucidated. Using a filtered near-infrared light source (Ifraray-A, model IRA-800, emission mostly between 700 and 1300 nm) Danno et al. [25] found a significant upregulation of MMP-2 (gelatinase) in cultured fibroblasts after exposure to infrared-A irradiation. Likewise, TGF-β1 secretion by cultured keratinocytes was enhanced by the irradiation. TGF-β1 has been shown to stimulate the production of MMP-2 while reducing the synthesis of MMP-1 and MMP-3 (stromelysin). Discordant with UV-based phototherapies, exposure of cultured human fibroblasts to wIRA at fluences of up to 1200 J/cm^2 did not cause systematic induction of MMP-1 expression [26]. It remains to be unravelled how these experimental findings can be reconciled with the observed clinical effects of wIRA in patients with SS or LS, since studies attempting to unravel its mode of action in diseased skin are so far lacking.

Currently, an explorative prospective bicentric intraindividual comparison study investigating the effects of wIRA in patients with morphea and sclerotic cutaneous GVHD is being performed at two phototherapy centers in Austria. For this, wIRA is being directed to a selected target area thrice weekly for 30 min over a total study period of 20 weeks. The primary endpoint of the study will be the change in skin thickness, as measured by high frequency ultrasound sonography (22 MHz) which is a sensitive and reliable tool for assessing the extent of cutaneous sclerosis. Secondary endpoints are treatment-induced changes in the modified Rodnan skin score, skin hardness (measured by durometry), range of motion and the patient global impression of change scale. Termination of the study and analysis of the data are expected for the second half of 2022.

In summary, the use of wIRA represents an exciting concept and strategy in the treatment of sclerosing skin disorders that often pose a therapeutic challenge. However, data on the effectiveness of wIRA remain scarce and further studies are required to further assess the future value and role of wIRA for managing these diseases.

18.2.3 Common Cutaneous Warts

Cutaneous warts are caused by infection of keratinocytes by human papillomaviruses (HPV). They most often occur in childhood with a prevalence rate of up to 33% among children between 6 and 12 years of age. Spontaneous regression is common, and a clearance rate of 50% has been reported in schoolchildren within an observation period of 1 year. Apart from watchful waiting, treatment options include chemical, physical and surgical removal, or immunostimulating agents. However, occasionally treatment-resistant disseminated cutaneous warts can be present in children and adults, particularly in the context of immunosuppression [27].

Evidence of a beneficial role of wIRA in the treatment of recalcitrant common warts on the hands and feet has been provided by a randomized, placebo-controlled trial on 80 patients that were divided into 4 groups of 20 patients each. After pre-treatment with salicylic acid and curettage, the patients received four different types of photodynamic therapy. *Group 1*: application of 20% 5-aminolaevulinic acid cream followed by irradiation with visible light (VIS) and wIRA; *group 2*: application of 20% placebo cream followed by irradiation with VIS and wIRA; *group 3*: application of 20% 5-aminolaevulinic acid cream followed by irradiation with VIS; *group 4*: application of placebo cream followed by irradiation with VIS. One to three PDT sessions were performed at 3-week intervals. Additional exposure to wIRA significantly increased the therapeutic response. In particular, the number of completely cured patients and vanished warts in the two wIRA groups 1 and 2 amounted to 42% and 72%, respectively, 18 weeks after termination of treatment, whereas the respective values for patients in group 3 and 4 were only 7% and 34%. These data indicate that wIRA might be a useful adjuvant measure for resolving treatment-resistant common warts [28].

18.2.4 Further Dermatological Indications for wIRA

A number of studies have shown that IR in conjunction with contact cooling can effectively and safely reduce facial skin laxity [29–32]. The underlying mechanisms are considered to be mainly heat-dependent. Dermal heating induces a breakdown of hydrogen bonds and a change in collagen structure with subsequent formation of new collagen. The generation of inflammatory responses leads to fibroblast proliferation and upregulation of collagen expression.

An interesting concept is the use of wIRA as a penetration enhancer for topically applied drugs. To this end, Otberg et al. [33] have been able to show an increased epidermal penetration depth of the hydrophilic dye fluorescein when applied immediately before or after irradiation of the skin with wIRA over 30 min. This effect was attributed to a wIRA-induced rise in hydration of the stratum corneum that was confirmed by laser scanning microscopy.

Importantly, wIRA may also be considered in photodynamic therapy (PDT) as an alternative light source to red-light emitting halogen or LED lamps. PDT is a highly effective and widely used treatment for patients with non-melanoma skin cancer and particularly field cancerization with multiple actinic keratoses. PDT is based on the topical application of a photosensitizer prodrug (5-aminolevulinic acid, 5-ALA, and methyl aminolaevulinate, MAL) which is preferentially metabolized in malignant cells to protoporphyrin IX (PP IX), within which it acts as a powerful photosensitizer. Subsequent illumination with PP IX activating wavebands (mostly red light with a peak around 630 nm) initiates photodynamic reactions that ultimately result in the destruction of malignant cells. The major side effect of PDT is pain during illumination which occasionally necessitates discontinuation of treatment. Two randomized controlled studies in patients with multiple actinic keratoses comparing PDT with a broadband VIS + wIRA radiator versus an LED lamp or an incoherent halogen light source have demonstrated that illumination with the VIS + wIRA device significantly lowered pain scores, while at the same time resulted in comparable clearance rates [34, 35].

18.3   Practical Considerations

Treatment procedures with wIRA are essentially simple. A device such as the hydrosun®750 radiator allows a homogeneous irradiation of a 25 cm in diameter treatment area. The distance between radiator exit and the skin is set at 30 cm and is assured through an attached holding rod. The beam is delivered in a perpendicular angle and irradiance at skin surfaces amounts up to 200 mW/cm² ($\pm 10\%$). The treatment usually lasts 20–30 min and generates a warm, most often pleasant feeling in the irradiated skin area. In case a patient complains about excessive heat, the distance to the radiator exit can be extended. Rarely, the heat feeling is perceived as pain and irradiation needs to be stopped. Special care should be taken in wound patients with impaired sensory perception, for example, due to diabetic polyneuropathy. However, despite its frequent use, there are as yet no reports on wIRA-induced skin burns. Although there is no evidence that accidental wIRA exposure might be harmful to the eyes, for safety reasons, the patients' eyes are protected by infrared radiation blocking goggles during the application period.

18.4   Conclusion and Future Outlook

In conclusion, wIRA is an interesting and promising (photo-)therapeutic modality for a heterogeneous group of dermatological skin disorders. wIRA is easy to use and has an excellent benefit-to-risk ratio. The treatment hardly causes any acute side effects and is not known to be associated with any long-term hazards. Thus, wIRA can be used across all age groups, in pregnant and breast-feeding women, in immune-competent and immune-compromised patients and in patients with a history of cancer. Given its safety, wIRA can also be performed as a home treatment. Future studies are required to shed more light on its mode of action and generate additional clinical data on its effectiveness and optimized protocols for treating skin disorders.

References

1. Hoffmann G. Clinical applications of water-filtered infrared-A (wIRA) - a review. Phys Med Rehab Kuror. 2017;27:265–74.
2. Hoffmann G. Principles and working mechanisms of water-filtered infrared-A (wIRA) in relation to wound healing. GMS Krankenhhyg Interdiszip. 2007;2:Doc54.
3. Mercer JB, de Weerd L. The effect of water-filtered infrared-A (wIRA) irradiation on skin temperature and skin blood flow as evaluated by infrared thermography and scanning laser Doppler imaging. Thermology Int. 2005;15(3):89–94.
4. Hartel M, Hoffmann G, Wente MN, et al. Randomized clinical trial of the influence of local water-filtered infrared A irradiation on wound healing after abdominal surgery. Br J Surg. 2006); Aug;93(8):952–60.
5. Singer D, Schröder M, Harms K, et al. Benefits of water-filtered as compared to conventional infrared radiation in neonatology. Z Geburtshilfe Neonatol. 2000;204:85–92.
6. Knels L, Valtink M, Piazena H, et al. Effects of narrow-band IR-A and of water-filtered infrared A on fibroblasts. Photochem Photobiol. 2016;92:475–87.
7. Daeschlein G, Alborova J, Patzelt A, et al. Kinetics of physiological skin flora in a suction blister wound model on healthy subjects after treatment with water-filtered infrared-A radiation. Skin Pharmacol Physiol. 2012;25:73–7.
8. Jung T, Höhn A, Piazena H, et al. Effects of water-filtered infrared A irradiation on human fibroblasts. Free Radic Biol Med. 2010;48:153–60.
9. Karu T. Primary and secondary mechanisms of action of visible to near-IR radiation on cells. J Photochem Photobiol B. 1999;49:1–17.
10. Hoffmann G, Hartel M, Mercer JB. Heat for wounds – water-filtered infrared-A (wIRA) for wound healing – a review. Ger. Med Sci. 2016;14:Doc08.
11. Winkel R, Hoffmann G, Hoffmann R. Water-filtered infrared-A (wIRA) promotes wound healing. Chirurg. 2014;85:980–92.
12. Hoffmann G. Improvement of wound healing in chronic ulcers by hyperbaric oxygenation and by water-filtered ultrared a induced localized hyperthermia. Adv Exp Med Biol. 1994;345:181–8.
13. Mercer JB, Nielsen SP, Hoffmann G, et al. Improvement of wound healing by water-filtered infrared-A (wIRA) in patients with chronic venous stasis ulcers of the lower legs including evaluation using infrared thermography. Ger. Med Sci. 2008;6:Doc11.
14. Schumann H, Calow T, Weckesser S, et al. Water-filtered infrared A for the treatment of chronic venous stasis ulcers of the lower legs at home: a randomized controlled blinded study. Br J Dermatol. 2010;165:541–51.
15. Hoffmann G. Water-filtered infrared-A (wIRA) in acute and chronic wounds. GMS Krankenhhyg Interdiszip. 2009;4:Doc12.
16. Hartel M, Illing P, Mercer JB, et al. Therapy of acute wounds with water-filtered infrared-A (wIRA). GMS Krankenhhyg Interdiszip. 2007;2:Doc53.
17. von Felbert V, Schumann H, Mercer JB, et al. Therapy of chronic wounds with water-filtered infrared-A (wIRA). GMS Krankenhhyg Interdiszip. 2008;2:Doc52.

18. Knobler R, Moinzadeh P, Hunzelmann N, et al. European dermatology forum S1-guideline on the diagnosis and treatment of sclerosing diseases of the skin, part 1: localized scleroderma, systemic sclerosis and overlap syndromes. J Eur Acad Dermatol Venereol. 2017;31:1401–24.

19. Knobler R, Moinzadeh P, Hunzelmann N, et al. European dermatology forum S1-guideline on the diagnosis and treatment of sclerosing diseases of the skin, part 2: Scleromyxedema, scleredema and nephrogenic systemic fibrosis. J Eur Acad Dermatol Venereol. 2017;31:1581–94.

20. Zeiser R, Blazar BR. Acute graft-versus-host disease - biologic process, prevention, and therapy. N Engl J Med. 2017;377:2167–79.

21. Foerster J, Fleischanderl S, Wittstock S, et al. Infrared-mediated hyperthermia is effective in the treatment of scleroderma-associated Raynaud's phenomenon. J Invest Dermatol. 2005;125:1313–6.

22. von Felbert V, Simon D, Braathen LR, et al. Treatment of linear scleroderma with water-filtered infrared-A irradiation. Hautarzt. 2007;58:923–4.

23. Kernland-Lang KH, Hunziker T. Treating fibrosis in morphea with water filtered infrared-A light. Eur J Pediatr Dermatol. 2010;20:49.

24. von Felbert V, Kernland-Lang K, Hoffmann G, et al. Irradiation with water-filtered infrared A plus visible light improves cutaneous scleroderma lesions in a series of cases. Dermatology. 2011;222:347–57.

25. Danno K, Mori N, Toda KI, et al. Near-infrared irradiation stimulates cutaneous wound repair: laboratory experiments on possible mechanisms. Photodermatol Photoimmunol Photomed. 2001;17:261–5.

26. Gebbers N, Hirt-Burri N, Scaletta C, et al. Water-filtered infrared-A radiation (wIRA) is not implicated in cellular degeneration of human skin. GMS Ger. Med Sci. 2007;5:Doc08.

27. Marini A, Niehues T, Stege H, et al. Plantar warts in twins after successful bone marrow transplantation for severe combined immunodeficiency. J Dtsch Dermatol Ges. 2006;4:417–20.

28. Fuchs SM, Fluhr JW, Bankova L. Photodynamic therapy (PDT) and waterfiltered infrared A (wIRA) in patients with recalcitrant common hand and foot warts. Ger. Med Sci. 2004;2:Doc08.

29. Tanaka Y, Tsunemi Y, Kawashima M, et al. Objective assessment of skin tightening in Asians using a water-filtered near-infrared (1,000-1,800 nm) device with contact-cooling and freezer-stored gel. Clin Cosmet Investig Dermatol. 2013;6:167–76.

30. Chan HH, Yu CS, Shek S, et al. A prospective, split face, single-blinded study looking at the use of an infrared device with contact cooling in the treatment of skin laxity in Asians. Lasers Surg Med. 2008;40:146–52.

31. Ruiz-Esparza J. Near painless, nonablative, immediate skin contraction induced by low-fluence irradiation with new infrared device: a report of 25 patients. Dermatol Surg. 2006;32:601–10.

32. Chua SH, Ang P, Khoo LSW, et al. Nonablative infrared skin tightening in type IV to V Asian skin: a prospective clinical study. Dermatol Surg. 2007;33:146–51.

33. Otberg N, Grone D, Meyer L, et al. Water-filtered infrared-A (wIRA) can act as a penetration enhancer for topically applied substances. GMS Ger. Med Sci. 2008;6:Doc08.

34. von Felbert V, Hoffmann G, Hoff-Lesch S, et al. Photodynamic therapy of multiple actinic keratoses: reduced pain through use of visible light plus water-filtered infrared A compared with light from light-emitting diodes. Br J Dermatol. 2010;163:607–15.

35. Giehl KA, Kriz M, Grahovac M, et al. A controlled trial of photodynamic therapy of actinic keratosis comparing different red light sources. Eur J Dermatol. 2014;24:335–41.

Rheumatism and wIRA Therapy

19

D. Vogler, G. Schmittat, and S. Ohrndorf

Abbreviations

axSpA	axial spondyloarthritis
BASDAI	Bath ankylosing spondylitis disease activity index
BASFI	Bath ankylosing spondylitis disease functional index
CDAI	Clinical disease activity index
CRP	C-reactive protein
CVI	Chronic venous insufficiency
FIQ	Fibromyalgia impact questionnaire
FM	Fibromyalgia
HAQ	Health assessment questionnaire
HT	Hyperthermia
KOOS	Knee injury osteoarthritis outcome score
NRS	Numeric rating scale
NSAID	Non-steroidal anti-inflammatory drugs
OA	Osteoarthritis
RA	Rheumatoid arthritis
TNFα	Tumour necrosis factor α
VAS	Visual analogue scale
VEGF	Vascular endothelial growth factor

D. Vogler · G. Schmittat · S. Ohrndorf (✉)
Department of Rheumatology and Clinical Immunology, Charité-Universitätsmedizin Berlin,
Campus Mitte, Humboldt-Universität zu Berlin, Freie Universität Berlin, Berlin, Germany
e-mail: sarah.ohrndorf@charite.de

© The Author(s) 2022
P. Vaupel (ed.), *Water-filtered Infrared A (wIRA) Irradiation*,
https://doi.org/10.1007/978-3-030-92880-3_19

19.1   Introduction

Rheumatologic disorders comprise various conditions having different etiologies and pathogeneses. The leading clinical symptoms are chronic joint pain and musculoskeletal impairment. With regard to pathogeneses, systemic autoimmune inflammatory diseases can be categorized as rheumatoid arthritis (RA), spondyloarthritis (e.g., axial spondyloarthritis, axSpA), connective tissue diseases and vasculitides. Rheumatic conditions such as osteoarthritis (OA) and fibromyalgia (FM) have no associated systemic inflammation.

The optimal treatment and management of rheumatologic disorders consist of non-pharmacological and pharmacological strategies. Physical therapy plays an important role in treatment algorithms and is therefore implemented in the relevant care guidelines [1–3]. The use of hyperthermia (HT) in physical therapy is a classical and developing therapeutic approach which can be applied in different forms. An established variant of HT is water-filtered infrared A (wIRA) therapy, which can be applied locally or systemically (whole-body). To date, local wIRA application has been tested in the context of rheumatological disorders in different entities (RA, axSpA, OA and FM), with whole-body wIRA treatment leading to pain reduction in patients with axSpA or FM [4, 5].

This chapter reviews the current state of research into the clinical effects of locally applied wIRA (using a wIRA radiator) in the field of rheumatism.

19.2   wIRA: Clinical Experiences in Rheumatology

19.2.1 Axial Spondyloarthritis (axSpA)

In 1996, Falkenbach et al. [6] published a clinical trial investigating the impact of wIRA on the cervical rotation mobility and sensation of pressure pain in the neck region of subjects with axSpA ($n = 11$) and subjects with degenerative disorders of the spine ($n = 11$). wIRA irradiation was applied as a monotherapy over 20 min with the irradiation field focused on the *vertebrum prominens*. Data were collected before, during and 10 min after the intervention. In both cohorts, the range of motion in transverse plane increased significantly. Using a pressure algometer, pain was quantified bilaterally on defined (trigger)-points of *musculus (m.) trapezius superior, m. supraspinatus,* and *m. infraspinatus.* Although significant changes in the sensitivity of pain during the intervention were not detected in either group, a trend towards an augmented level of sensitivity was described. The authors assumed that the improved cervical mobility was due to a modified elasticity of collagen in tissue triggered by wIRA irradiation and not an alleviation of pain.

In 2019, Xu et al. [7] investigated the effects of wIRA treatment on sacroiliitis in patients with active axSpA. The pharmacological therapy of the exclusively male probands ($n = 120$) consisted of methotrexate and non-steroidal anti-inflammatory drugs (NSAIDs). The patients were split randomly into two groups. The interventional group received regional wIRA therapy focused on the sacroiliac joints twice daily for 20 min each in a sequence of 5 days. After an interval of 24 hours, wIRA therapy was switched to the control group (crossover design). Significant decreases in morning stiffness and pain, as measured with VAS (visual analogue scale) scores (0–100 mm) and the Bath Ankylosing Spondylitis Disease Activity Index (BASDAI), a validated questionnaire to assess disease-specific disease activity, were observed after the intervention. The following blood serum data were additionally assessed: levels of C-reactive protein (CRP) declined significantly under wIRA treatment and increased after completion. Levels of vascular endothelial growth factor (VEGF) only showed a slight downward trend. An increase in the resistance index of sacro-iliac joint assessed by ultrasonography may be interpreted as a sign of attenuated inflammation.

In 2020, a prospective randomized controlled trial evaluating the effects of serially applied wIRA irradiation on patients with an active axSpA was reported by Klemm et al. [8], allowing only pharmacological therapy with NSAIDs. In the context of a 7-day multimodal rheumatologic treatment, the intervention group ($n = 36$), in comparison with the control group ($n = 35$), also received wIRA irradiation twice daily for 30 min (a total of 12 applications). The radiation field encompassed the lower thoracic and lumbar area. A numeric rating scale (NRS) demonstrated a significant reduction of pain (primary outcome parameter) in the intervention group, with about 75% of the treated cohort reducing their pain medication after the completion of the trial. Approximately one-third of the treated patients discontinued their NSAID medication. The authors related these findings to a significant reduction of the levels of tumour necrosis factor α (TNFα) in the wIRA group after the intervention. As secondary outcome parameters, BASDAI and Bath ankylosing spondylitis disease functional Index (BASFI), a validated questionnaire to assess disease-specific functionality, were suggestive of beneficial effects. However, no statistically significant differences in these indices were found between the groups. According to the authors, the design of the trial could have influenced this outcome in terms of a bias due to the multimodal rheumatologic treatment for all probands. Furthermore, BASDAI and BASFI are regarded as tools detecting differences particularly in longer time periods. No adverse or severe adverse events were documented.

19.2.2 Osteoarthritis (OA)

Osteoarthritis (OA) was one of the first rheumatologic disorders for which the analgesic effects of wIRA were tested. In 1992, the first experiences of locally applied wIRA in patients with gonarthrosis ($n = 52$) or coxarthrosis ($n = 63$) with pain as leading symptom were reported by Goltermann (extracted from [9]). This study also included subjects with non-rheumatological disorders such as lumbago. Therapy with anti-rheumatic agents, glucocorticoids or painkillers was exclusion criteria. For the study, patients were treated for 20–35 min on a total of 10 occasions at intervals of 1 or 2 days. About one-third were regarded as responders, as defined as at least considerable reduction of pain post-interventional. Worsening pain under therapy was reported by one patient with gonarthrosis and two patients with coxarthrosis.

In the same year, positive effects of wIRA (for 20 min three to five times per week on 10–20 occasions) in reducing pain for patients ($n = 26$) with degenerative musculoskeletal alterations such as gonarthrosis were presented by Scherf et al. (extracted from [9]). Subjects with non-rheumatological disorders were also included, analogous to Goltermann. Outcomes and findings were based on the subjective assessment of the investigators.

In 1995, Merle et al. reported two case series of patients with osteoarthritis of the knee ($n = 10$) and hand ($n = 10$) treated with wIRA therapy (extracted from [9]). A control group received conventional, unfiltered infrared irradiation. A defined exclusion criterion was secondary OA caused by, for example, inflammatory rheumatologic diseases. The knee irradiation in both groups was applied twice weekly for 30 min on 10 occasions. The treatment regime of the hands was approximately twice weekly for 20 min on 12 occasions. NSAIDs could be taken as required. The intensity of pain, which was measured using a rating scale ($0 =$ no pain to $6 =$ unbearable pain), reduced in the treated group in comparison to the control group. The requirement for painkillers also declined in the treated group. However, the low number of cases in this study requires that its findings are regarded as explorative.

To re-evaluate and confirm the effects of wIRA on gonarthrosis, Schuester et al. [10] designed a randomized controlled trial, the results of which were published in 2020. In this study, patients ($n = 54$) were required to irradiate their predominant knee at home for 30 days for at least 60 min per day. The control group ($n = 54$) continued their standard therapy. The wIRA intervention significantly reduced pain under stress and improved quality of life, as quantified using the VAS score (VAS 0–100 mm), with twice as many subjects in the intervention group (20 vs. 10) stating that they could walk pain-free for an unlimited distance post-intervention. The Knee Injury Osteoarthritis Outcome Score (KOOS) in all its categories showed a trend to improvement, albeit without being statistically significant. No substantial changes in additional outcome parameters, such as the range of motion and the length of one leg stand, were observed. The intake of analgesics (NSAIDs) was not monitored. Two female subjects undergoing wIRA therapy stopped therapy because of increasing pain. Chronic venous insufficiency (CVI), one of their common comorbidities, was reported as the trigger for pain. The discontinuation of treatment led to rapid recovery without consequences. This adverse event is remarkable and was discussed as an exclusion criterion by the authors.

19.2.3 Fibromyalgia

In a controlled observational study, Krüger et al. [11] addressed the effects of serial exercise plus wIRA therapy in patients with fibromyalgia (FM), with the control group undergoing exercise therapy alone. Patients received 12 treatment sessions of 30 min each over 4 weeks. Clinical effects were measured using the Fibromyalgia

Impact Questionnaire (FIQ), a validated measurement of health status in FM. wIRA irradiation significantly reduced pain and increased overall well-being.

19.2.4 Current Research Activities

We are currently investigating the effectiveness of applying wIRA to both hands of patients with osteoarthritis, non-inflammatory arthralgia and recent-onset arthritis in an observational study. In this study, adult subjects received wIRA for 30 min, three times a week (15 min from palmar and dorsal, respectively) over 4 weeks. Anti-inflammatory therapy (e. g., glucocorticoids) is one of the exclusion criteria. The following outcome parameters are evaluated: patients' global, physicians' global, patients' pain (each VAS 0–100 mm), duration of morning stiffness, tender joints, swollen joints, clinical disease activity index (CDAI) and the self-reported functional score HAQ (Health Assessment Questionnaire). Musculoskeletal ultrasound in grey-scale and power Doppler are also being performed. Preliminary data on patients with hand OA ($n = 14$), and non-inflammatory arthralgia ($n = 2$), predominantly females, reveal a reduction of mean (SD) patients' global from 52 mm (25) to 36 mm (27; $p = 0.003$), physicians' global from 16 mm (9) to 12 mm (8; $p < 0.001$), and patients' pain from 46 mm (26) to 32 mm (24; $p = 0.008$) from baseline (BL) to week 4. No positive effect of wIRA on the duration of morning stiffness has been detected {mean (SD) 21.8 min (29.5) at BL, 22.2 min (31.5) after 4 weeks}. The number of tender/swollen joints only tends to be reduced. CDAI was significantly reduced from 13.0 (7.7) at BL to 9.8 (8.0) after 4 weeks ($p = 0.001$). In addition, HAQ was significantly reduced from 0.7 (0.5) at BL to 0.5 (0.4) at week 4 ($p < 0.001$) (Abstract submitted to DGRh, 2021). The study and further inclusion of eligible subjects is on-going. The researchers intend to compare the effects of wIRA in the three different aforementioned conditions.

19.3 Discussion and Summary

Rheumatologic diseases are predominantly chronic with potential progressive courses which cover a broad field of different conditions. Joint pain is a leading symptom and the core therapeutic effects to deliver include pain reduction, functionality improvements and a deceleration of disease progression. A multimodal therapy including pharmacological and non-pharmacological treatment options is favoured. The chronic aspect of rheumatologic diseases often requires long-term therapies. Therefore, compliance and therapy adherence are required. In this context, the easy handling (portable wIRA irradiator), safety aspects and lack of adverse events upon wIRA treatment should be considered.

Referring to the above studies and considering the aforementioned aspects, locally applied wIRA reveals therapeutics benefits in the field of rheumatologic disorders, and thus can be recommended as an additive treatment option. Especially in patients with axSpA, OA and FM, wIRA therapy applied locally and serially leads to a strong relief of pain.

wIRA significantly reduces lower back pain in axSpA and sacroiliitis. The findings of Klemm et al. [8] that NSAID intake is reduced after wIRA therapy suggests it might help to minimize the side-effects of long-term NSAID therapy, and be especially appropriate for patients with contraindications for NSAIDs. Locally applied wIRA also reduces levels of the acute-phase protein CRP and the proinflammatory cytokine TNFα. These findings confirm those of Tarner et al. [12] who have reported decreasing TNFα levels after mild whole-body HT induced by wIRA. Taken together, these findings indicate that a disease modifying capacity on its own is at play, and that wIRA could act as a useful complement to TNFα-inhibitors for treating axSpA.

In OA of the hands, knees and hips, the first explorative studies that were already performed in the 1990s reported pain reduction after wIRA treatment. More recently, Schuester et al. [10] confirmed these findings and also demonstrated an increased quality of life after wIRA therapy. Merle et al. (extracted from [9]) reported on a reduced demand for analgesic medication after wIRA treatment; however, these findings need to be validated in a larger study. As worsening pain temporally related to wIRA was reported occasionally in patients with OA of the knee/hip [9, 10]; it is necessary to be careful with patient selection. In two cases, retrospective chronic venous insufficiency has been considered as a causative trigger.

Irradiation with wIRA was also an effective therapy in patients with FM and pain, a key symptom in this disease. Multimodal combination therapies are necessary as FM is difficult to treat. The good safety and good tolerability of wIRA makes it an excellent candidate for combination therapies with standard approaches.

19.4 Limitations

The number of trials investigating the effects of locally applied wIRA in rheumatologic disorders is limited so far, and their level of evidence differs. Additional limitations are the lack of standardization in the treatment protocols (optimal intensity, e.g., frequency, duration and course of treatment for each disorder need to be defined), and the lack of follow-ups make it difficult to assess beneficial effects of wIRA in the longer term. Additionally, head-to-head studies of local wIRA therapy and other thermal interventions are necessary in order to generate robust comparative evidence.

19.5 Outlook

Other rheumatologic disorders should be considered for wIRA therapy. Beneficial effects on patients with secondary Raynaud's phenomenon (RP) in the context of systemic sclerosis could be possible and the value of wIRA as adjuvant therapy to help reduce the frequency, duration or intensity of Raynaud attacks could be envisioned. Foerster et al. [13] found positive effects of mild whole-body hyperthermia induced by wIRA irradiation on scleroderma-associated RP. Furthermore, positive trends for skin manifestation and arthralgia have been reported. A case study of a 6-year-old girl with progressive linear morphea affecting the left upper extremity by von Felbert et al. [14] demonstrated therapeutic success after wIRA therapy in terms of softening sclerotic skin lesions and reducing functional impairment. The capacity to deliver wIRA locally with a radiator in children underlines the tolerability of the treatment. Evaluating the effects of wIRA on patients with sclerosing skin changes requires further research. Raynaud's phenomenon also occurs in other connective tissue diseases, such as systemic lupus erythematosus (SLE) or dermatomyositis (DM), which might increase photosensitivity of the skin as a potential contradiction to wIRA therapy. The possible influence of local and whole-body hyperthermia on proven and possible influences on the network of the mucosal and systemic immune system has been considered [15], but needs to be further evaluated.

References

1. Kolasinski SL, Neogi T, Hochberg MC, Oatis C, Guyatt G, Block J, et al. 2019 American College of Rheumatology/Arthritis Foundation guideline for the management of osteoarthritis of the hand, hip, and knee. Arthritis Care Res (Hoboken). 2020;72(2):149–62.
2. Ward MM, Deodhar A, Gensler LS, Dubreuil M, Yu D, Khan MA, et al. 2019 update of the American College of Rheumatology/spondylitis Association of America/Spondyloarthritis research and treatment network recommendations for the treatment of ankylosing spondylitis and nonradiographic axial Spondyloarthritis. Arthritis Rheumatol. 2019;71(10):1599–613.
3. Schneider M, Baseler G, Funken O, Heberger S, Kiltz U, Klose P, et al. Management der frühen rheumatoiden Arthritis. Z Rheumatol. 2020;79(1):1–38.
4. Lange U, Müller-Ladner U, Dischereit G. Wirkung iterativer Ganzkörperhyperthermie mit wassergefilterter Infrarot-A-Strahlung bei ankylosierender Spondylitis – eine kontrollierte, randomisierte, prospektive Studie. Aktuelle Rheumatologie. 2017;42(02):122–8.
5. Walz J, Hinzmann J, Haase I, Witte T. Ganzkörperhyperthermie in der Schmerztherapie. Schmerz. 2013;27(1):38–45.
6. Falkenbach HD, Werny F, Gütl S. Wassergefilterte Infrarot-A-Bestrahlungen bei Morbus Bechterew und degenerativen Wirbelsäulenver-änderungen: Effekte auf Beweglichkeit und Druckschmerzhaftigkeit. Water-filtered infrared A radiation in ankylosing spondylitis and in degenerative diseases of the spine: effects on mobility and pain on pressure. Österr Z Phys Med. 1996;6:96–102.
7. Xu J, Deng Y, Yu C-Y, Gao Z-M, Yang X-R, Zhang Q, et al. Efficacy of wIRA in the treatment of sacroiliitis in male patients with ankylosing spondylitis and its effect on serum VEGF levels. J Orthop Surg Res. 2019;14(1):313.
8. Klemm P, Eichelmann M, Aykara I, Hudowenz O, Dischereit G, Lange U. Serial locally applied water-filtered infrared A radiation in axial spondyloarthritis – a randomized controlled trial. Int J Hyperth. 2020;37(1):965–70.
9. Vaupel P, Krüger W, editors. Wärmetherapie mit wassergefilterter Infrarot-A-Strahlung : Grundlagen und Anwendungsmöglichkeiten. 2nd. ed. Stuttgart: Hippokrates; 1995.
10. Schuester L, Liebl ME, Stroux A, Reißhauer A. Wassergefiltertes Infrarot A (wIRA) bei Gonarthrose – eine prospektive randomisierte kontrollierte Studie. Physikalische Medizin, Rehabilitationsmedizin, Kurortmedizin.
11. Krüger S, Lipski A, Jahr S, Kujath K, Mathiske-Schmidt K, Reißhauer A. Serielle wassergefilterte Infrarot A Bestrahlung mit Fahrradergometrie (Hydrosun®) bei Fibromyalgiepatienten. Physikalische Medizin, Rehabilitationsmedizin, Kurortmedizin. 2008;18(04):A12.

12. Tarner IH, Müller-Ladner U, Uhlemann C, Lange U. The effect of mild whole-body hyperthermia on systemic levels of TNF-alpha, IL-1beta, and IL-6 in patients with ankylosing spondylitis. Clin Rheumatol. 2009;28(4):397–402.
13. Foerster J, Fleischanderl S, Wittstock S, Storch A, Meffert H, Riemekasten G, et al. Infrared-mediated hyperthermia is effective in the treatment of scleroderma-associated Raynaud's phenomenon. J Invest Dermatol. 2005;125(6):1313–6.
14. von Felbert V, Simon D, Braathen LR, Megahed M, Hunziker T. Behandlung einer linearen Sklerodermie mit wassergefilterter Infrarot-A-Strahlung. Hautarzt. 2007;58(11):923–4.
15. Hylander BL, Repasky EA. Temperature as a modulator of the gut microbiome: what are the implicationsand opportunities for thermal medicine? Int J Hyperth. 2019;36:83–9.

Water-Filtered Infrared A Irradiation in Axial Spondyloarthritis: Heat for Lower Back Pain

P. Klemm, I. Aykara, and U. Lange

Abbreviations

ASAS	Assessment of SpondyloArthritis International Society
ASDAS	Ankylosing spondylitis disease activity score
axSpA	axial Spondyloarthritis
BASDAI	Bath ankylosing spondylitis disease activity index
BASFI	Bath ankylosing spondylitis functionality index
BAS-G	Bath ankylosing spondylitis global score
bDMARD(s)	Biological disease modifying anti-rheumatic drug(s)
CG	Control group
DMARD(s)	Disease modifying anti-rheumatic drug(s)
EULAR	European league against rheumatism
IG	Intervention group
IL	Interleukin
MRCT	Multimodal rheumatologic complex treatment
NGF	Nerve growth factor
NRS	Numeric rating scale
NSAIDs	non-steroidal anti-inflammatory drugs
nr-axSpA	non-radiographic axSpA
r-axSpA	radiographic axSpA
sl-wIRA	serial locally applied wIRA
TNF-α	Tumor necrosis factor α

P. Klemm · I. Aykara · U. Lange (✉)
Department of Rheumatology, Clinical Immunology, Osteology and Physical Medicine, Justus-Liebig-University Giessen, Campus Kerckhoff, Bad Nauheim, Germany
e-mail: u.lange@kerckhoff-klinik.de

© The Author(s) 2022
P. Vaupel (ed.), *Water-filtered Infrared A (wIRA) Irradiation*,
https://doi.org/10.1007/978-3-030-92880-3_20

20.1 Introduction

Axial spondyloarthritis (axSpA) is a chronic inflammatory rheumatic disease mainly affecting the axial skeleton [1] with a prevalence of 9–30 per 10,000 in the general population, and an incidence of about 3.1 per 100,000/year [2, 3]. Although patients with axSpA typically present with chronic back pain and stiffness of the pelvis and lower back, any part of the spine and even the peripheral joints can be affected [1]. AxSpA leads to an increased morbidity and mortality, and affected patients often experience a loss of function as most patients develop structural changes of the axial skeleton at some point in their lives [1, 2]. The term "axSpA" thereby includes patients who have already developed structural and radiologically assessable damage (radiographic axSpA, r-axSpA, formerly called ankylosing spondylitis) and patients without such damage (non-radiographic axSpA, nr-axSpA) [1]. Since axSpA is a chronic, non-curable disease with potential for a severe disease progression, lifelong pharmacological therapy is common [1, 4]. Treatments aim to maximize health-related quality of life by controlling symptoms and inflammation, preventing progressive structural damage, preserving/normalizing function and social life [4]. Regarding pharmacological treatment, patients with active axSpA are initially treated with non-steroidal anti-inflammatory drugs (NSAIDs). For patients with inadequate responses to NSAIDs, biological disease modifying anti-rheumatic drug (bDMARD) therapy can be started [1, 4]. Innovations and advances in disease modifying anti-rheumatic drugs (DMARDs) over the last two decades have led to the so-called "biologic era" which has delivered effective pharmacological therapy for rheumatic diseases, and especially for axSpA [5]. Nonetheless, current data from the German Collaborative Arthritis Centers show that a significant proportion of patients with axSpA continue to have moderate to high disease activity despite these pharmacological treatments [6]. Concerning trends in outcomes for axSpA, two aspects can be considered. For one, the proportion of patients with good functional status has increased from 36% in 2000 to 49% in 2012 in Germany. On the other side, more than 50% of patients with axSpA continue to experience at least a limited functional status [7]. In addition, periods of flares (clinical worsening) and remission are common for inflammatory rheumatic diseases, in general, and are frequent in axSpA [8]. The term "flare" is poorly defined and often interpreted differently by rheumatologists and patients and has not been well investigated [9]. However, a definition for a clinically relevant exacerbation in axSpA which has recently been established for use in clinical trials based on the Ankylosing Spondylitis Disease Activity Score (ASDAS) [8] may encourage further research and promote reproducibility. Nevertheless, flares seem to occur quite frequently. About 74% of patients primarily treated with NSAIDs [10] and 25% of patients primarily treated with bDMARDs report at least one flare [11], both within a 3-month-period. Although not always long-lasting (>3 days), flares are related to a decrease in physical activity and well-being [11]. In addition, as flares remain quite common even under (stable) bDMARD-therapy [11], not every flare can lead to a change in pharmacological treatment. Therefore, recommendations by the Assessment of SpondyloArthritis International Society (ASAS)/European League Against Rheumatism (EULAR) for the management of axSpA clearly recommend a combination of non-pharmacological and pharmacological treatment for optimal management [4]. In non-pharmacological treatment, physical therapy (PT) interventions play a central role in the treatment algorithm of axSpA [12, 13].

The use of hyperthermia in physical medicine, in particular in axSpA in the form of whole-body hyperthermia (WBH) applications, such as mud baths, low-dose radon exposure in combination with WHB, overheating baths, and water-filtered infrared A irradiation (wIRA-WBH), have been shown to reduce pain and disease activity [14–18]. Additionally, the use of WBH in treating axSpA has an effect on pro- and anti-inflammatory cytokines [17–19].

wIRA is a special form of infrared irradiation in the range of 780–1400 nm with high tissue penetration and low thermal load on the skin surface, which is easy to apply and contact-free [20]. wIRA has both temperature-dependent and non-thermal effects, the latter not associated with relevant thermal energy transfer and/or relevant temperature changes [20].

Based on the positive effects of wIRA-WBH in axSpA [16], we have used locoregional wIRA (serial locally applied wIRA, or sl-wIRA) on the back to achieve positive effects in axSpA. Therefore, we investigated the effects of sl-wIRA on (1) pain levels, (2) disease activity and functionality, (3) levels of molecular markers of disease activity, and (4) dosage of non-steroidal anti-inflammatory drug (NSAID) [21].

20.2   Trial Design

To evaluate the effects of sl-wIRA on the back of patients with axSpA, we conducted a prospective monocentric randomized controlled trial with an assessor-blinded parallel group design. Participants were randomly assigned in a 1:1 ratio to one of two treatment groups using simple randomization procedures (computerized random numbers). All patients aged 18–80 with axSpA fulfilling the ASAS classification criteria [22] receiving stable NSAID therapy or stable non-pharmacological therapy for at least 4 weeks prior to treatment with moderate disease activity defined by a Bath Ankylosing Spondylitis Disease Activity Index (BASDAI) of four to seven receiving an inpatient 7-day multimodal rheumatologic complex treatment (MRCT) were eligible [21].

Both the intervention group (IG) as well as the control group (CG) received a 7-day MRCT in an inpatient setting. MRCT is a specific concept of German inpatient care which focuses on physical therapy in addition to occupational therapy, behavioral therapy, and patient education for patients with rheumatic diseases suffering from exacerbated pain and functional impairment [23, 24]. The 7-day MRCT delivered 11 h of different MRCT modalities to each patient, with every modality being applied for a duration of 30 min. In total, 22 applications

(7× physiotherapy, 3× pain processing strategies, 7× classic massage, 3× electrotherapy, 2× patient disease training program) were delivered to each patient. In addition, the IG received standardized sl-wIRA treatment of the back (2 applications daily [morning/afternoon] for 30 min for 6 days totaling in 12 applications) using a Hydrosun®750 radiator. Irradiation was applied vertically in an irradiation field of 25 cm encompassing the lower thoracic and lumbar area in prone position.

20.3 Trial Outcomes

A total of 71 patients were recruited and completed the trial; all of them could be analyzed (35 patients in the IC and 36 patients in the CG) [21]. The mean age was 51 years with a mean disease duration of 5.9 years. Disease activity, disease-related functional capacity, and disability between the groups were comparable (Table 20.1).

20.3.1 Effects of wIRA on Lower Back Pain

wIRA treatment led to a significant between-group difference in pain after the intervention (95% confidence interval (CI), -2.8 to -0.8, $p = 0.006$). The IG experienced a significant improvement of -1.6 ± 0.3 (mean $\pm$ standard error [SE]) from baseline to after the intervention (95% CI, -2.2 to -0.9, $p < 0.001$), whereas the control group experienced a nominal improvement of -0.3 ± 0.2 (95% CI, -0.8 to 0.1, $p = 0.088$) (Table 20.2). Furthermore, an onset of a significant analgesic effect of sl-wIRA treatment could be seen immediately after two applications, on the evening of day 1 in the IG, with a significant between-group difference. Subsequently, significant differences in the IG (before and after treatment) and between groups were found in each comparison. Analgesic effects did not vanish after night rest at day 2 and cumulatively increased as pain values progressively decreased at each reading (Table 20.3).

Table 20.1 Patient and disease characteristics at baseline (values are means $\pm$ SD)

	Intervention group ($n = 36$)	Control group ($n = 35$)
Age (years)	51.7 ± 10.8	51.1 ± 10.2
Disease duration (years)	5.8 ± 4.2	6.1 ± 4.5
Sex (female/male)	24 (66%) / 12 (34%)	24 (68%) / 11 (32%)
HLA-B27 positivity	30 (83%)	32 (91%)
BASDAI	4.8 ± 1.8	4.6 ± 2.1
BASFI	4.1 ± 2.2	4.5 ± 2.6
NSAIDs	34 (94%)	32 (91%)

BASDAI bath ankylosing spondylitis disease activity index, *BASFI* bath ankylosing spondylitis functional index, *NSAIDs* non-steroidal anti-inflammatory drugs.

Table 20.2 Change in pain levels (Numeric Rating Scala, or NRS) between baseline and after-trial completion. Mean ± standard deviation and [min; max] are displayed for values at certain time points. Differences are displayed using mean ± standard error

	Baseline	After intervention	Difference	p-value (95% CI)
IG (n = 36)	4.1 ± 2.4 [0;8]	2.6 ± 2.0 [0;7]	−1.6 ± 0.3	< 0.001 (−2.2 to −0.9)
CG (n = 35)	4.8 ± 2.5 [1;9]	4.4 ± 2.2 [1;8]	−0.3 ± 0.2	0.088 (−0.8 to 0.1)
p-value (95% CI)		0.006 (−2.8 to −0.8)		

IG intervention group, *CG* control group, *CI* confidence interval.

Table 20.3 Onset and development of sl-wIRA effects on pain levels. Pain levels (NRS) were assessed at days 1, 2, 5 and 6 before and after treatment (2 applications of wIRA on the lower back per day, 12 applications in total). Mean ± standard deviation and [min;max] are displayed

	Intervention group (n = 36)	Control group (n = 35)	p-value**
Baseline (day 1 before treatment)	4.1 ± 2.4 [0;8]	4.8 ± 2.5 [1;9]	
Day 1 after treatment	3.5 ± 2.2 [0;8]	4.7 ± 2.3 [1;9]	
Difference (p-value*)	−0.7 ± 1.2 [−3;4] (p < 0.001)	−0.1 ± 0.6 [−1;1] (p < 0.405)	p < 0.001
Day 2 before treatment	3.9 ± 2.2 [0;8]	4.8 ± 2.2 [1;8]	
Day 2 after treatment	3.3 ± 2.2 [0;7]	4.8 ± 2.2 [1;9]	
Difference (p-value*)	−0.6 ± 1.1 [−3;2] (p < 0.005)	−0.0 ± 0.7 [−1;1] (n.s.)	p < 0.007
Day 5 before treatment	3.6 ± 2.3 [0;8]	4.8 ± 2.1 [1;8]	
Day after treatment	3.1 ± 2.2 [0;7]	4.5 ± 2.1 [1;8]	
Difference (p-value*)	−0.5 ± 0.9 [−3;1] (p = 0.003)	−0.3 ± 0.9 [−2;2] (p = 0.032)	(n.s.)
Day 6 before treatment	3.3 ± 2.4 [0;8]	4.6 ± 2.3 [1;9]	
Day 6 after treatment (trial completion)	2.6 ± 2.0 [0;7]	4.4 ± 2.2 [1;8]	
Difference (p-value*)	−0.7 ± 1.0 [−3;1] (p < 0.0005)	−0.2 ± 0.6 [−1;1] (n.s.)	p < 0.023

*p-values of the Wilcoxon test for intra-group differences to compare two related samples.
**p-values of the Mann–Whitney test for between-group differences in differences between both treatment arms.

20.3.2   Effects of wIRA on Disease Activity and Functional Impairment in axSpA Patients

Both the IG and the CG experienced a significant reduction of disease activity, as measured by BASDAI, whereas only patients in the IG experienced a significant improvement in functionality, as measured by BASFI. There was no significant difference between the IG and the CG in BASFI nor BASDAI after trial completion. BAS-G, which reflects the effect of axSpA on the patient's well-being, was significantly changed in the IG with a mean difference (±SD) of −0.5 ± 1.1 (p = 0.006), whereas a significant difference was just missed in the CG (p = 0.051) (Tables 20.4 and 20.5).

Table 20.4 Change in functionality and disease activity between baseline and after-trial completion

		T0 (baseline)	T1 (after trial completion)	Difference	p-value (Wilcoxon test)
BASFI	IG (n = 36)	4.1 ± 2.2	3.7 ± 2.2	−0.4 ± 0.9	0.004
	CG (n = 35)	4.5 ± 2.6	4.1 ± 2.5	−0.4 ± 1.3	0.055
BASDAI	IG (n = 36)	4.8 ± 1.8	4.2 ± 1.8	−0.6 ± 1.1	0.004
	CG (n = 35)	4.6 ± 2.1	4.1 ± 2.3	−0.5 ± 1.0	0.007

BASDAI bath ankylosing spondylitis disease activity index, *BASFI* bath ankylosing spondylitis functionality index, *IG* intervention group, *CG* control group, *axSpA* axial spondyloarthritis.

Functionality was measured using BASFI, disease activity was measured using BASDAI. Mean ± standard deviation and [min; max] is displayed. BASDAI is a validated tool for assessing disease activity of axSpA and contains six questions determining fatigue, back and joint pain, pain at the tendons and morning stiffness. The BASDAI ranges from 0 = no disease activity to 10 = maximal disease activity with a score of >4 indicating active disease. BASFI is a validated tool to determine functional restrictions due to axSpA using 10 questions related to everyday activities with a BASFI score of 0 indicating no restriction and a score of 10 indicating poorest functionality.

Table 20.5 Course of BAS-G. Mean ± standard deviation and [min;max] are displayed for values at certain time points. Differences are displayed using mean ± standard error

	T0 (baseline)	T1 (after trial completion)	Difference	p-value (Wilcoxon test)
IG (n = 36)	5.8 ± 2.1 [0.0; 10.0]	5.3 ± 2.0 [0.0; 8.5]	−0.5 ± 0.18 [−3.0; 2.0]	0.006 (−0.89 to −0.16)
CG (n = 35)	5.3 ± 2.7 [2.0; 12.0]	4.4 ± 1.8 [1.0; 8.0]	−1.0 ± 0.56 [−9.0; 3.0]	0.051 (−2.4 to −0.12)
p-value			(n.s.) (−0.02 to 1.8)	

20.3.3 Effects of wIRA on Pro- and Anti-Inflammatory Cytokines

TNF-α levels were only significantly reduced between baseline and trial completion in the IG, and there was a significant difference in measured TNF-α levels between the IG and CG. There were no physiologically relevant or statistically significant changes in serum levels of pro-inflammatory (IL-1 and IL-6) and anti-inflammatory cytokines (IL-10) either within or between the two groups.

20.3.4 Effects of wIRA on Concomitant Use of Analgesics

Twenty-six (76%) of patients in the IG decreased their NSAID intake after trial completion (at day 7). Out of these 26, 10 (29.4%) opted to completely stop NSAID usage at day 7. In contrast, only one patient of the CG decreased NSAID intake.

20.3.5 Adverse Effects

No adverse or severe adverse events were recorded in both groups.

20.4   Discussion

To the best of our knowledge, this is the first randomized controlled trial to investigate the effects of sl-wIRA on the progressive onset and development of pain and a range of other clinical parameters and cytokine levels as molecular markers of inflammatory processes in patients with axSpA [21].

20.4.1 Discussion of Study Data

sl-wIRA as part of a 7-day MRCT significantly reduced pain levels and disease activity and improved functionality. TNF-α levels significantly decreased. Compared to the control group, auxiliary sl-wIRA led to significant benefits in terms of pain reduction ($p = 0.006$). Whereas the control group showed a non-significant pain reduction of -0.3 (mean), the intervention group experienced a change in pain levels of -1.6 (mean) ($p < 0.0005$) in this 6-day-trial.

wIRA application is a rapid acting and effective method to significantly reduce pain in axSpA. The significant analgesic effect is already measurable after only two applications and increases with further treatment. The treatment group showed a significant improvement in pain and BAS-G in comparison to the non-treatment group with only six treatment days involving two applications per day. Baseline BASDAI (mean: 4.8 IG and 4.6 CG), BASFI (mean: 4.1 IG and 4.5 CG), and pain levels (mean: 4.1 IG and 4.8 CG) were elevated as only patients with active axSpA were eligible for this trial. Since flares, although poorly defined outside of clinical trials [9], are common in axSpA patients treated primarily with bDMARDs [11] and in patients treated with NSAIDs [10], sl-wIRA treatment seems to be a good alternative to changing pharmacological therapy. A complementary and easy-to-apply wIRA treatment that can be performed in an outpatient setting seems to be suitable for initial treatment with a focus on a quick pain reduction, especially when flare duration is variable. In addition, wIRA can be easily "dosed" by varying (1) the irradiation distance and thus the irradiance and treatment field as well as (2) the duration of the irradiation. Pain reduction leads to improved physiotherapeutic mobilization, ultimately resulting in an improvement in quality of life. In addition, 76% of patients in the IG decreased their dosages of NSAIDs after completion of the trial to varying extent, with some even stopping NSAID therapy. Although it cannot be stated how long patients continued with the reduced dosage, potential side effects of NSAID could be minimized for at least 1 day.

20.4.2 Additional Pathophysiological Aspects

The rapid onset of pain relief lasting for up to 6 days is based on thermal and non-thermal effects. The *thermal effect* results from increased blood flow and improved elimination of accumulated metabolites, such as pain mediators, as well as an increased metabolic rate due to the increased tissue temperature. The *non-thermal effect* results from a direct effect on cellular structures and cells as well as an altered skeletal muscle tension with consecutive pain reduction [20]. The pro-inflammatory cytokines IL-1ß, IL-6, and TNF-α play a central role in both the inflammatory process and the inflammation induced pain [25]. Local nociceptive reactions involve peripheral polymodal nociceptors expressing glycoprotein 130 (gp 130) which plays a role in cytokine signaling [26, 27]. Proinflammatory cytokines also induce systemic effects. For example, IL-6 and PGE_2 are regulators of the hepatic synthesis of C-reactive protein (CRP) [25]. A distinction between hyperalgesic mediators, e.g., prostaglandins, IL-1, -6, -8, TNF-α, and analgesic mediators, such as IL-1, -4, -10, -13, needs to be made. Cytokine interactions are prominent during inflammatory pain. In the early stage, hyperalgesic mediators dominate, whereas at the same time analgesically active cytokines are induced by the immune system [26, 27]. A drop of these mediators may reduce depolarization of the peripheral nociceptors due to reduced input from ascending neurons in the cortical pain matrix, and therefore enhance a consecutive decrease in pain sensation.

During inflammation, the nociceptors of the joints are sensitized to mechanical stimuli and usually mute sensory C-fibers become mechanosensitive [28]. A decrease in inflammatory mediators could thus influence this process.

Proinflammatory cytokines induce the production of nerve growth factor (NGF) [28] which activates and sensitizes tropomysin receptor kinase (TrkA)-positive sensitive neurons to mechanical, chemical, and thermal stimuli and changes the properties of Aδ fibers (sensitization). A blockade of NGF-TrkA causes a reduction of skeletal pain [28]. It is possible that a decrease of the proinflammatory cytokines reduces the NGF production with consecutive desensitization of TrkA-positive-sensitive neurons. It might therefore be that the significant reduction ($p = 0.001$) of TNF-α in the intervention group from (mean) 8.8 pg/mL (baseline) to 5.8 pg/mL (after-trial completion) with a significant difference between the IG and the CG ($p = 0.01$) is of importance, even though no significant changes in the cytokines IL-1, -6, and -10 after sl-wIRA treatments for 6 days were detected.

The change in TNF-α levels in the intervention group could possibly explain the profound effect of the intervention on pain in this study. In a model of knee inflammation for example, reduced TNF-α levels have been shown to have antinociceptive effects [26]. These effects resulted from a neuronal site of action rather than from a reduction of inflammation. As the effects on TNF-α appeared only in the intervention group, they are probably related to sl-wIRA treatment. In the context of this study, we consider the temperature-dependent effects of wIRA to be particularly important. In addition, previous studies have shown whole-body hyperthermia [14, 15, 17] and whole-body wIRA hyperthermia [16, 19] to influence levels of pro- and anti-inflammatory cytokines, whereas whole-body wIRA-HT also induced changes in TNF-α levels [16, 19].

In this study, there was a significant reduction in disease activity, as measured by BASDAI, in both the IG and CG, whereas only the IG showed a significant increase in functionality capacity, as measured by BASFI. However, there were no significant differences between both groups. Since only patients with axSpA on NSAID therapy with a BASDAI between 4 and 7 correlating to active disease (moderate to high disease activity) were eligible to participate, we considered it unethical to test against placebo without any additional active treatment in addition to baseline NSAID therapy. Therefore, all patients received a 7-day MRCT, which provided each patient with a high volume (22 units) of physical therapy modalities and were shown to be effective in treating axSpA in a 14-day program [24]. While this choice was for the benefit of the patient and may have led to no dropouts in this trial, it may have influenced outcomes in these secondary parameters of disease activity (BASDAI) and functionality (BASFI). The more so as the trial period only lasted 7 days, and BASDAI and BASFI were designed as disease-specific outcome measures to assess differences over a longer period of time and are normally assessed in routine care once every 12 weeks.

Regarding non-pharmacological treatment in axSpA, although physical therapy interventions play a central role [4], its potential is often not exploited in everyday practice [6]. In this study, eligibility criteria similar to those used in randomized controlled trials for pharmacological treatments were used (BASDAI >4 under NSAID therapy and DMARD naïve) [29]. It could be shown that an enhanced additive physical therapy reduced pain and disease activity and improved physical function. Therefore, additive and or enhanced physical therapy should be considered for every patient with axSpA who has responded poorly pharmacological treatment and can, in some cases at least, be preferred to pharmacological therapy escalation.

20.5   Summary

This sl-wIRA trial shows that locoregional applied hyperthermia in patients with axSpA is an effective treatment option to reduce pain in axSpA with rapid onset and a cumulative beneficial effect with each use as shown over 6 days. Moreover, the pain reduction thus achieved leads to reduced pain medication, beneficial effects on inflammation, disease activity, and functional capacity. Therefore, it could be a valid option to effectively treat patients with axSpA in addition to pharmacological therapy.

References

1. Sieper J, Poddubnyy D. Axial spondyloarthritis. Lancet. 2017;390:73–84.
2. Sieper J, Braun J, Dougados M, Baeten D. Axial spondyloarthritis. Nat Rev Dis Primers. 2015;1:15013.
3. Wang R, Ward MM. Epidemiology of axial spondyloarthritis: an update. Curr Opin Rheumatol. 2018;30:137–43.
4. Van Der Heijde D, Ramiro S, Landewé R, et al. 2016 update of the ASAS-EULAR management recommendations for axial spondyloarthritis. Ann Rheum Dis. 2017;76:978–91.
5. Godfrin-Valnet M, Prati C, Puyraveau M, et al. Evaluation of spondylarthritis activity by patients and physicians: ASDAS, BASDAI, PASS, and flares in 200 patients. J Bone Spine. 2013;80:393–8.
6. Albrecht K, Huscher D. Verordnen wir ausreichend Physikalische Medizin? Aktuelle Daten aus der Kerndokumentation der Arbeitsgemeinschaft Regionaler Kooperativer Rheumazentren. Akt Rheumatol. 2017;42:118–21.

7. Huscher D, Thiele K, Rudwaleit M, et al. Trends in treatment and outcomes of ankylosing spondylitis in outpatient rheumatological care in Germany between 2000 and 2012. RMD Open. 2015;1:e000033.
8. Molto A, Gossec L, Meghnathi B, et al. An assessment in SpondyloArthritis International Society (ASAS)-endorsed definition of clinically important worsening in axial spondyloarthritis based on ASDAS. Ann Rheum Dis. 2018;77:124–7.
9. Keat ACS. Axial spondyloarthritis flares - whatever they are. J Rheumatol. 2017;44:401–3.
10. Jacquemin C, Maksymowych WP, Boonen A, Gossec L. Patient-reported flares in ankylosing spondylitis: a cross-sectional analysis of 234 patients. J Rheumatol. 2017;44:425–30.
11. Jacquemin C, Molto A, Servy H, et al. Flares assessed weekly in patients with rheumatoid arthritis or axial spondyloarthritis and relationship with physical activity measured using a connected activity tracker: a 3-month study. RMD Open. 2017;3:e000434.
12. Dagfinrud H, Hagen KB, Kvien TK. Physiotherapy interventions for ankylosing spondylitis. Cochrane Database Syst Rev. 2008;1:CD002822. https://doi.org/10.1002/14651858. CD002822.pub3.
13. Perrotta FM, Musto A, Lubrano E. New insights in physical therapy and rehabilitation in axial Spondyloarthritis: a review. Rheumatol Ther. 2019;6:479–86.
14. Dischereit G, Goronzy JE, Müller-Ladner U, et al. Effects of serial mud baths on inflammatory rheumatic and degenerative diseases. Z Rheumatol. 2019;78:143–54.
15. Dischereit G, Neumann N, Müller-Ladner U, et al. The impact of serial low-dose radon hyperthermia exposure on pain, disease activity and pivotal cytokines of bone metabolism in ankylosing spondylitis – a prospective study. Akt Rheumatol. 2014;39:304–9.
16. Lange U, Müller-Ladner U, Dischereit G. Effectiveness of whole-body hyperthermia by mild water-filtered infrared A radiation in ankylosing spondylitis – a controlled, randomised. Prospective Study Akt Rheumatol. 2017;42:122–8.
17. Moder A, Hufnagl C, Lind-Albrecht G, et al. Effect of combined low-dose radon-and hyperthermia treatment (LDRnHT) of patients with ankylosing spondylitis on serum levels of cytokines and bone metabolism markers: a pilot study. Int J Low Radiat. 2010;7:423–35.
18. Lange U, Dischereit G. Effects of different iterative whole-body hyperthermia on pain and cytokines in rheumatic diseases: a current review. Akt Rheumatol. 2018;43:479–83.
19. Tarner IH, Müller-Ladner U, Uhlemann C, Lange U. The effect of mild whole-body hyperthermia on systemic levels of TNF-alpha, IL-1beta, and IL-6 in patients with ankylosing spondylitis. Clin Rheumatol. 2009;28:397–402.
20. Vaupel P, Krüger W, editors. Wärmetherapie mit wassergefilterter Infrarot-A-Strahlung. Stuttgart: Hippokrates; 1992.
21. Klemm P, Eichelmann M, Aykara I, et al. Serial locally applied water-filtered infrared A radiation in axial spondyloarthritis – a randomized controlled trial. Int J Hyperthermia. 2020;37:965–70.
22. Rudwaleit M, van der Heijde D, Landewe R, et al. The development of assessment of SpondyloArthritis international society classification criteria for axial spondyloarthritis (part II): validation and final selection. Ann Rheum Dis. 2009;68:777–83.
23. Klemm P, Hudowenz O, Asendorf T, et al. Multimodale rheumatologische Komplexbehandlung bei rheumatoider Arthritis – eine monozentrische Retrospektivanalyse. Z Rheumatol. 2019;78:136–42.
24. Klemm P, Hudowenz O, Asendorf T, et al. Evaluation of a special concept of physical therapy in spondyloarthritis: German multimodal rheumatologic complex treatment for spondyloarthritis. Clin Rheumatol. 2020;39:1513–20.
25. Rittner HL, Brack A, Stein C. Pain and the immune system: friend or foe? Anaesthesist. 2002;51:351–8.
26. Boettger MK, Hensellek S, Richter F, et al. Antinociceptive effects of tumor necrosis factor α neutralization in a rat model of antigen-induced arthritis: evidence of a neuronal target. Arthritis Rheum. 2008;58:2368–78.
27. Kulkarni B, Bentley DE, Elliott R, et al. Arthritic pain is processed in brain areas concerned with emotions and fear. Arthritis Rheum. 2007;56:1345–54.

28. Peuker E. Neuroanatomische Grundlagen des Gelenkschmerzes. Akt. Rheumatology. 2016;41:300–5.
29. Sieper J, van der Heijde D, Dougados M, et al. Efficacy and safety of adalimumab in patients with non-radiographic axial spondyloarthritis: results of a randomised placebo-controlled trial (ABILITY-1). Ann Rheum Dis. 2013;72:815–22.

Part VII

Clinical Practice: Infectiology

Water-Filtered Infrared A (wIRA) Irradiation: Novel Treatment Options for Chlamydial Infections

21

J. Kuratli, H. Marti, C. Blenn, and N. Borel

Abbreviations

Akt	Stress kinase
C.	*Chlamydia*
CXL	Corneal cross-linking
dpi	Days post infection
EBs	Elementary bodies (extracellular, infectious form of *Chlamydia*)
ERK1/2	Extracellular signal-regulated kinases 1/2
HCjE	Human conjunctival epithelial cells
HeLa	Human cervical cancer cells (adenocarcinoma)
hpi	hours post infection
IL-6	Interleukin 6
IL-8	Interleukin 8
LC-3B	Autophagy marker
MIF/GIF	Macrophage migration inhibiting factor (MIF), glucosylation inhibiting factor (GIF)
PDT	Photodynamic therapy
pi	post infection
RBs	Reticulate bodies (intracellular, metabolically active and dividing form of *Chlamydia*).
RANTES	Regulated upon activation, normal T Cell expressed, and presumably secreted (also called CCL5 for chemokine [C-C motif] ligand 5)
SAFE strategy	Acronym for actions in trachoma treatment and elimination programs: Surgery, Antibiotics, Facial Cleanliness, and Environmental improvement

J. Kuratli · H. Marti · C. Blenn · N. Borel (✉)
Department of Pathobiology, Vetsuisse-Faculty, Institute of Veterinary Pathology, University of Zurich, Zurich, Switzerland
e-mail: nicole.borel@uzh.ch

© The Author(s) 2022
P. Vaupel (ed.), *Water-filtered Infrared A (wIRA) Irradiation*,
https://doi.org/10.1007/978-3-030-92880-3_21

247

Serpin E1	Serpin Family E member 1, also known as PAI-1 (plasminogen activator inhibitor 1)
STI	Sexually transmitted infection
Vero cells	African green monkey kidney cells
WHO	World Health Organization

21.1 The Effect of wIRA on *Chlamydia*

21.1.1 Introducing *Chlamydia*

Only few bacterial species can claim to be as famous as the chlamydiae, which gained their notoriety as being a cause of sexually transmitted infections (STI) in humans and as the 'koala bug' known to contribute to the extinction of free-living koalas in some regions of Australia [1, 2]. However, these are not the only examples of the *Chlamydiaceae* family being a threat to both animal and human health. To date, 14 different *Chlamydia* species have been reported to infect various mammals, birds, and reptiles [2]. A common feature of all these chlamydial species is the obligate intracellular lifestyle involving infection of the cell by the infectious elementary bodies (EBs), and their transformation into reticulate bodies (RBs) inside a vacuole termed inclusion. After several rounds of replication by binary fission, RBs transform back into EBs and exit the cells by extrusion or cell lysis [1]. In contrast to this specialized growth cycle, the range of hosts for individual chlamydial species is highly variable. Whereas *Chlamydia (C.) trachomatis* almost exclusively infects humans to cause an STI or the chronic eye disease trachoma [1], the 'koala bug' is primarily represented by *C. pecorum*, which is also known to infect ruminants and pigs [2].

Generally, these chlamydial infections are treatable with antibiotics such as azithromycin and tetracycline. However, some chlamydial species have developed resistance strategies, both naturally acquired and in vitro [3]). Therefore, alternative and preferably non-chemical therapy strategies are needed to prevent widespread emergence of antibiotic resistance in the *Chlamydiaceae* family. Considering these aspects, wIRA is an excellent candidate as a supportive therapy for difficult-to-treat chlamydial infections such as trachoma. Moreover, investigating the effect of wIRA on *Chlamydia* growth can also serve as a model for the effect of wIRA on other, slow-growing, intracellular bacteria such as *Mycobacterium ulcerans* [4].

21.1.2 Establishing an in vitro Model for wIRA Treatment of Chlamydiae

In vitro models are commonly used to determine the effect of new treatments on the viability of bacteria. As a result of their obligate intracellular lifestyle, in vitro models involving *Chlamydia* require the use of cell cultures for infection, which in turn allows an investigator to assess whether treatment has any negative impact on the cells.

For wIRA treatment *in vitro*, we use a wIRA radiator with attached light probes allowing treatment of specific cultures in a 24-well plate format (Fig. 21.1a). Initial wIRA-treatment studies used two different cell lines: Vero cells, a permanent cell line derived from African green monkey kidney cells, and HeLa cells, a human cervical cancer cell line. Prior to chlamydial infection, any potential impact of wIRA on the host cells must be evaluated. A resazurin viability assay and expression/activation of various molecular markers of stress and autophagy/apoptosis, specifically the stress kinases Akt, p38, and ERK1/2, the autophagy marker LC-3B, as well as cleaved Caspases 7 and 9 (markers of apoptosis) have consistently shown that wIRA has no negative impact on the viability of either cell line (Fig. 21.1b) regardless of irradiances used ranging from 620 to 3700 W/m^2 [5]. This confirms that wIRA does not damage *in vitro* cultured cells upon treatment [5].

wIRA treatment can be applied either on the infectious, extracellular (EB) chlamydial form or on the intracellular dividing (RB) form within inclusions. Studies have shown that the anti-chlamydial activity of wIRA is effective in both an *in vitro* animal model consisting of Vero cells infected with the porcine *C. pecorum* strain 1710S, and in an in vitro human genital model for which HeLa cells are infected with serovar E (genital serovar) of *C. trachomatis* [5, 6]. Treatment of EBs with wIRA prior to infection strongly reduces the infectivity of chlamydiae in both models (Fig. 21.1c). Furthermore, a single application of wIRA toward the end of the chlamydial lifecycle (40 hours post infection, hpi), when fully developed chlamydial inclusions are present, reduces the amount of infectious progeny by approximately 40% (Fig. 21.1d). This effect is even more pronounced following repeated irradiation over time (24 hpi, 36 hpi, and 40 hpi), resulting in a reduction by almost 75% in the human genital model. Ultrastructural morphology after wIRA treatment reveals a reduction of total bacterial bodies per inclusion as well as severe disruption of the chlamydial developmental stages (Fig. 21.1e) [5].

The anti-chlamydial activity of wIRA is promising and calls for further investigations and elucidation of potential mechanisms. Initial analyses indicate the relevance of thermal effects which might be, at least in part, responsible for the chlamydial reduction [5]. However, experiments in temperature-controlled settings also show that non-thermal effects of wIRA might be equally important for the anti-chlamydial effect [6]. In conclusion, wIRA has an anti-chlamydial effect *in vitro* that is independent of the infection model and does not compromise host cell health. Furthermore, initial insights into the working mechanism demonstrate that thermal effects do not fully explain the impact of wIRA on the chlamydiae.

21.2   Insights into wIRA-Induced Anti-Chlamydial Mechanisms *in vitro*

21.2.1 Challenges for Elaborating wIRA Mechanisms in Chlamydia Infection Models

Investigating potential mechanisms underpinning the anti-chlamydial effects of wIRA *in vitro* is challenging: Obligate intracellular bacteria like *Chlamydia* depend

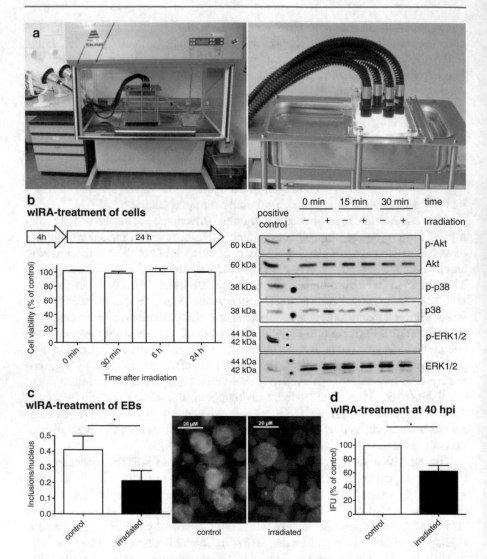

Fig. 21.1 Establishing an in vitro irradiation model for *Chlamydia*. Figure modified from [5]. Water-filtered infrared-A irradiation in combination with visible light inhibits acute chlamydial infection. PLoS One 9. https://doi.org/10.1371/journal.pone.0102239. (**a**) Shown is the wIRA setup (left panel) with a close-up of the six light probes (right panel). (**b**) The results of the resazurin assay after 4 h of wIRA treatment on HeLa cells demonstrate that the cell viability is not affected by irradiation (left panel), and stress kinase markers are not activated 0, 15, and 30 min following wIRA irradiation of HeLa cells for 20 min (right panel). (**c**) The number of inclusions per nucleus was counted following irradiation of EBs for 20 min and compared to the non-irradiated control (*left panel*). Representative immunofluorescence images are displayed in the *right panel*: Green = chlamydial inclusions; blue = nuclei of HeLa cells (DAPI staining). (**d**) Infectious progeny following 20-min irradiation of infected cells at 40 hpi is expressed as inclusion forming units (IFU), represented as % of the non-irradiated control. (**e**). The effect of three-fold irradiation (20 min at 24, 36, and 40 hpi) is shown on an ultrastructural level by transmission electron microscopy and subsequent determination of the average number of bacteria per chlamydial inclusion comparing the non-irradiated control with wIRA-treated *Chlamydia* (*left panel*). Representative images are displayed on the *right* showing the severe disruption of chlamydial developmental stages within an inclusion

e
Repeated wIRA treatment (24 hpi, 36 hpi and 40 hpi) of infected cells

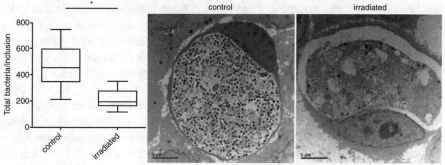

Fig. 21.1   (continued)

on host cells and their development cycle cannot be studied in cell-free systems. Therefore, the anti-chlamydial impact of wIRA could originate from a prokaryotic and/or eukaryotic response. First, thermal effects have to be separated from non-thermal influences using appropriate experimental settings such as tightly controlled temperature settings (e.g. temperature-controlled water bath, [5, 6]). Furthermore, the wavelength spectrum might impact irradiation results. Irradiation wavelengths ranging from 400 to 1400 nm are more efficient in reducing extracellular chlamydial forms than wavelengths ranging from 780 to 1400 nm [6]. Furthermore, the anti-chlamydial activity of wIRA is "dose-dependent" (higher irradiances are more effective), but independent of the infectious dose [5, 6].

Extracellular chlamydial forms (EBs) can be irradiated before any contact with the cell monolayer by irradiating an EB suspension which is added to the monolayer *after* irradiation. The anti-chlamydial activity of wIRA in this setting is primarily caused by direct interactions between wIRA and bacterial EB structures. These anti-chlamydial effects of wIRA could be mediated by modifying the EB surface proteins and limiting the potential of EB to enter host cells and form the inclusions which produce the next generation of infectious EBs. Results showing a reduced ratio of inclusions/host cells in irradiated vs. control conditions from [5] favor this hypothesis (Fig. 21.1c). However, specific bacterial target proteins have not been investigated or identified to date.

Alternatively, it is possible that irradiated EBs differentiate less effectively into RBs after entering the host cells and that a reduction in division events induced by unknown mechanisms reduces the number of infectious particles in inclusions.

A single irradiation of infected host cells with wIRA at 40 hpi reduces chlamydial infectivity to 62.9% of controls ($\approx$40% reduction) [5]. At 40 hpi, chlamydial inclusions are matured and primarily contain EBs which can infect new host cells. At this stage, anti-chlamydial effects on bacterial progeny are most likely caused by irradiation damage of EBs within mature inclusions (thereby leading to the same hypotheses as stated above). However, this hypothesis awaits confirmation.

Interestingly, treatment of infected cells with wIRA 24, 36, 40 hpi reduces infectious progeny by 75% compared to approximately 40% following a single treatment at 40 hpi [5]. These findings indicate that biological effects can be increased by repeated treatments and that the full anti-chlamydial efficiency of wIRA is not reached after a single treatment. Irradiation at three time points means that chlamydial inclusions are irradiated at different stages of the development (Fig. 21.2). At 24 hpi, inclusions mainly contain dividing RBs, whereas at later time points, mixtures of RBs and EBs (or mainly EBs) are present. The difference between three wIRA treatments and a single treatment could therefore also arise from different susceptibilities of chlamydial developmental stages, meaning that, for example, growing inclusions are more vulnerable to irradiation than mature inclusions. Transmission electron microscopy analysis of triple-irradiated inclusions have revealed that the ratio of chlamydial development stages does not change upon irradiation, but that the overall number of chlamydial particles within an inclusion are reduced by about 50% [5]. This supports the hypothesis that irradiation of chlamydial inclusions interacts with the efficiency of chlamydial development such as

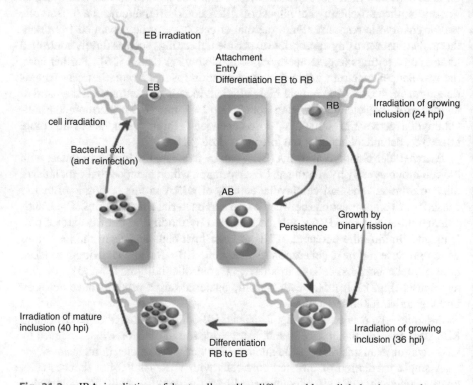

Fig. 21.2 wIRA irradiation of host cells and/or different chlamydial developmental stages: Figure modified from [4]. wIRA-hyperthermia as a treatment option for intercellular bacteria, with special focus on Chlamydiae and Mycobacteria. Int J Hyperthermia. 2020; 37(1): 373–383. https://doi.org/10.180/02656736.2020.1751312. PMID: 32319834. Figure 21.2 summarizes the experimental approach to investigate anti-chlamydial wIRA effects during the *Chlamydia trachomatis* life cycle. wIRA irradiation displays anti-chlamydial activity on EB/RB bacterial stages as well as on host cells/*Chlamydia* combinations

the division of RBs and RB to EB differentiation. Experiments to investigate the most effective time point for wIRA irradiation during the chlamydial life cycle are currently being performed.

Surprisingly, irradiation of host cells prior to infection (total of four irradiations at 8, 6, 3, and 0 h prior to infection) is sufficient to reduce subsequent chlamydial infectivity by about 35%, independent of the wavelength spectrum [7]. Furthermore, combining the irradiation of EBs and host cells before infection enhances the anti-chlamydial effects of wIRA and leads to a maximum reduction in subsequent infectivity of 87% [7]. These findings indicate that the effects of irradiation on bacterial and cellular structures must act synergistically. One major limitation in testing all the above-mentioned hypotheses is that anti-chlamydial effects can only be investigated in a combined host-*Chlamydia* system. Theoretically, irradiated bacterial structures could interact with host cell structures or pathways and irradiated host cells could impact non-irradiated bacteria. This hinders the identification of specific irradiation target structures in bacteria and/or host cells. The future will show, how (and if) the observed anti-chlamydial mechanisms can be investigated in more detail.

21.2.2 The Impact of Cellular Cytokines on the Working Mechanism of wIRA

Cytokines are inflammatory products secreted by host cells after infection. *Chlamydia*-infected cells (without irradiation) and irradiated cells (without chlamydial infection) exhibit a similar cytokine secretion pattern, including the secretion of IL-6, IL-8, RANTES, MIF/GIF, and Serpin E1 [5]. This might indicate that chlamydial infection and wIRA irradiation similarly trigger the host immune response and might result in the increased resistance of host cells to a chlamydial infection [7] if they are treated with wIRA prior to infection.

Kuratli et al. [8] investigated the impact of IL-6, IL-8, and RANTES cytokine secretion from HeLa cells during triple wIRA treatment (24, 36, and 40 hpi). Interestingly, impaired cytokine production or secretion does not influence the anti-chlamydial effects of wIRA-irradiation [8], indicating that wIRA-mediated effects are independent of these cytokines.

Inflammatory responses of the host immune system are typically required to clear ongoing infections. However, in the case of *Chlamydia,* inflammatory responses are known to mediate negative infection sequelae such as pelvic inflammatory disease or ocular scarring in trachoma [1]. For potential future in vivo wIRA applications, the observation that wIRA acts independently from host cell cytokine secretion is of utmost importance as this would indicate that wIRA treatment remains effective, even when the host immune system is impaired. In contrast, treatment of chlamydial infections by antibiotics is hypothesized to negatively impact the development of a protective host immune response, as described by the so-called "arrested immunity hypothesis" [9]. However, the fact that cytokine release by the host cell is not impaired by wIRA irradiation [5] indicates that consequences like the arrested immunity hypothesis after wIRA irradiation are unlikely.

21.2.3 Other Cellular and Tissue Effects of wIRA

Based on current literature, we conclude that host cell cytokines are unlikely to be involved in the anti-chlamydial effect of wIRA. Future investigations are needed to elucidate alternative potential targets or pathways in the working mechanism. Kuratli and Borel [10] have presented an overview on studies about wIRA or irradiation with similar wavelengths spectra, putting them into the context of potential future treatments of patients with trachoma [10], whereas a recent review specifically discusses the effects of wIRA on obligate intracellular bacteria, namely *C. trachomatis* and *Mycobacterium ulcerans* (causing Buruli ulcer, [4]).

The effects of wIRA have been intensively investigated in several clinical applications outside of infectious diseases by other authors (reviewed in [10]). Known in vivo effects include increases in oxygen partial pressure, temperature, and tissue blood flow in the irradiated area. However, the mechanistic pathways at a cellular level which allow physical properties of wIRA irradiation to be "transduced" into biological systems are still not fully understood. The current major hypothesis includes cytochrome c (a mitochondrial membrane protein involved in the respiratory chain) as the primary photo-acceptor which serves as the key molecule for the resulting light action mechanisms [11].

21.3 wIRA and *Chlamydia* in the Ocular Model: A Success Story

21.3.1 Trachoma in Humans: Why Do We Need wIRA?

Blinding trachoma, caused by ocular strains of *C. trachomatis*, remains the most common cause of infectious blindness worldwide ([12], WHO-Trachoma, http://www.who.int/topics/trachoma/en/) and is a neglected tropical disease which particularly affects children. Trachoma develops as a sequela of recurrent *C. trachomatis* infections of the conjunctival epithelium triggering fibrosis and scarring of the conjunctiva and leading to trichiasis and corneal opacity with blindness [1]. In the past few years, a number of global health organizations have aimed to eliminate blinding trachoma by the year 2020 (SAFE strategy by the WHO). The SAFE strategy includes surgery for trichiasis, antibiotic treatment (azithromycin as primary frontline antibiotic) for active trachoma, facial cleanliness, as well as environmental improvement [1]. As of January 2020, although 13 countries have achieved elimination goals ([12] WHO-Trachoma, http://www.who.int/topics/trachoma/en/), the disease is not yet eradicated on a global scale, and so far no vaccine is available. The current strategy for treatment and prevention measurements could highly profit from additional non-chemical interventions that limit disease, reduce transmission, and prevent re-infections. wIRA has not only proven its efficacy on mature chlamydial inclusions (disease) but also on extracellular infectious stages, the elementary bodies (EBs), and transmission limitation (re-infection). wIRA radiators are easy-to-use devices that do not require specific environmental conditions or skilled medical personnel; they can even be used in remote areas without a power supply. Their use in remote villages as an ambulant therapy could bring treatments closer to the affected communities. This motivated our group to explore the use of wIRA in trachoma models in vitro and in vivo.

21.3.2 Preliminary In Vitro Steps

A suitable in vitro model to evaluate the anti-chlamydial effect of wIRA involves human conjunctival epithelial cells (HCjE) and *C. trachomatis* strain HAR-36, an ocular serotype B [7]. A reduction of more than 50% in fully developed mature chlamydial inclusions (40 hpi) can be achieved using a single wIRA treatment of 30 min ($2100 \, W/m^2$). This could be theoretically transferred into an in vivo setting which could reduce the chlamydial load in the conjunctiva, at least partially. Repetition of the wIRA treatment in human patients, for example daily, could further reduce the chlamydial load. The wIRA treatment of EBs alone renders them less infectious and might reduce transmission of the extracellular chlamydial stages in the in vivo setting. The lower prevalence of *C. trachomatis* EBs in the environment might also reduce transmission events and lead to fewer inclusions formed in conjunctival epithelial cells. Even more encouraging are the results of the combined treatment of EBs and HCjE cells with wIRA prior to chlamydial infection. It can be hypothesized that wIRA irradiation of non-infected cells might pre-condition cells to be more resistant to the initial infection or be more effective in subsequent chlamydial clearance. Four times irradiation of HCjE prior to infection (8 h, 6 h, 3 h, and 0 h) reduces the chlamydial burden when non-irradiated EBs are added by around 35% of the control. Infection of irradiated HCjE cells with irradiated EBs results in the most pronounced reduction of chlamydial load (70–87%), thereby suggesting that wIRA protects cells from infection. It would be of great importance to understand the host cell factors that are involved in the anti-chlamydial effect of wIRA. These promising in vitro results encouraged a transition of work into an in vivo setting, the guinea pig model of inclusion conjunctivitis.

21.3.3 Promising In Vivo Results

The guinea pig model of inclusion conjunctivitis examines the effect of wIRA in a *C. caviae* conjunctival infection model [13]. The major advantage of this model is that it assesses wIRA in a complex tissue (the conjunctiva) instead of previous in vitro studies on cell monolayers. Chlamydial inclusions are formed in the conjunctival epithelium and inflammatory cells are recruited to the epithelium and underlying stroma after infection. Thus, the effect of wIRA on inflammatory processes can also be studied in this model. As expected, and in accordance with previous in vitro studies, repeated treatment for 30 min each (day 2 and 4 pi, $2100 \, W/m^2$) is more effective in reducing chlamydial load and ocular pathology than a single treatment (day 2). Over an observation period of 21 days, wIRA reduces the ocular pathology score (days 7 and 14 pi) and the chlamydial conjunctival load (days 2, 4, 7, and 14 pi). The latter denotes a reduction in infectious EBs, and therefore reflects a reduced re-infection and transmission. At 21 dpi, chlamydial inclusions in conjunctival epithelial cells are less numerous in treated guinea pigs and the acute inflammatory response is dampened (lower number of polymorphonuclear neutrophils), suggesting that wIRA can even reduce inflammation. Of importance, the ocular and systemic immune response normally present following *C. caviae* infection is not suppressed by wIRA treatment. In conclusion, wIRA might be capable to reducing trachoma transmission and pathology of ocular chlamydial infections in human patients. These promising findings confirm the results of previous in vitro studies [5–8] and encourage further investigations for the application of wIRA in the field of trachoma therapeutics. In a very recent report [14] possible, other fields of application have been outlined.

21.3.4 Future Plans and Outlook

wIRA can reduce the chlamydial burden in vitro and in vivo by affecting mature inclusions as well as by reducing infectious EBs. In the future, wIRA treatment of trachoma patients could be applied by irradiation of the *C. trachomatis*-infected conjunctiva through a closed eyelid, thereby reaching the infected area (inner conjunctival lining) without harming the deeper structures of the eye such as the vitreous body or the retina, or resulting in corneal damage [4]. Ocular safety studies are needed to exclude deleterious effects of wIRA on sensitive ocular structures, such as the cornea, lens, vitreous body, and retina [4]. Moreover, short-term irradiation protocols including various irradiances would be preferable to apply wIRA in the clinical setting. Future in vitro and in vivo studies aim to investigate the daily application of wIRA to further reduce chlamydial load. Of potential benefit would be to shorten the irradiation time from 30 to 10 min while retaining anti-chlamydial efficacy in view of treatment protocols suitable for children, the main age group affected by trachoma. Enhancement of the anti-chlamydial activity might be achieved by combining wIRA with photodynamic substances (e.g., hypericin) as photodynamic therapy (PDT). PDT using Riboflavin and UV-A therapy, called corneal cross-linking (CXL), has been implemented as treatment for keratoconus in human patients and to treat infectious keratitis in animal and human patients [15, 16]. Similar approaches are envisaged for wIRA, but necessitate a step back to elaborate this idea further in the in vitro model.

References

1. Jordan S, Nelson D, Geisler W. *Chlamydia trachomatis* infections. In: Tan M, Hegeman JH, Sütterlin C, editors. *Chlamydia* biology: from genome to disease. Norfolk: Caister Academic Press; 2020. p. 1–30.
2. Sachse K, Borel N. Recent advances in epidemiology, pathology and immunology of veterinary chlamydiae. In: Tan M, Hegeman JH, Sütterlin C, editors. *Chlamydia* biology: from genome to disease. Norfolk: Caister Academic Press; 2020. p. 403–28.

3. Sandoz KM, Rockey DD. Antibiotic resistance in Chlamydiae. Future Microbiol. 2010;5:1427–42.
4. Borel N, Sauer-Durand AM, Hartel M, et al. WIRA: hyperthermia as a treatment option for intracellular bacteria, with special focus on Chlamydiae and mycobacteria. Int J Hyperthermia. 2020;37:373–83.
5. Marti H, Koschwanez M, Pesch T, et al. Water-filtered infrared A irradiation in combination with visible light inhibits acute chlamydial infection. PLoS One. 2014;9(7):e102239.
6. Marti H, Blenn C, Borel N. The contribution of temperature, exposure intensity and visible light to the inhibitory effect of irradiation on acute chlamydial infection. J Photochem Photobiol B. 2015;153:324–33.
7. Rahn C, Marti H, Frohns A, et al. Water-filtered infrared A reduces chlamydial infectivity *in vitro* without causing *ex vivo* eye damage in pig and mouse models. J Photochem Photobiol B. 2016;165:340–50.
8. Kuratli J, Pesch T, Marti H, et al. Water filtered infrared A and visible light (wIRA/VIS) irradiation reduces *Chlamydia trachomatis* infectivity independent of targeted cytokine inhibition. Front Microbiol. 2018;9:2757.
9. Brunham RC, Rekart ML. The arrested immunity hypothesis and the epidemiology of *Chlamydia* control. Sex Transm Dis. 2008;4:53–4.
10. Kuratli J, Borel N. Perspective: water-filtered infrared-A-radiation (wIRA) – novel treatment options for chlamydial infections? Front Microbiol. 2019;10:1053.
11. Passarella S, Karu T. Absorption of monochromatic and narrow band radiation in the visible and near IR by both mitochondrial and non-mitochondrial photoacceptors results in photobiomodulation. J Photochem Photobiol B. 2014;140:344–58.
12. WHO. Trachoma. Geneva: WHO; 2020.
13. Inic-Kanada A, Stojanovic M, Miljkovic R, et al. Water-filtered infrared A and visible light (wIRA/VIS) treatment reduces *Chlamydia caviae*-induced ocular inflammation and infectious load in a Guinea pig model of inclusion conjunctivitis. J Photochem Photobiol B. 2020;209:111953.
14. Gazel D, Demirbakan H, Erinmez M. *In vitro* activity of hyperthermia on swarming motility and antimicrobial susceptibility profiles of *Proteus mirabilis* isolates. Int J Hyperthermia. 2021;38(1):1002–12. https://doi.org/10.1080/02656736.2021.1943546.
15. Randleman JB, Khandelwal SS, Hafezi F. Corneal cross-linking. Surv Ophthalmol. 2015;60(6):509–23.
16. Gallhoefer NS, Spiess BM, Guscetti F, et al. Penetration depth of corneal cross-linking with riboflavin and UV-A (CXL) in horses and rabbits. Vet Ophthalmol. 2016;19(4):275–84.

Safety of Water-Filtered Infrared A (wIRA) on the Eye as a Novel Treatment Option for Chlamydial Infections

22

A. Frohns and F. Frohns

Abbreviations

Akt	Serine/threonine kinase
aPDT	Antimicrobial photodynamic therapy
DAPI	4′,6-Diamidino-2-phenylindole
ELISA	Enzyme-linked immunosorbent assay
ERK1/2	Extracellular signal-regulated kinases 1/2
GCL	Ganglion cell layer
HSP70	Heat shock protein 70
HSP90	Heat shock protein 90
INL	Inner nuclear layer
IR-A	Infrared-A
NfκB	Nuclear factor 'kappa-light-chain-enhancer' of activated B-cells
ONL	Outer nuclear layer
p38	Mitogen activated protein kinases
ROS	Reactive oxygen species
SAPK/JNK	Stress-activated protein kinases/Jun amino-terminal kinases
UVA	Ultraviolet-A
VIS	Visible light

A. Frohns (✉) · F. Frohns
Department of Plant Membrane Biophysics, Technical University of Darmstadt, Darmstadt, Germany

© The Author(s) 2022
P. Vaupel (ed.), *Water-filtered Infrared A (wIRA) Irradiation*,
https://doi.org/10.1007/978-3-030-92880-3_22

22.1   The Eye as a Highly Sensitive Structure for Thermal Interventions

Temperature is of utmost importance for all biological functions, with temperature changes in tissues influencing the kinetics of biological processes and consequently slowing or accelerating metabolism. Non-physiological increases in temperature in tissues can result in protein denaturation and cell death and thus contribute to the onset of pathological changes.

Eyes are considered to be the most vulnerable to even small temperature changes for the following reasons. Some of the inner posterior parts of the eye lack sufficient blood flow for the removal of excess heat, whereas the anterior part is only temporarily covered by the eyelid as a protective skin layer [1]. Hence, environmental conditions such as humidity, airflow and thermal radiation can have a massive impact on ocular temperature and contribute to pathological changes in the eye. For this reason, the safety of medical treatments which induce temperature changes in the eye, including water filtered infrared-A (wIRA) irradiation, require special attention. However, direct temperature measurements in the interior of the human eye are technically challenging and almost impossible. Up to now, in vivo temperature measurements of the interior eye is confined to animal experiments and often involve potentially damaging invasive or direct contact-based procedures or is limited to simulated eye models [2].

22.2   Histological Structures of the Eye and Their Contribution to Thermal Regulation of the Ocular Compartments

The human eye is a complex organ consisting of several histological compartments having different biological properties and a complex geometry (Fig. 22.1). In the posterior part of the eye, the outermost layer consists of the sclera. The sclera is a white coloured, protective layer containing mainly collagen and some elastic fibers. Beneath the sclera lies the choroid, which is the vascular layer of the eye and supplies the underlying retina layer. The choroid has the highest blood flow in the body, and this is believed to protect the retina from heat stress [3]. Together with the sclera, the choroid can contribute to convective heat transport in the ocular compartments [4]. During this process, the blood absorbs energy from warmer regions and releases it to cooler regions and vice versa. The retina is the photoreceptive tissue of the eye and is believed to be highly thermosensitive. Although it is also vascularized, the contribution to its own temperature regulation is much lower when compared to the choroid [5]. The sclera in the anterior part of the eye becomes transparent – the cornea. This avascular tissue is constantly wetted by tear fluid and, together with other ocular compartments, contributes to the refraction of light that gives the eye its optical power. The conjunctiva, a highly vascularized tissue that lines the inside of the eyelids and covers the sclera, can contribute to the regulation of the corneal temperature [6]. Although not a direct component of the eye, the eyelid also significantly contributes to the temperature regulation of the cornea by blinking during the waking cycle and by constantly covering it during sleep [1]. The lens, as part of the anterior eye, is a transparent biconvex structure surrounded by vitreous humour which, with the cornea, contributes to

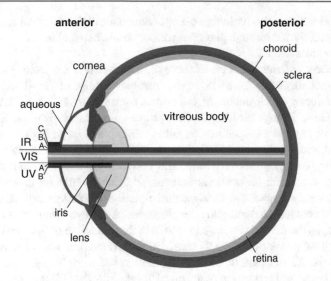

Fig. 22.1 Transmission of light through the compartments of the human eye. Infrared (IR) C: >3000 nm, B: 1400–3000 nm, A: 780–1400 nm, visible light (VIS): 400–780 nm, ultraviolet (UV) A: 315–400 nm, B: <315 nm

the refraction of light on the photosensitive retina. The lens lacks vascularization and is well known to be a highly temperature-sensitive structure. The vitreous body is a transparent gelatinous mass consisting of 98–99% water that fills the inner space between the lens and the retina. The vitreous membrane, which consists of collagen, separates the vitreous body from the other parts of the eye. The high amount of water in the vitreous body gives this structure a high 'heat storing' potential.

In summary, the eye comprises various structures that can function as heat sinks or as heat stores. With the cornea, the lens and the retina, the eye is therefore comprised of highly temperature-sensitive tissues. Accordingly, exposure to elevated temperatures risks impairment of visual perception. Regarding which elements of the electromagnetic spectrum interact with the eye, it is known that visible light ($\approx$ 400–780 nm) and infrared-A (780–1400 nm) pass through all the thermosensitive layers of the eye before reaching the photosensitive retina (Fig. 22.1) [7]. Although a small amount of ultraviolet-A radiation can still penetrate to the retina, most of the shorter wavelengths <400 nm and the longer wavelengths >1400 nm are absorbed by the cornea and the lens. This is of importance to all medical applications that are based on radiation and can result in photothermal reactions in the ocular structures. As a consequence, treating chlamydial eye infections using wIRA irradiation requires a detailed analysis of the thermal effects occurring in the eye.

22.3   Effects of Radiation-Induced Photothermal and Photochemical Events on Ocular Structures

Considering wIRA as a potential treatment option for chlamydial eye infections, it is important to note that in recent studies, this approach is most effective when using wIRA-irradiation (780–1400 nm) in combination with visible light (VIS) in the range of 400–780 nm. Both of these components have been described to potentially damage ocular tissues through photothermal or photochemical reactions, depending on exposure time and energy [8].

As the most anterior structure of the eye, the *cornea* is particularly exposed to temperature changes and radiation. In the infrared-A range of 780–1400 nm which is delivered during wIRA treatment, the cornea transmits up to 96% of the incoming radiation. Thus, damage resulting in immediate pain, vascularization, and eventually a loss of corneal transparency requires the application of high irradiances of infrared radiation to the cornea [9]. For the VIS part of the electromagnetic spectrum, the high energy short-wave blue light between 415 and 455 nm is considered to be the most harmful for ocular structures, and thereby also for the cornea. Blue light can severely impact the survival and function of corneal cells and promote pathological changes, including the development of dry eye syndrome [10].

The lens, as the second structure involved in the refraction of light and contributing to the visual power of the eye, is sensitive to infrared irradiation and exposure to thermal stress. As an example, cataract formation has been frequently observed in humans exposed to high levels of infrared irradiation (>1400 nm) such as glassblowers or ironworkers [11]. Cataract formation associates with clouding of the lens and is, on the molecular level, caused by the disturbed arrangement of crystalline proteins which are the major components of the lens [12]. However, it is assumed that infrared-induced cataract formation is not only caused by the direct heating of the lens but also by the indirect heating of neighbouring ocular structures [9]. For this reason, wIRA may contribute to cataract formation by indirect heating of adjacent ocular structures, even if the wavelengths of 780–1400 nm are not absorbed by the lens. With regard to a combined therapy involving wIRA and VIS components, it should also be noted that blue light has been shown to induce the production of reactive oxygen species (ROS) in the mitochondria of lens epithelial cells, which may also promote the development of cataracts [10].

The retina, as the innermost layer of the posterior eye, converts light stimuli into the nerve signals to the brain, and thereby provides visual capacity. This nervous tissue is probably the most complicated in terms of its sensitivity to thermal and visual stimulation. Infrared radiation that is transmitted through the transparent ocular structures to the retina is not absorbed by the retina itself, but by the adjacent cells of the so-called retinal pigment epithelium [9]. Consequently, thermal injury of retinal cells does not occur directly, but by indirect heating from the pigment epithelium. The induction of thermal damage depends on multiple factors such as the pupil size, the exposure duration, the nature and spectral distribution of the radiation source, as well as the rate of energy delivery. In this context, the exposure time inversely correlates with the radiation power that is necessary to damage the retina. With regard to the threshold of a non-critical temperature increase, a rise of 10 °C above the body temperature will produce permanent damage to the retina and also the underlying choroid by inducing protein denaturation. However, even thermal effects significantly below this limit can alter gene expression in the retina and adjacent pigment epithelium, and therefore risk long-term tissue damage [13, 14]. In addition to the possible hyperthermia effects of wIRA treatment in ocular structures, attention must also be paid to the phenomenon of retinal damage if light of the visible spectrum is included. Photochemical reactions caused by light stress can lead to the degeneration of specific cell types in the whole retina [15]. For this, the visual pigment rhodopsin, which is localized in the light-sensitive photoreceptor cells, plays a decisive role. Rhodopsin regulates the conversion of optical stimuli into the electrochemical signals which initiate the visual cascade via a cycle of changes in the protein configuration. Overloading this cycle by delivering a continuous light stress degenerates the photoreceptors and can lead to a degeneration of the entire retina, and thus to blindness. Since the absorption maximum of rhodopsin lies within the range of 500 nm, blue light represents the most critical photochemical action spectrum for inducing retinal damage [10]. Although blue light has a clear negative effect on the retina, the red light directly adjacent to the wIRA spectrum may have a protective effect on this tissue. For example, wavelengths of 670 nm have been shown to counteract white light-induced lipid oxidation in photoreceptors and their degeneration [16]. In addition, it may contribute to the reduced inflammatory processes in mice with age-related macular degeneration and enhance neuroprotective effects by retinal cells [17–20].

In summary, the possible severe impact of thermal and light-based therapies on different compartments of the eye, and thereby impaired vision needs to be considered. This also includes the anti-chlamydial therapy with wIRA alone or in combination with VIS.

22.4   Effect of wIRA on the Eye: Ex Vivo Models

22.4.1   Temperature Effects of wIRA on Pig Eyes Ex Vivo

Given the risks of thermal exposure to ocular structures, we considered it necessary to gain a better understanding of the development of the thermal field in the eye during wIRA irradiation as a prerequisite for its subsequent application within the framework of therapeutic treatment approaches. For this, we established an experimental model which allowed us to reproducibly study temperature changes in the cornea and the vitreous body of isolated, perfused pig eyes during exposure to different wIRA irradiances [21]. Pig eyes were chosen as they are similar in size to human eyes and have similar histological and physiological features. Briefly, the experimental model involves the perfusion of whole pig eyes with Krebs solution via the ciliary artery and the placement of the eyes within a temperature-regulated water bath which mimics blood flow and the physiological environment of the eye (Fig. 22.2a). The cornea was not covered by the water bath but constantly washed with Krebs solution to mimic tear flow. Finally, temperature development was measured using two temperature probes that were placed on the cornea and within the vitreous body of the eyes.

In this ex vivo study, the perfused pig eyes were irradiated with a spectrum of 595–1400 nm for 30 min with irradiances of 100, 210, 370 and 500 mW/cm^2 (Fig. 22.2b). Before irradiation was started, the vitreal and corneal temperature was

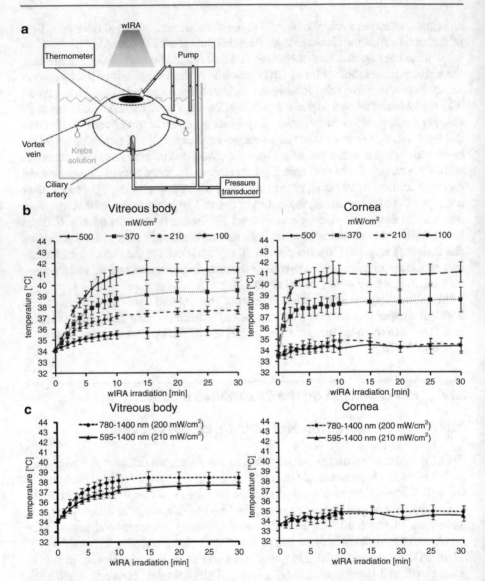

Fig. 22.2 Temperature measurements during wIRA irradiation of perfused pig eyes (modified from [21]). (**a**) Pig eyes were placed in a water bath and perfused with Krebs solution via the ciliary artery. Temperature probes were placed on top of the cornea and inside the vitreous body during wIRA irradiation. (**b** and **c**) Temperature measurements during wIRA treatment in the vitreous body (left panel) and on the cornea (right panel). Initial temperature was set to ≈34 °C before eyes were irradiated. (**b**) Eyes were irradiated with different wIRA irradiances (500, 370, 210 and 100 mW/cm²) (595–1400 nm) for 30 min. During irradiation, an irradiance-dependent temperature increase (except for 100 and 210 mW/cm² in the cornea) is shown, with a rapid rise in the first 10 min before reaching a plateau. (**c**) Eyes were irradiated with either wavelengths of 595–1400 nm at an irradiance of 210 mW/cm² or wavelengths of 780–1400 nm at an irradiance of 200 mW/cm². In the vitreous body, a mild but significant lower temperature increase was shown upon irradiation with 595–1400 nm compared to wIRA alone (780–1400 nm). The corneal temperature generally shows a slight increase without any differences between the irradiation spectrum of 595–1400 nm and 780–1400 nm

adjusted to 34 °C, which has been reported to be the physiological temperature of pig eyes [22]. As expected, the measured temperature significantly increased with increasing irradiances, before reaching a plateau after 10 min. The temperature of the vitreous body was 41.3 °C (± 0.7 °C) after an irradiance of 500 mW/cm^2. In contrast, the temperature after treatment at 100 mW/cm^2 was 35.8 °C (± 0.4 °C). Contrary to the results in the vitreous body, corneal temperatures only increased after treatments at irradiances of 370 and 500 mW/cm^2 (38.6 °C ± 1.13 °C; 41.13 °C ± 0.93 °C, respectively).

Since visible light in a range of 380–780 nm has been shown to contribute to the increase in intra-well temperatures during in vitro experiments, we examined the impact of the 780–1400 nm spectrum on temperature development in the vitreous body and cornea [23]. For this measurement, an irradiance of 200 mW/cm^2 was used. This corresponds with the irradiance of 210 mW/cm^2 when the visible part (595–780 nm) is included. However, irradiation for 30 min led to significantly lower temperatures in the vitreous body, including the visual component (37.6 °C ± 0.3 °C), than irradiation with wIRA alone (38.4 °C ± 0.7 °C) (Fig. 22.2c). In contrast, the temperature in the cornea did not exceed 35 °C and was the same for irradiation at 595–1400 nm and 780–1400 nm.

In conclusion, our results show a wIRA-irradiance-dependent increase in the temperature of ocular structures, which is more pronounced in the vitreous body than on the cornea. These findings are consistent with the fact that the vitreous body represents a closed system in which excess heat accumulates and is difficult to be removed. Even more important with respect to the use of wIRA against chlamydial eye infections, our results showed that the temperature increase after treating with a therapy-relevant irradiance of 210 mW/cm^2 did not exceed physiological temperatures for both the cornea and the vitreous body. This therapy-relevant irradiance has also been shown to be effective in reducing chlamydial infectivity in vitro and in vivo [21, 24, 25].

Hence, wIRA exposure of ocular structures at moderate irradiances represents a promising approach for treating chlamydial infections, and thus for the prevention of trachoma-induced blinding diseases without increasing ocular temperatures to non-physiological levels.

22.4.2 Impact of wIRA on the Mouse Retina Ex Vivo

The wIRA-irradiance-dependent temperature increase in the vitreous body of pig eyes might suggest that structures adjacent to the vitreous body, such as the retina, are also heated up during irradiation. Since the retina is a heat- and radiation-sensitive tissue, we investigated the expression of heat- and stress-induced proteins in retinal explants of adult mice. For this, we incubated mouse retina explants at 37 °C or 40 °C for 30 min in the presence or absence of wIRA (595–1400 nm) at an irradiance of 100 mW/cm^2, after which we analysed the levels of phosphorylated stress kinases p38, Akt, Erk1/2 and SAPK/JNK by ELISA and found no significant changes immediately (0 h), 3 h or 24 h following treatment (Fig. 22.3a). Consistent with this

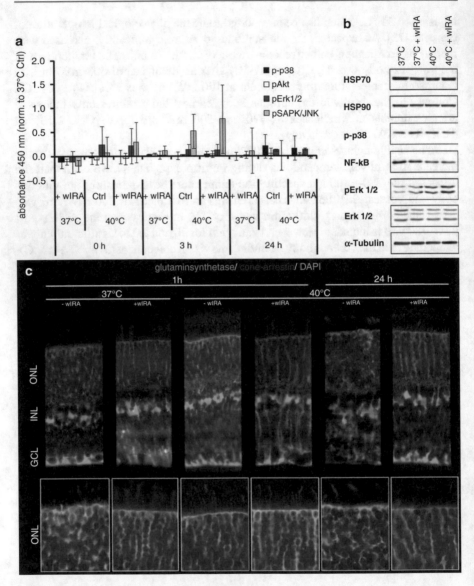

Fig. 22.3 wIRA effects on the mouse retina. Explants of adult mouse retina were incubated at 37 °C (Ctrl = control) or 40 °C in cell culture media in the presence and absence of wIRA (595–1400 nm) using an irradiance of 100 mW/cm². (**a**, modified from [21]) Levels of phosphory-lated stress proteins (p-p38, pAkt, pErk1/2, pSAPK/JNK) were analysed by ELISA, immediately (0 h), 3 h or 24 h after wIRA irradiation. Neither hyperthermia alone nor in combination with wIRA induces any significant changes in protein levels. (**b**) Western blot analyses of HSP70, HSP90, p-p38, NfκB, pErk 1/2 and Erk 1/2 showed no changes in expression 3 h after the treat-ments. α-Tubulin serves as loading control. (**c**) Immunolabeling of cell type specific markers (glu-tamine synthetase (green) = Müller glia cells, cone arrestin (red) = cones) in mouse retina sections. Cell nuclei were stained with DAPI (blue) in all retinal layers (ONL-outer nuclear layer, INL-inner nuclear layer, GCL-ganglion cell layer). Regardless of treatment, all immunolabeling patterns after 1 h and 24 h were similar

observation, Western blot analysis for stress-induced proteins HSP70, HSP90, p-p38, NfκB, pErk 1/2 and Erk 1/2 showed no changes in expression levels 3 h after treatment (Fig. 22.3b). In addition, immunolabeling for cell type specific retina markers (glutamine synthetase for Müller glia cells, cone arrestin for cones) to evaluate maintenance of the retina structure indicated no changes in their expression patterns 1 h or 24 h after hyperthermia or a combination of hyperthermia and wIRA (Fig. 22.3c).

Consequently, our analysis showed that the heat- and radiation-sensitive retina is unaffected by wIRA exposures using an irradiance of 100 mW/cm² in terms of activation of stress proteins and maintenance of the retinal structure. Together with the results of the temperature measurements, these findings support the use of wIRA irradiation as a novel and safe therapeutic approach for treating chlamydial infections.

22.5   Outlook

wIRA may be a promising future therapy for the treatment of chlamydial infections of the eye, as has been suggested by various in vitro studies [21, 26]. However, for clinical delivery, it is essential to ensure the safety of the ocular structures that are exposed to wIRA irradiation during treatment. In our ex vivo pig and mouse model experiments, we have been able to obtain the first evidence that wIRA is likely to be safe [21]. Recently, the first in vivo study also demonstrated the efficacy of wIRA for the treatment of chlamydial infections in guinea pig eyes, a well-established model for trachoma-like diseases [25]. In our accompanying in vivo study into the safety of wIRA irradiation on ocular structures in guinea pig eyes, we have also obtained promising results and have excluded the possibility of adverse side-effects due to wIRA exposure (work in progress). Nevertheless, the effects of wIRA irradiation on *Chlamydia* and ocular structures need to be investigated in more detail and optimized for clinical application in humans. In order to further increase the efficacy of wIRA in terms of chlamydial reduction, the use of photosensitizers (e.g., indocyanine green) could be a promising possibility, since these compounds have been shown to improve the effectiveness of antimicrobial photodynamic therapy (aPDT) [27]. Such approaches also require parallel studies on the mode of action, applicability and safety of the used photosensitizers, both in vitro and in vivo. For this reason, we are currently conducting initial safety studies on human conjunctival cells, by investigating the impact of the photosensitizer indocyanine green during wIRA-based aPDT.

References

1. Gokul KC, Gurung DB, Adhikary PR. Thermal effects of eyelid in human eye temperature model. J Appl Math Informatics. 2014;32(56):649–63.
2. Regal S, Troughton J, Delattre R, et al. Changes in temperature inside an optomechanical model of the human eye during emulated transscleral cyclophotocoagulation. Biomed Opt Express. 2020;11(8):4548–59.
3. Parver LM, Auker C, Carpenter DO. Choroidal blood flow as a heat dissipating mechanism in the macula. Am J Ophthalmol. 1980;89(5):641–6.

4. Flyckt VMM, Raaymakers BW, Lagendijk JJW. Modelling the impact of blood flow on the temperature distribution in the human eye and the orbit: fixed heat transfer coefficients versus the Pennes bioheat model versus discrete blood vessels. Phys Med Biol. 2006;51(19):5007–21.
5. Geiser MH, Bonvin M, Quibel O. Corneal and retinal temperatures under various ambient conditions: a model and experimental approach. Klin Monatsblätter Augenheilkunde. 2004;221(5):311–4.
6. Itokawa T, Suzuki T, Okajima Y, et al. Correlation between blood flow and temperature of the ocular anterior segment in normal subjects. Diagnostics. 2020;10(9):695.
7. Ivanov IV, Mappes T, Schaupp P, et al. Ultraviolet radiation oxidative stress affects eye health. J Biophotonics. 2018;11:e201700377.
8. Youssef PN, Sheibani N, Albert DM. Retinal light toxicity. Eye. 2011;2011(25):1–14.
9. Voke J. Radiation effects on the eye part 1: infrared radiation effects on ocular tissue. Optom Today. 1999;9:22–8.
10. Zhao ZC, Zhou Y, Tan G, et al. Research progress about the effect and prevention of blue light on eyes. Int J Ophthalmol. 2018;11(12):1999–2003.
11. Vos JJ, van Norren D. Thermal cataract, from furnaces to lasers. Clin Exp Optom. 2004;87(6):372–6.
12. Aly EM, Mohamed ES. Effect of infrared radiation on the lens. Indian J Ophthalmol. 2011;59(2):97–101.
13. Wakakura M, Foulds WS. Response of cultured Müller cells to heat shock - an immunocytochemical study of heat shock and intermediate filament proteins in response to temperature elevation. Exp Eye Res. 1989;48(3):337–50.
14. Sekiyama E, Saint-Geniez M, Yoneda K, et al. Heat treatment of retinal pigment epithelium induces production of elastic lamina components and antiangiogenic activity. FASEB J. 2012;26(2):567–75.
15. Różanowska M, Sarna T. Light-induced damage to the retina: role of rhodopsin chromophore revisited. Photochem Photobiol. 2005;81(6):1305–30.
16. Rutar M, Natoli R, Albarracin R, et al. 670-nm light treatment reduces complement propagation following retinal degeneration. J Neuroinflammation. 2012;9:257.
17. Begum R, Powner MB, Hudson N, et al. Treatment with 670 nm light up regulates cytochrome C oxidase expression and reduces inflammation in an age-related macular degeneration model. PLoS One. 2013;8(2):e57828.
18. Albarracin R, Eells J, Valter K. Photobiomodulation protects the retina from light-induced photoreceptor degeneration. Invest Ophthalmol Vis Sci. 2011;52:3582–92.
19. Albarracin R, Valter K. 670 nm red light preconditioning supports Müller cell function: evidence from the white light-induced damage model in the rat retina. Photochem Photobiol. 2012;88(6):1418–27.
20. Heinig N, Schumann U, Calzia D, et al. Photobiomodulation mediates neuroprotection against blue light induced retinal photoreceptor degeneration. Int J Mol Sci. 2020;21(7):2370.
21. Rahn C, Marti H, Frohns A, et al. Water-filtered infrared A reduces chlamydial infectivity *in vitro* without causing *ex vivo* eye damage in pig and mouse models. J Photochem Photobiol B. 2016;165:340–50.
22. Landers MB, Watson JS, Ulrich JN, et al. Determination of retinal and vitreous temperature in vitrectomy. Retina. 2012;32(1):172–6.
23. Marti H, Blenn C, Borel N. The contribution of temperature, exposure intensity and visible light to the inhibitory effect of irradiation on acute chlamydial infection. J Photochem Photobiol B. 2015;153:324–33.
24. Kuratli J, Pesch T, Marti H, et al. Water filtered infrared A and visible light (wIRA/VIS) irradiation reduces *chlamydia trachomatis* infectivity independent of targeted cytokine inhibition. Front Microbiol. 2018;9:2757.
25. Inic-Kanada A, Stojanovic M, Miljkovic R, et al. Water-filtered infrared A and visible light (wIRA/VIS) treatment reduces *chlamydia caviae*-induced ocular inflammation and infectious load in a Guinea pig model of inclusion conjunctivitis. J Photochem Photobiol B. 2020;209:111953.

26. Marti H, Koschwanez M, Pesch T, et al. Water-filtered infrared A irradiation in combination with visible light inhibits acute chlamydial infection. PLoS One. 2014;9(7):e102239.
27. Al-Ahmad A, Tennert C, Karygianni L, et al. Antimicrobial photodynamic therapy using visible light plus water-filtered infrared-A (wIRA). J Med Microbiol. 2013;62:467–73.

Part VIII
Recommended Readings

Molecular and Cellular Mechanisms of Water-Filtered IR

23

Michael R. Hamblin

23.1 Infrared Radiation

Electromagnetic radiation is a form of energy propagation through space that travels at a constant speed in the form of waves or particles; light and radio waves, for instance, are types of radiation. Solar radiation reaching the earth, also known as the *electromagnetic spectrum*, exhibits a dual nature as it acts both like a wave and a particle travelling in packets of energy (*photons*) which propagate through space at the speed of light (2.998×10^8 m/s) [1–3]. The energy of electromagnetic radiation is quantified by the number of electron volts (eV) (1 eV describes the energy gained by an electron subjected through a potential difference of 1 Volt) [3]. The wavelike properties of electromagnetic radiation are described by the relationship of velocity (c) to wavelength (λ) (the distance between two consecutive peaks of a wave) and frequency (v) (number of cycles per second, or Hertz, Hz), expressed in the formula Eq. (23.1) [1].

$$c = \lambda v \tag{23.1}$$

Regarding photons, the energy carried is described by Planck's eq. 23.2:

$$E = hv \tag{23.2}$$

where E is the energy (given in Joule [J]); v is the frequency (Hz), and h is Planck's constant (6.626×10^{-34} J·s). In both equations, the energy associated to the electromagnetic radiation is directly proportional to its frequency and inversely proportional to wavelength, meaning that longer wavelengths result in lower energy and vice versa [1].

M. R. Hamblin (✉)
Laser Research Centre, Faculty of Health Science, University of Johannesburg, Doornfontein, South Africa

Radiation Biology Research Center, Iran University of Medical Sciences, Tehran, Iran

© The Author(s) 2022
P. Vaupel (ed.), *Water-filtered Infrared A (wIRA) Irradiation*,
https://doi.org/10.1007/978-3-030-92880-3_23

The spectrum of electromagnetic radiation ranges from 290 nm to more than 1000,000 nm [4] and is generally divided into seven regions of decreasing wavelength (or increasing energy and frequency). The common designations, as shown in Fig. 23.1, are radio waves, microwaves, infrared (IR), visible light, ultraviolet, X-rays and gamma rays [2].

Infrared radiation constitutes the waveband longer than 0.7 μm and up to 1000 μm. Corresponding frequencies and quantum energies are from the range 300 GHz–385 THz to 1.2 meV–1.6 eV, respectively [5]. Historically, infrared radiation has been divided into three bands, the definition of which differs across industries. The International Commission on Illumination (CIE) indicates the following nomenclature and ranges: IR-A (0.7–1.4 μm); IR-B (1.4–3 μm); IR-C (3–1000 μm) [6]. Alternatively, the International Standard Organization (ISO) 20,473 provides the following definitions: near-IR as 0.78–<3 μm; mid-IR ≥3–<50 μm; and far-IR, or FIR, ≥50–<1000 μm [7]. In this review, we will be using the CIE definition.

All matter (solid, liquid, gas) can absorb as well as emit energy in the form of electromagnetic radiation [8]. The absorption of energy in the visible region of the spectrum excites electrons in molecular bonding orbitals to a higher quantum energy state; this energy is either converted into heat (vibrational energy), and lost as emitted infrared radiation (radiative heat), or alternatively is emitted as visible light of a longer wavelength (fluorescence). For wavelengths in the infrared region, the energy is directly absorbed by molecular vibrational levels and later emitted as infrared radiation. For an object with a temperature T (Kelvin) and a surface area (A), the radiative heat transfer in a time t is given by the Stefan–Boltzmann law of radiation (Eq. 23.3), where P is net radiated power, e is emissivity, A is radiating area, T is

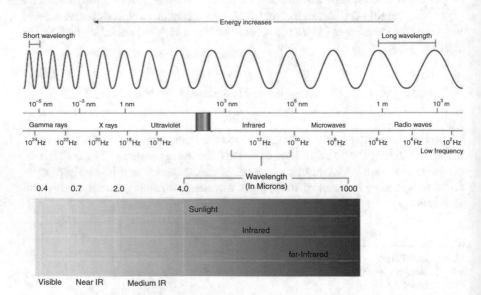

Fig. 23.1 Electromagnetic spectrum and infrared radiation. IR-A (0.7 μm–1.4 μm); IR-B (1.4 μm–3 μm); IR-C (3 μm–1000 μm). λ wavelength, ν frequency, *UV* ultraviolet

temperature of radiator, σ is Boltzmann's constant ($\sigma = 5.6703 \times 10^{-8}$), and T_c are the temperature of the surrounding matter [9].

$$P = e\sigma A\left(T^4 - T_C^4\right) \tag{23.3}$$

Although electromagnetic radiation occurs at all temperatures above absolute zero, the amount of energy (heat) an object can radiate depends greatly on the difference in temperature between the systems involved. In fact, energy transfer occurs from high to lower temperature bodies. It is also important to note that due to the First Law of Thermodynamics, the internal energy of all systems involved in the radiation (emitter or receiver) changes as a consequence of the energy transfer (energy can neither be created nor destroyed) [10] . Within molecules, internal energy can be stored in two main ways, either by exciting the electronic quantum energy levels to a higher state or by increasing the vibrational, rotational and translational energy levels of the bonds or molecules. Depending on the amount of energy transferred, radiation can be divided into ionizing and non-ionizing. Non-ionizing radiation (ultraviolet or visible light) transfers enough energy to the receiver to excite the electron in the highest occupied molecular orbital to the lowest unoccupied molecular orbital. By contrast, the energy carried by ionizing electromagnetic radiation is strong enough to entirely remove tightly bound electrons from an atom or molecule [3]. Ionizing radiation causes damage to biological matter and living cells; for instance, radiotherapy with high-energy radiation such as x-rays or gamma-rays is used to destroy tumor cells. Infrared is a type of non-ionizing radiation whose absorption leads to changes in the vibrational and rotational energy levels of molecules and bonds [5, 11]. All types of infrared radiation (IR-A, IR-B, IR-C) increase the temperature of the absorbing matter, which extent depends on the power density of the radiation, the absorption coefficient of the material, and the rate of energy lost by emission, convection, or conduction.

23.2   Photobiomodulation

Photobiomodulation (PBM) therapy employs the application of relatively low power levels of red or near-infrared (NIR) radiation to the human body [12]. The overall goal is to treat and heal wounds and injuries, reduce pain and inflammation, regenerate damaged tissue, and protect tissue at risk of dying. Recent studies have made significant advances in understanding the mechanisms of action of PBM [13]. It has long been realized that the cellular powerhouses, called mitochondria, function as major photoreceptors for light of these specific wavelengths (red and NIR). It appears that organs that are particularly rich in mitochondria respond very well to PBM. The photons are absorbed by chromophores present in the mitochondria, and cytochrome c oxidase (unit IV in the respiratory chain) is a leading candidate for this role. The mitochondrial membrane potential is raised and oxygen consumption and ATP generation are increased. Signaling pathways are triggered and transcription factors are activated, leading to fairly long-lasting effects after relatively brief exposure of the tissue to light.

The stimulation of mitochondrial metabolism by PBM can have important biological effects, beyond the simple increase in cellular ATP supplies. Let us consider stem cells and progenitor cells. Stem cells whether they are hemopoietic or mesenchymal in nature are relatively quiescent cells that inhabit hypoxic stem cell niches, which vary depending on the tissue or organ of origin [14]. One of the most important hypoxic niches for stem cells is the bone marrow [15]. Because stem cells are intended to survive for the entire lifespan of the organism, they must take exceptional care to avoid DNA damage that could introduce mutations that could cause cancer. The most common cause of this DNA damage is the oxidative stress produced by reactive oxygen species (ROS). ROS such as hydrogen peroxide and superoxide anion are a natural by-product of aerobic respiration and oxidative phosphorylation (OXPHOS), which takes place in the mitochondria. Because stem cells live in a niche with a low pO_2 environment, their mitochondrial metabolism is skewed toward glycolysis and away from OXPHOS. However, under the influence of PBM, the mitochondrial electron transport chain is stimulated toward OXPHOS [16], which tends to produce ROS to induce stem cell differentiation and enhanced motility [17]. When the stem cells emerge from their hypoxic niche in search of higher oxygen concentrations to support their altered mitochondrial metabolism, they will be exposed to many cues and chemokines that direct them to sites of tissue injury or degeneration, where they can then fulfill their regenerative roles [18].

Another very important function of PBMT is its anti-inflammatory effect [19]. The mechanism for this is based upon the division of many types of human immune cells into two completely different phenotypes. This division is most often seen in monocyte/macrophage cells that can either be the M1 or the M2 phenotype [20]. The M1 phenotype is pro-inflammatory in function, with secretion of cytokines, such as tumor necrosis factor-α (TNF-α), interleukin-1 (IL-1), IL-6, IL-12, and type I interferons (IFN). M1 macrophages are involved in inflammatory responses by producing chemokine ligands, such as chemokine (C-X-C motif) ligands 1–3 (CXCL1–3), CXCL5, and CXCL8–10 [21]. They also produce nitric oxide and ROS to kill microbial cells. On the other hand, M2 macrophages show high phagocytosis capacity, produce extracellular matrix (ECM) components, secrete proangiogenic and chemotactic factors, and IL-10 [22]. M2 macrophages can clear apoptotic cells, and can mitigate the inflammatory response to promote wound healing [23]. One key difference between M1 and M2 macrophages involves arginine metabolism [24]. M1 macrophages express inducible nitric oxide synthase, which metabolizes arginine to nitric oxide (NO) and citrulline, while M2 macrophages express arginase, which hydrolyzes arginine to ornithine and urea. It was recently discovered that another major difference between M1 and M2 macrophages involves the mitochondrial metabolism [25]. M1 macrophages rely mainly on cytosolic glycolysis, while M2 macrophages are more dependent on mitochondrial OXPHOS. It has been shown in several studies that PBM can switch the macrophage polarization state away from the M1 and toward the M2 phenotype [26–28]. Therefore, the hypothesis is that PBM switches the mitochondrial metabolism from glycolysis to OXPHOS, thus turning M1 into M2 macrophages and producing the beneficial anti-inflammatory and wound healing effects.

A third biological effect of PBM is involved in pain. Mitochondrial dysfunction has recently been appreciated to be a major factor involved in a variety of painful conditions. These painful conditions include neuropathic pain [29], myalgic encephalomyelitis [30], tendinopathy [31], chemotherapy-induced peripheral neuropathy [32], trigeminal neuralgia [33], and intervertebral disc degeneration [34]. The hypothesis is that the widespread use of PBM to treat painful conditions, especially chronic pain which does not respond to opioid analgesics, could be based on improving the mitochondrial function and normalizing the mitochondrial membrane potential.

23.3 Heat Sensitive Ion Channels

Over recent years, a large number of stimulus-sensitive ion channels have been identified in all life forms, including humans, called transient receptor potential (TRP) channels. TRP channels were first discovered in 1969 in the "transient receptor potential" mutant (trp-mutant) strain of the fruit fly *Drosophila melanogaster* [35]. Since then, nine separate families have been proposed which are divided into two groups. Group 1 contains TRPC, TRPV, TRPVL, TRPA, TRPM, TRPS, and TRPN, while group 2 contains TRPP and TRPML [36]. TRPs are relatively non-selective ion channels allowing passage of Ca^{2+}, Mg^{2+}, and Na^+ ions. TRP channels can be activated by a wide range of stimuli, including pain, temperature (heat and cold), molecules associated with different tastes, pH, pressure, stretching, vibration, and visible light [37]. There is considerable overlap between different individual TRP family members in terms of which stimulus they can respond to [38].

One of the most interesting sub-family of TRP channels is the TRPV (vanilloid) group [39]. TRPV1 was the first TRP channel to be discovered in humans and was identified as the receptor for capsaicin (the active ingredient in hot chili peppers) [40]. The same group showed that TRPV1 could be activated by a modest temperature increase ($\approx$43 °C) [41]. Later studies described three different TRPV channels that were also heat sensitive, TRPV2 ($\approx$52 °C), TRPV3 ($\approx$33 °C), and TRPV4 (28–44 °C) [42]. These TRPV channels are widely expressed in neurons but are also expressed in other organs, such as tongue, bladder, kidneys, skin, inner ear, and endothelial cells [42]. The expression of TRPV1 in the skin is responsible for the clinically useful topical application of a capsaicin-containing cream as a pain-relieving treatment [43]. TRPV channels are mainly found in the plasma membrane of cells but have also been found to be present in the mitochondrial membrane, particularly in non-neuronal cells [44].

One interesting involvement of TRPV channels concerns the production of nitric oxide. It has long been realized that both IR therapy and PBMT produce vasodilation in the skin and increased blood flow, which has been attributed to increased nitric oxide production. There are many sources of NO in the human body, with the principle ones being the three isoforms of nitric oxide synthase (NOS), inducible (iNOS), endothelial (eNOS), and neuronal (nNOS), as well as dissociation from stores such as hemoglobin and myoglobin, and reduction of nitrite to nitric oxide

[45]. Miyamoto et al. showed that activation of TRPV3 in the skin triggered the production of nitric oxide from nitrite that was independent of NOS activity [46].

There is a field of research based on pulsed infrared laser stimulation of neurons (INS) [47]. This technique employs the delivery of circa 1 ms pulses of infrared radiation to depolarize the neuronal membrane and generate an action potential. The mechanism of INS is due to the transient and localized heating caused by absorption of IR radiation by water causing a local temperature increase of between 3.8 and 6.4 °C [48]. It was originally designed to be more versatile than using electrical stimulation, in that it does not require any implantation of wires, but still has good spatial resolution because the laser spot can be 100–400 μm in diameter. When the technique of optogenetics (which uses the introduction of a genetically engineered channel-rhodopsin ion channel into specific neurons using the spatially controlled delivery of virus) became widespread [49], it was realized that INS did not require any genetic modification, and could therefore be more practical for human use [50]. In fact a fiberoptic array for multiple channel INS of the brain has been described [51].

There are two main mechanisms that have been proposed to explain how INS actually works at the level of the axon. The most popular mechanism involves TRPV channels (and particularly TRPV4) being stimulated to produce intracellular calcium changes [52]. The second mechanism involves altering the electrical capacitance of the cell membrane by producing a rapid local increase in the temperature of water, thus depolarizing the target cell [53].

23.4   Infrared-Emitting Fabrics and Garments

There are several ways to deliver infrared radiation for therapeutic use, varying from heat lamps, saunas, and water-filtered IRA (wIRA), all of which require an external power source, to infrared-emitting materials that rely solely on body heat as a source of power [5, 54]. *Bioceramic* describes a specific type of mineral material that emits IR-C radiation at body temperature, and which can produce biological effects on the tissue, particularly when worn in close contact with the body for extended periods of time [55, 56]. While the power density emitted by these fabrics is very small when compared to electrically powered IR sources, this is compensated by the fact that garments and patches can be worn for extended periods of time (hours or days), while lamps or saunas are usually only used for minutes at a time. Bioceramic materials are produced by a combination of polymers with ceramic-containing mineral oxides, such as silicon dioxide (SiO_2), aluminium oxide (Al_2O_3), and titanium dioxide (TiO_2) [5]. In industrial applications, these minerals are often used in the construction of firebricks and gas mantles. In domestic kitchens, the use of a clay cooking pot is often preferred to a metal cooking pot, because of its ability to emit more infrared radiation at lower temperatures. There have been some attempts to characterize the properties of these infrared-emitting fabrics in the laboratory, including reflectance, transmittance, and emissivity. Emissivity is a measure of how much radiation (7.5–14 μm) an object can absorb and emit compared with a black body (a body that absorbs and emits all radiation falling in it), whose emissivity is defined as 1.0 [57]. Emissivity is a surface phenomenon, therefore nanoparticles or microparticles (which have a large ratio of surface area to mass) are considered to be the most efficient configuration for emitting infrared radiation compared to bulk ceramic material. Anderson et al. utilized Fourier transform infrared spectroscopy to measure the spectral optical properties of textile fabrics woven with varying percentages of ceramic particle-bearing polymeric fibers and found that the emissivity of polyester fabric can be engineered controllably via the inclusion of ceramic microparticles within the fabric fibers [58, 59].

In general, the mechanism of action of infrared radiating materials is to absorb heat energy from the body (radiation, convection, and conduction) and maintain the temperature at sufficiently high levels to be able to re-emit the IR-C energy back to the body with a broad peak centered at 10 μm, according to the Stefan–Boltzmann law [5, 60].

The effects of infrared-emitting ceramics on skin blood flow have been investigated by analyzing the changes observed on several biomarkers. For instance, in a study conducted on 153 healthy individuals wearing shirts containing ceramics compared with standard polyester shirts, changes in arterial oxygen saturation and transcutaneous partial pressure of oxygen ($tcPO_2$) were measured [61]. Similar findings were observed in another study which found increased blood flow (measured as $tcPO_2$ changes) and improved muscular performance (measured as mean hand grip strength) [60]. The benefits of infrared on blood circulation were supported further by a study on patients with Raynaud's syndrome, where reduced pain and disability of the arm, shoulder, and hand were recorded after wearing infrared-emitting gloves [62]. The topical use of compressive infrared-emitting ceramic containing socks reduced edema and pain in the feet compared with control socks [63].

Other studies have used infrared-emitting nanoparticles incorporated into apparel, such as gloves, socks, belts, or patches, to provide an easy and practical application of therapeutic IR [56, 64]. Bagnato et al. evaluated the efficacy of an IR-C emitting plaster in the treatment of knee osteoarthritis (OA) in a randomized, placebo-controlled clinical study [65]. Loturco et al. investigated the effects of IR-C-emitting non-compressive pants on indirect markers of exercise-induced muscle damage and physical performance recovery in soccer players [64]. The use of IR-C emitting socks showed a beneficial effect on chronic foot pain resulting from diabetic neuropathy or other disorders [66]. The efficacy of an IR-C-emitting sericite (a common mineral) belt in patients with primary dysmenorrhea was evaluated over three menstrual cycles (and 2 follow-up cycles) by Lee et al. in a multicentre, randomized, double-blind, placebo-controlled trial ($n = 104$) [67]. Lai et al. used a IR-C emitting neck device to partly reduce muscle stiffness in chronic neck pain [68]. These infrared-emitting materials (ceramics and fabrics) are well tolerated, and the only side effect that was occasionally reported was skin irritation and itching (which disappeared within a few days without treatment) [62, 67].

23.5 Application to Water-Filtered IR-A

It is interesting to compare the two treatments discussed above (PBM and IR emitting bioceramics) with wIRA. The big difference of course is that PBM and bioceramics were designed to produce no detectable heating effect in the tissue. wIRA is very different, in that it was originally designed to produce therapeutic tissue heating. Mild hyperthermia (39 °C– 43 °C) has long been known to be an effective adjuvant in cancer treatment, and the main question is what is the best approach to increase the temperature of the tumor to a therapeutically effective level, without causing unacceptable side effects either to the whole body or to surrounding normal tissue? The wIRA device (hydrosun, Müllheim, Germany) can focus the IR radiation onto a discrete region of the body and is basically a modern sophisticated version of an infrared heat lamp. The big unanswered question is to what extent do the medical benefits of wIRA depend on biological processes that do not require measurable tissue heating to be stimulated? By now everybody will accept that PBMT using red or NIR radiation (or indeed blue and green wavelengths) can produce biological effects by a *photochemical mechanism* as opposed to a *photothermal mechanism*. In contrast, it would appear that IR emitting fabrics cannot carry out a photochemical effect because they do not emit light, neither can they carry out a thermal effect because the temperature of the tissue is not increased to a measurable effect. The only solution to this dilemma is the concept of IR energy absorption by nanostructured water clusters that could alter the protein conformation at the nanoscale [69]. The concept of nanostructured water was introduced by Gerald Pollack, who observed the build-up of an "exclusion zone" on certain types of hydrophobic surfaces immersed in water [70]. In fact Pollack called this phenomenon of interfacial water "the fourth phase of water' [71]. Pollack has also suggested many ways that this interfacial water could be involved in cells and in human biology [72, 73].

Certainly, wIRA does cause a measurable increase in the tissue temperature. This fact does not exclude the possibility of a similar alteration in protein conformation occurring at the same time. The activation of heat-sensitive TRP channels is the main hypothesis to explain the beneficial effects of IR-emitting fabrics, and it is only reasonable to expect this to occur to an even greater extent with the application of wIRA. Future studies should examine the role of TRP channels in the biological activity of wIRA, especially those applications related to wound healing, and the reduction of pain and inflammation.

Funding and Conflict of Interest MRH was supported by US NIH Grants R01AI050875 and R21AI121700. MRH declares the following potential conflicts of interest. Scientific Advisory Boards: Transdermal Cap Inc., Cleveland, OH; Hologenix Inc. Santa Monica, CA; Vielight, Toronto, Canada; JOOVV Inc., Minneapolis-St. Paul MN; Consulting; USHIO Corp, Japan; Sanofi-Aventis Deutschland GmbH, Frankfurt/Main, Germany.

References

1. Percuoco R. Plain radiographic imaging. In: Marchiori DM, editor. Clinical imaging. 3rd ed. St Louis: Mosby; 2014. p. 1–43.
2. Funk RK, Stockham AL, Laack NNI. Basics of radiation therapy. In: Herrmann J, editor. Clinical cardio-oncology. Amsterdam: Elsevier; 2016. p. 39–60.
3. Elliott DA, et al. Radiation therapy. In: Bell RB, Fernandes RP, Andersen PE, editors. Oral, head and neck oncology and reconstructive surgery. Amsterdam: Elsevier; 2018. p. 268–90.
4. Barolet D, Christiaens F, Hamblin MR. Infrared and skin: Friend or foe. J Photochem Photobiol B. 2016;155:78–85.

5. Vatansever F, Hamblin MR. Far infrared radiation (FIR): its biological effects and medical applications. Photonics Lasers Med. 2012;4:255–66.
6. International Commission on Illumination (CIE). 17–580 infrared radiation, http://eilv.cie.co.at/term/580.
7. International Organization for Standardization (ISO). ISO 20473:2007 optics and photonics — Spectral bands, https://www.iso.org/standard/39482.html; 2007.
8. Meseguer J, Pérez-Grande I, Sanz-Andrés A. Spacecraft thermal control. In: Meseguer J, Pérez-Grande I, Sanz-Andrés A, editors. Thermal radiation heat transfer. New York: Woodhead Publishing; 2012. p. 73–86.
9. Dorofeyev IA, Vinogradov EA. Fluctuating electromagnetic fields of solids. Phys Rep. 2011;504:75–143.
10. Bergman TL, Lavine AS, Incropera FP, De Witt DP. Fundamentals of heat and mass transfer. 7th ed. New York: John Wiley & Sons; 2011.
11. Schieke SM, Schroeder P, Krutmann J. Cutaneous effects of infrared radiation: from clinical observations to molecular response mechanisms. Photodermatol Photoimmunol Photomed. 2003;19:228–34.
12. Chung H, Dai T, Sharma SK, et al. The nuts and bolts of low-level laser (light) therapy. Ann Biomed Eng. 2012;40:516–33.
13. De Freitas LF, Hamblin MR. Proposed mechanisms of Photobiomodulation or low-level light therapy. IEEE J Sel Top Quantum Electron. 2016;22:7000417.
14. Suessbier U, Nombela-Arrieta C. Assessing cellular hypoxic status in situ within the bone marrow microenvironment. Methods Mol Biol. 2019;2017:123–34.
15. Szade K, Gulat GS, Chan CKF, et al. Where hematopoietic stem Cells live: the bone marrow niche. Antioxid Redox Signal. 2018;29:191–204.
16. Martins MD, Silveira FM, Martins MAT, et al. Photobiomodulation therapy drives massive epigenetic histone modifications, stem cells mobilization and accelerated epithelial healing. J Biophotonics. 2021;14(2):e202000274. https://doi.org/10.1002/jbio.202000274.
17. Ludin A, Gur-Cohen S, Golan K, et al. Reactive oxygen species regulate hematopoietic stem cell self-renewal, migration and development, as well as their bone marrow microenvironment. Antioxid Redox Signal. 2014;21:1605–19.
18. Yin Y, Li X, He XT, et al. Leveraging stem cell homing for therapeutic regeneration. J Dent Res. 2017;96:601–9.
19. Hamblin MR. Mechanisms and applications of the anti-inflammatory effects of photobiomodulation. AIMS Biophys. 2017;4:337–61.
20. Vergadi E, Ieronymaki E, Lyroni K, et al. Akt signaling pathway in macrophage activation and M1/M2 polarization. J Immunol. 2017;198:1006–14.
21. Lu C-H, Lai C-Y, Yeh D-W, et al. Involvement of M1 macrophage polarization in endosomal toll-like receptors activated psoriatic inflammation. Mediators Inflamm. 2018;2018:3523642. https://doi.org/10.1155/2018/3523642.
22. Rőszer T. Understanding the mysterious M2 macrophage through activation markers and effector mechanisms. Mediators Inflamm. 2015;2015:816460. https://doi.org/10.1155/2015/816460.
23. Novak ML, Koh TJ. Macrophage phenotypes during tissue repair. J Leukoc Biol. 2013;93:875–81.
24. Rath M, Müller I, Kropf P, et al. Metabolism via arginase or nitric oxide synthase: two competing arginine pathways in macrophages. Front Immunol. 2014;5:5. https://doi.org/10.3389/fimmu.2014.00532.
25. Liu Y, Xu R, Gu H, et al. Metabolic reprogramming in macrophage responses. Biomark Res. 2021;9:1. https://doi.org/10.1186/s40364-020-00251-y.
26. Reis VP, Paloschi MV, Rego CMA, et al. Photobiomodulation induces murine macrophages polarization toward M2 phenotype. Toxicon. 2021;198:171–5.
27. de Brito Sousa K, Rodrigues MFSD, de Souza SD, et al. Differential expression of inflammatory and anti-inflammatory mediators by M1 and M2 macrophages after photobiomodulation with red or infrared lasers. Lasers Med Sci. 2020;35:337–43.

28. Li K, Liang Z, Zhang J, et al. Attenuation of the inflammatory response and polarization of macrophages by photobiomodulation. Lasers Med Sci. 2020;35:1509–18.
29. Dai C-Q, Guo Y, Chu X-Y. Neuropathic pain: the dysfunction of Drp1, mitochondria, and ROS homeostasis. Neurotox Res. 2020;38:553–63.
30. Toogood PL, Clauw DJ, Phadke S, Hoffman D. Myalgic encephalomyelitis/chronic fatigue syndrome (ME/CFS): where will the drugs come from? Pharmacol Res. 2021;165:105465. https://doi.org/10.1016/j.phrs.2021.105465.
31. Zhang X, Eliasberg CD, Rodeo SA. Mitochondrial dysfunction and potential mitochondrial protectant treatments in tendinopathy. Ann N Y Acad Sci. 2021;1490:29–41.
32. Doyle TM, Salvemini D. Mitochondrial dysfunction and chemotherapy-induced neuropathic pain. Neurosci Lett. 2021;760:136087.
33. Ravera S, Colombo E, Pasquale C, et al. Mitochondrial bioenergetic, Photobiomodulation and trigeminal branches nerve damage, What's the connection? A review. Int J Mol Sci. 2021;22:4347.
34. Saberi M, Zhang X, Mobasheri A. Targeting mitochondrial dysfunction with small molecules in intervertebral disc aging and degeneration. GeroScience. 2021;43:517–37.
35. Cosens DJ, Manning A. Abnormal Electroretinogram from a drosophila mutant. Nature. 1969;224:285–7.
36. Li H. TRP Channel classification. Adv Exp Med Biol. 2017;976:1–8.
37. Emir TLR. Neurobiology of TRP channels. Boca Raton: CRC Press; 2017.
38. Kirkwood NK, Albert JT. Sensory transduction: confusing the senses. Curr Biol. 2013;23:R22–3.
39. Seebohm G, Schreiber JA. Beyond hot and spicy: TRPV channels and their pharmacological modulation. Cell Physiol Biochem. 2021;55:108–30.
40. Caterina MJ, Schumacher MA, Tominaga M, et al. The capsaicin receptor: a heat-activated ion channel in the pain pathway. Nature. 1997;389:816–24.
41. Caterina MJ, Rosen TA, Tominaga M, et al. A capsaicin-receptor homologue with a high threshold for noxious heat. Nature. 1999;398:436–41.
42. Wetsel WC. Sensing hot and cold with TRP channels. Int J Hyperthermia. 2011;27:388–98.
43. Chrubasik S, Weiser T, Beime B. Effectiveness and safety of topical capsaicin cream in the treatment of chronic soft tissue pain. Phytother Res. 2010;24:1877–85.
44. Juárez-Contreras R, Méndez-Reséndiz KA, Rosenbaum T, et al. TRPV1 channel: a noxious signal transducer that affects mitochondrial function. Int J Mol Sci. 2020;21:8882.
45. Tejero J, Shiva S, Gladwin MT. Sources of vascular nitric oxide and reactive oxygen species and their regulation. Physiol Rev. 2019;99:311–79.
46. Miyamoto T, Petrus MJ, Dubin AE, Patapoutian A. TRPV3 regulates nitric oxide synthase-independent nitric oxide synthesis in the skin. Nat Commun. 2011;2:369.
47. Chernov M, Roe AW. Infrared neural stimulation: a new stimulation tool for central nervous system applications. Neurophot. 2014;1:011011.
48. Wells J, Kao C, Konrad P, et al. Biophysical mechanisms of transient optical stimulation of peripheral nerve. Biophys J. 2007;93:2567–80.
49. Deisseroth K. Optogenetics: 10 years of microbial opsins in neuroscience. Nat Neurosci. 2015;18:1213–25.
50. Richardson RT, Ibbotson MR, Thompson AC, et al. Optical stimulation of neural tissue. Healthc Technol Lett. 2020;7:58–65.
51. Chernov MM, Friedman RM, Roe AW. Fiberoptic array for multiple channel infrared neural stimulation of the brain. Neurophotonics. 2021;8(2):025005. https://doi.org/10.1117/1.NPh.8.2.025005.
52. Albert ES, Bec JM, Desmadryl G, et al. TRPV4 channels mediate the infrared laser-evoked response in sensory neurons. J Neurophysiol. 2012;107:3227–34.
53. Shapiro MG, Homma K, Villarreal S, et al. Infrared light excites cells by changing their electrical capacitance. Nat Commun. 2012;3:376. https://doi.org/10.1038/ncomms1742.
54. Tsai SR, Hamblin MR. Biological effects and medical applications of infrared radiation. J Photochem Photobiol B. 2017;170:197–207.

55. Leung TK. In vitro and in vivo studies of the biological effects of bioceramic (a material of emitting high performance far-infrared ray) irradiation. Chin J Physiol. 2015;58:147–55.
56. Nunes RFH, Cidral-Filho FJ, Flores LJF, et al. Effects of far-infrared emitting ceramic materials on recovery during 2-week preseason of elite futsal players. J Strength Cond Res. 2020;34:235–48.
57. Romanovsky AA. The thermoregulation system and how it works. In: Romanovsky AA, editor. Handbook of clinical neurology. Amsterdam: Elsevier; 2018. p. 3–43.
58. Pooley MA, Anderson DM, Beckham HW, Brennan JF, et al. Engineered emissivity of textile fabrics by the inclusion of ceramic particles. Opt Express. 2016;24:10556–64.
59. Anderson DM, Fessler JR, Pooley MA, et al. Infrared radiative properties and thermal modeling of ceramic-embedded textile fabrics. Biomed Opt Express. 2017;8:1698–711.
60. Gordon IL, Casden S, Vangel M, Hamblin MR. Effect of shirts with 42% Celliant™ fiber on tcPO$_2$ levels and grip strength in healthy subjects: a placebo-controlled clinical trial. J Text Sci Eng. 2019;9:403.
61. Washington K, Wason J, Thein MS, et al. Randomized controlled trial comparing the effects of far-infrared emitting ceramic fabric shirts and control polyester shirts on transcutaneous PO$_2$. J Text Sci Eng. 2018;8:349.
62. Ko GD, Berbrayer D. Effect of ceramic-impregnated "thermoflow" gloves on patients with Raynaud's syndrome: randomized, placebo-controlled study. Altern Med Rev. 2002;7:328–35.
63. Sakugawa AADS, Conrado LAL, Villaverde AB, Munin E. Antiedematous effect promoted by occlusion of legs with compressive socks containing infrared-emitting ceramic particulates. Photobiomodul Photomed Laser Surg. 2020;38:51–6.
64. Loturco I, Abad CCC, Nakamura FY, et al. Effects of far infrared rays emitting clothing on recovery after an intense plyometric exercise bout applied to elite soccer players: a randomized double-blind placebo-controlled trial. Biol Sport. 2016;33:277–83.
65. Bagnato GL, Miceli G, Atteritano M, et al. Far infrared emitting plaster in knee osteoarthritis: a single blinded, randomised clinical trial. Reumatismo. 2012;64:388–94.
66. York RMB, Gordon IL. Effect of optically modified polyethylene terephthalate fiber socks on chronic foot pain. BMC Complement Altern Med. 2009;9:10. https://doi.org/10.118 6/1472-6882-9-10.
67. Lee CH, Roh J-W, Lim C-Y, et al. A multicenter, randomized, double-blind, placebo-controlled trial evaluating the efficacy and safety of a far infrared-emitting sericite belt in patients with primary dysmenorrhea. Complement Ther Med. 2011;19:187–93.
68. Lai Y-T, Chan H-L, Lin S-H, et al. Far-infrared ray patches relieve pain and improve skin sensitivity in myofascial pain syndrome: a double-blind randomized controlled study. Complement Ther Med. 2017;35:127–32.
69. Sommer AP, Haddad MK, Fecht H-J. Light effect on Water viscosity: implication for ATP biosynthesis. Sci Rep. 2015;5:12029.
70. Sharma A, Adams C, Cashdollar BD, et al. Effect of health-promoting agents on exclusion-zone size. Dose Resp. 2018;16:1559325818796937.
71. Pollack GH. Fourth phase of water: beyond solid, liquid & vapor. Oxford: Ebner and Sons, Blackwells; 2013.
72. Pollack GH, Cameron IL, Wheatley DN. Water and the cell. Amsterdam: Springer; 2007.
73. Pollack GH. Cells, gels and the engines of life: A new, unifying approach to cell function. Oxford: Ebner and Sons, Blackwells; 2001.

wIRA-Related Research and Medical Applications: Cornerstones and Further Reading of Interest

24

Jan-Olaf Gebbers and Peter Vaupel

This chapter intends to fuel the readers' discussion on wIRA applications, inspires further research and draws the readers' attention to (a) some highlights of therapies that have delivered proven beneficial effects, (b) interesting basic research, and (c) the extensive breadth of wIRA applications that have been studied in an increasingly active area of research, as well as the clinical trials in different fields of medicine. Nevertheless, basic research on the nature and possible implementations of wIRA must considered and be continued. Of course, given the large amount of information in this area, it has only been possible to highlight some of them that might be of particular interest, and which might address often raised questions.

Two essential items concerning water-filtered IR should be stressed. First, this kind of irradiation is the natural energy transfer of the sun using 60–80% of its radiation energy. Sun energy is the base of the development/evolution of multicellular organisms on earth, and thus is the life conserving energy. In most parts of the earth, solar infrared (IR) radiation reaches the surface after passing through a humid atmosphere as water-filtered infrared (exceptions are arid zones like deserts). wIRA of the radiators described and nearly exclusively used in the aforementioned studies, almost 100% emulates the sun's radiation on the earth. It can therefore be considered as an "artificial sun radiator" which is strictly limited to IR (without any UV), particularly on IR-A, which has deep-reaching, transcutaneous impacts without critically over-heating the skin surface. In other words, the wIRA radiator (syn.: wIRA-irradiator) almost perfectly imitates the solar IR reaching the Earth's surface.

J.-O. Gebbers (✉)
Lucerne, Switzerland

P. Vaupel (✉)
Department of Radiation Oncology, University Medical Center, University of Freiburg, Freiburg/Breisgau, Germany
e-mail: vaupel@uni-mainz.de

wIRA should *not* be seen as an *alternative therapeutic approach* in medicine rather as an effective *adjuvant-based therapeutic measure.*

References	Essence
1. Basics	

– Vaupel, et al. Strahlenther Onkol. 1991; 167: 353
  – Vaupel, et al. Strahlenther Onkol.1992; 168: 633
  – Vaupel, Krüger. Stuttgart: Hippokrates Verlag, 1st ed. ISBN 3–37,773-1076-x
	– First descriptions of water-filtered infrared-A (wIRA) irradiation as a novel technique to therapeutically heat superficial tumors (preclinical studies)
	– Comprehensive review of wIRA applications: Basics and preclinical applications

– Kelleher et al. Int J Hyperthermia. 1995; 11: 241 https://doi.org/10.3109/02656739509022460	– First description of changes in therapeutically relevant parameters of the tumor microenvironment upon wIRA
– Seegenschmiedt et al. Strahlenther Oncol. 1996; 172	– First retrospective analysis of combined wIRA and radiotherapy of superficial cancers in the clinical setting
– Vaupel, Krüger, Stuttgart: Hippokrates Verlag, 2nd ed; 1995 ISBN 3–7773–1196-0	– Comprehensive review of wIRA applications: Basics, pre-clinical and clinical applications
– Kelleher et al. Int J Hyperthermia 1999; 15: 467 https://doi.org/10.1080/026567399285468 – Kelleher et al. Br J Cancer. 2003; 89: 405–2333 https://doi.org/10.1038/sj.bjc.6601036 https://doi.org/10.1038/sj.bjc.6601457	– First descriptions of enhanced efficacy of photodynamic therapy (PDT) in combination with wIRA irradiation
– Piazena et al. Int J Hyperthermia 2019; 36: 938 https://doi.org/10.1080/02656736.2019.1655594	– The formation of thermal fields within the skin and subcutis upon wIRA irradiation of piglets was studied in terms of the thermotherapy of superficial cancers and local infections of thermosensible microbial pathogens. Findings confirmed the high relevance of wIRA-hyperthermia based therapies to humans
– Piazena et al. Int J Hyperthermia 2020; 37: 887 https://doi.org/10.1080/02656736.2020.1792562	– An experimental study by the European Society for Hyperthermic Oncology (ESHO) which reports the criteria for superficial hyperthermia to be comparable with those reported for the in vivo setting in the abdominal wall and also in patients with recurrent breast cancer. The potential of wIRA heating for adequate treatment of cancers that have spread to the skin and subcutis were therefore confirmed for the clinical setting

(continued)

(continued)

References	Essence
– Multhoff et al., Chap. 10 (this book)	– This is the first article to comprehensively consider the *immunobiological consequences* of tissue warming by wIRA in tumors. The chapter covers the interdependencies of tumor physiology, immunology, and hyperthermia (HT) and describes the "cooperation" between the presence and development of protective anti-tumor immunity and HT
– Biena et al. Pharmaceutics. 2021; 13: 1147	– This extensive review highlights hyperthermia as being an essential part of the current, most promising combination therapies for cancer (chemotherapy, radiotherapy, PDT, surgery, immunotherapy in various combinations)
– van Rhoon et al. Adv Drug Deliv Rev. 2020;163–164;145–156 https://doi.org/10.1016/j.addr.2020.03.006	– This chapter provides an in-depth discussion of hyperthermia as a chemosensitiser of tumors and its capacity to enhance the efficacy of chemotherapy. It also considers the tumor temperatures that are required for optimal thermochemotherapy
– Karu TI. Int Union Biochem Mol Biol Life 2010; 62: 607 https://doi.org/10.1002/iub.359	– This review discusses the current knowledge in photobiology and medicine relating to the influence of monochromatic, quasi-monochromatic, and broad-band radiation of red-to-near infrared (IR-A), as part of the solar spectrum, on mammalian cells and human skin. The role of cytochrome c oxidase as a photoacceptor and photosignal transducer, and its photosensitivity are highlighted and considers ATP as a critical signaling molecule.
– Hartel et al. Br J Surg. 2006; 93: 952 https://doi.org/10.1002/bjs.5429	– Reports on the first randomized clinical trial showing that wIRA improves surgical wound healing and lowers postoperative pain
2. Oncology/Radiation Biology	
– Notter et al. Int J Hyperthermia 2017; 33: 227 https://doi.org/10.1080/02656736.2016.1235731	– Delivery of the first highly promising results reporting on thermography-controlled wIRA combined with hypofractionated re-irradiation of large recurrent breast cancers
– Notter et al. Cancers. 2020; 12: 606 https://doi.org/10.3390/cancers12030606	– Using this combined modality, this study which evaluated the therapeutic outcome in 200 patients reports high overall clinical response rates and low toxicity
– Notter et al. Cancers. 2021; 13: 3911 https://doi.org/10.3390/cancers12030606	– This chapter proposes that combined wIRA-hyperthermia (wIRA-HT) and re-irradiation (re-RT) should be considered for (a) adjuvant treatment of radiation-associated angiosarcoma of the breast (RAASB) after surgery of local recurrence and (b) for definitive treatment of non-resectable RAAS

(continued)

References	Essence
– Heselich et al. Photochem Photobiol. 2012; 88: 135 https://doi.org/10.1111/j,1751-1097,2011.01031.x	– Reports that combining nonthermal NIR with clinically/biologically relevant X-ray doses leads to genomic instability, elevated risks of mitotic catastrophes, increased ROS generation, and an impaired repair of DNA double-strand break, all of which suggest that this combined approach may increase the efficacy of radiotherapy
– König et al. Photochem. Photobiol B. 2018; 178: 115 https://doi.org/10.1111/j,1751-1097,2011.01031.x	– Reports that exposure to NIR modulates cellular responses to X-rays in human full thickness skin models and indicates that exposure to NIR prior to treatment can reduce the required effective X-ray dosages
– Zschaeck et al. Oral Oncol. 2021; 116: 105240 https://doi.org/10.1016/j.oraloncology.2021.105240	– Shows that fever-range whole body hyperthermia (WHB) improves tumor oxygenation in vivo and can therefore increase the radiosensitivity to subsequent irradiations of head and neck squamous cell carcinomas without an excess of toxicity
3. Nanomedicine	
– Hainfeld et al. Nanomedicine. 2014; 10: 1609 https://doi.org/10.1016/j.nano.2014.05.006.	– Gold nanoparticles are known to enhance the efficacy of X-rays, resulting in tumor heating and ablation, as well as the absorbance of wIRA. Studying this dual property in a highly radio-resistant subcutaneous squamous cell carcinoma in mice revealed that the dose required to control 50% of the tumors could be reduced by a factor of >3.7
4. Psychiatry	
– Janssen et al. JAMA Psychiatr. 2016; 73: 789 https://doi.org/10.1001/jamapsychiatry2016.1031	– Major depressive disorders were treated in a randomized clinical trial which included sham-treated controls. A single session of WBH using wiRA resulted a significant antidepressant effect within 1 week of treatment which persisted for 6 weeks after treatment. Based on these findings, this therapeutic concept is currently being followed at three universities in Germany and Switzerland (see Chap. 12 in this book)
5. Wound healing	
– Hartel et al. Ann Surg. 2013; 258: 887 https://doi.org/10.1097/SLA.0000000000000235	– A prospective randomized study showing that preoperative wIRA reduces wound infections and postoperative pain
– Schumann et al. Br J Dermatol. 2011; 165: 541 https://doi.org/10.1111/j.1365-2133.2011.10410.x	– Patients with chronic venous stasis lower leg ulcers were treated with compression therapy, debridement, adhesive wound dressing, and 30 min wIRA irradiation or VIS (as control). Several essential symptoms significantly improved in the wIRA group

(continued)

(continued)

References	Essence
– Mercer et al. Ger Med Sci. 2008; 21: 6 PMID: 19675738	– wIRA irradiation of patients with chronic venous ulcers of the lower leg resulted in complete or nearly complete healing in most cases, a general reduction of pain and need for analgesics
– Tanaka et al. Australasian J Dermatol. 2018; 59: e87 https://doi.org/10.1111/ajd.12604	– Reports an upregulated expression of La ribonucleoprotein domain family member 6 and collagen type I gene following wIRA at 10 J/cm^2 in a 3-dimensional model of human epidermal tissue using DNA microarray and real-time PCR, thereby demonstrating the ability of NIR irradiation to stimulate type I collagen production
– von Felbert et al. GMS Krankenhaushyg Interdiszip. 2008; 5: 2 PMID: 20204086; PMCDC2831243	– This randomized controlled study demonstrates that wIRA irradiation of patients with chronic venous ulcers of lower legs accelerated the healing process (18 vs. 42 days until complete wound closure; residual ulcer area: 0.4 cm^2 vs. 28 cm^2) and reduced the requirement of analgesics
6. Dermatology	
– Fuchs et al. Ger Med Sci. 2004; 2 PMID: 19675691	– Treatment of verrucae vulgares, a significant problem in immunosuppressed patients, using PDT (5-ALA as photosensitizer) and wIRA delivered strong positive effects in this first prospective randomized controlled blinded study of recalcitrant warts. The findings suggest that other HPV-related neoplasia such as oral verrucous hyperplasia or cervical intraepithelial dysplasia should be explored as possible indications for this treatment modality
– von Felbert. Dermatology. 2011; 222: 347 https://doi.org/10.1159/000329024	– A series of patients with cutaneous scleroderma lesions, a chronic inflammatory disease leading to skin sclerosis, dysmorphism, contractures and movement restrictions were treated with wIRA. This approach led to a marked improvement which persisted during a long-term follow-up in 7 of 10 patients
– Knels et al. Photochem Photobiol. 2016; 92: 475 https://doi.org/10.1159/000329024	– An in vitro assay studied the therapeutic benefits of wIRA for wound healing in chronic diabetic skin lesions. For this, the effects of wIRA on 3 T3 fibroblast cultures with and without Glyoxal (causing a diabetic metabolic state) were examined. wIRA-reduced apoptotic cell numbers and more mitochondria showed a well-polarized MMP. This study underlines the immediate positive effects of wIRA, particularly on mitochondria

(continued)

(continued)

References	Essence
– Gebbers N, et al. Ger Med Sci. 2007; 14: 5 PMID: 19675716	– Infrared-induced skin damage, as communicated by some authors, has led to widespread confusion. This chapter documents that wIRA does not cause cellular degeneration of human skin, even at high irradiances. These high irradiances neither induce cell death or an MMP-1 mRNA overexpression (both of which are readily induced by UV-A irradiation)
7. Neonatology	
– Singer et al. Z Geburtshilfe Neonatol. 2000; 204: 85 https://doi.org/10.1055/s-2000-10202	– This chapter reports on the advantages of wIRA over conventional infrared irradiation in neonatology using comparative physical means of irradiances in several clinically applied IR sources. Clinical observations on the protective effect of wIRA in incubator nursing and primary care of preterm neonates were evident
8. Infectiology	
– Borel et al. Int J Hyperthermia. 2020; 37: 373 https://doi.org/10.1080/02656736.2020.1751312	– The emergence of antibiotic-resistant bacteria urgently requires the development of alternative, non-chemical treatments. This chapter presents recent research on reducing the infectious burden of thermosensitive bacteria such as *mycobacterium ulcerans* and *chlamydia trachomatis* using wIRA. *M. Ulcerans* causes chronic necrotizing skin disease (Buruli ulcer) and *C. trachomatis* infection of the ocular conjunctiva results in blinding trachoma. Both infections belong to the neglected tropical diseases and exhibit similar geographical distributions. Results of previous in vitro and in vivo studies have revealed wIRA to be a promising therapeutic tool against these bacteria
	– wIRA irradiation of other bacterial species such as *mycobacterium tuberculosis, Leishmania, Shigella, listeria monoytogenes,* dermatophytes, *Propionibacterium acnes,* and *helicobacter pylori* should therefore also be tested
– Marti et al. PLos One. 2014; 9: e10223 https://doi.org/10.1371/journal.pone.0102239	– This seminal in vitro study showed, for the first time, that wIRA- irradiation inhibits acute chlamydial infection
– Inic-Kanada et al. J Photochem Photobiol B. 2020; 209: 111953 https://doi.org/10.1016/j.jphotobiol.2020.111953	– This in vivo study evaluated the influence of wIRA (2100 W/m^2) in single or double treatments on the infectivity and bacterial load of *chlamydia caviae* and its ocular pathology in Guinea pigs. A marked decrease of infectivity was found, particularly in the double treated eyes. Importantly, no irradiation-related pathologies were microscopically detected in the follow-up period

(continued)

(continued)

References	Essence
– Oleg et al. Med Laser Appl. 2006; 21: 251 https://doi.org/10.1016/j.mla.2006.07.002	– This chapter comprehensively discusses the potential and problems of photodynamic therapy (PDT) against intracellular pathogens. Success depends on selecting the optimal approach for parasite killing while inflicting little or no host tissue damage: Short photosensitizer incubation time (1–5 min), low concentration of photosensitizer (0.1–1 μM), irradiance not exceeding 50 mW/cm^2, a relatively low fluence (<5–10 J/cm^2), and more than 3 PDT treatments
– Gelfand et al. FASEB J. 2019; 33: 3074 https://doi.org/10.1096/fj.201801095R	– This pilot trial tested a "near IR laser vaccine" adjuvant approach for safety, tolerability, and cutaneous immune cell trafficking. As the epidermis contains a large population of antigen-presenting cells (Langerhans cells, MHC class II), it is conceivable that wIRA could stimulate this population and promote an immunologically relevant trafficking of antigen to the regional lymph nodes

9. Ophthalmology

– Rahn et al. J Photochem Photobiol B. 2016; 165: 340 https://doi.org/10.1016/j.jphotobiol.2016.11.001	– This study reports that wIRA reduces chlamydial infectivity in vitro without causing ex vivo eye damage in pig and mouse models
– Nelidova et al. Science. 2020: 368:1108 https://doi.org/10.1126/science.aaz5887	– This study reports on enabling NIR sensitivity in a blind human retina by restoring light sensitivity using tunable NIR sensors. This approach may supplement or restore visual function in patients with regional retinal degeneration. Mammalian or snake transient receptor potential (TRP) channels were expressed in light-insensitive retinal cones in a mouse model of retinal degeneration, and NIR-induced sensitivity was induced using gold nanorods bound to temperature-sensitive TRP channels. NIR stimulation increased activity in cones, ganglion cell layer neurons, and cortical neurons and enabled mice to perform a learned light-driven behavior. Responses to different wavelengths were tuned by nanorods of different lengths and to different radiant powers using engineered channels with different temperature thresholds. TRP channels were targeted to human retinas, which allowed the postmortem activation of different cell types by NIR

(continued)

(continued)

References	Essence
10. Rheumatology	
– Schuester et al. Phys Med Rehab Kuror. 2021 https://doi.org/10.1055/a-1349-1482	– Treatment of patients with gonarthrosis, the world's most common joint disease, with wIRA in a prospective double blind controlled study resulted in a statistically proven efficacy with marked pain reduction and an improved life quality
– Xu et al. Orthop Surg Res. 2019; 14: 313 https://doi.org/10.1186/s13018-019-1322-7	– Patients with sacroiliitis and ankylosing spondylitis (AS) were treated with wIRA in a randomized controlled trial using a cross-over design. Treatment markedly decreased AS activity index (BASDAI), pain, morning stiffness, and CRP levels during treatment paralleled pain reduction ($p < 0.018$). Levels of serum VEGF were not affected
– Klemm et al. Int J Hyperthermia. 2020; 37: 965 https://doi.org/10.1080/02656736.2020.1804079	– Patients with axial spondyloarthritis were treated using serially applied, localized wIRA. The study group rapidly noted a reduction of pain and the consumption of NSAID after completion of the trial. Possible changes in TNF-α levels are discussed